# FUNDAMENTALS OF CLINICAL OPHTHALMOLOGY:
## PAEDIATRIC OPHTHALMOLOGY

**Fundamentals of Clinical Ophthalmology series**

Cataract Surgery
*Edited by David Garty*

Glaucoma
*Edited by Roger Hitchins*

Paediatric Ophthalmology
*Edited by Anthony Moore*

Plastic and Oribital Surgery
*Edited by Richard Collin and Geoffrey Rose*

Uveitis
*Edited by Susan Lightman and Hamish Towler*

Cornea
*Edited by Douglas Coster*

Neuro-ophthalmology
*Edited by James Acheson and Paul Riordan-Eva*

Scleritis
*Edited by Paul McCluskey*

Strabismus
*Edited by Frank Billson*

# FUNDAMENTALS OF CLINICAL OPHTHALMOLOGY: PAEDIATRIC OPHTHALMOLOGY

Edited by

ANTHONY MOORE
*Consultant Ophthalmic Surgeon*
*Addenbrooke's Hospital NHS Trust, Cambridge, UK*
*and Moorfields Eye Hospital, London, UK*

*Series Editor*
SUSAN LIGHTMAN
*Department of Clinical Ophthalmology,*
*Institute of Ophthalmology/Moorfields Eye*
*Hospital, London, UK*

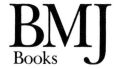

First published in 2000
by BMJ Books, BMA House, Tavistock Square,
London WC1H 9JR

www.bmjbooks.com

Unless stated otherwise in captions, all figures are reproduced
courtesy of Anthony Moore, Addenbrooke's Hospital Trust.

**British Library Cataloguing in Publication Data**

A catalogue record for this book is available from the British Library

ISBN 0–7279–1203–8

Typeset by Phoenix Photosetting, Chatham, Kent
Colour separation by Tenon & Polert Colour Scanning Ltd
Printed and bound in China by Tenon & Polert

# Contents

# Contributors

**Louise Allen**
Senior Registrar
Department of Ophthalmology
Addenbrooke's Hospital NHS Trust
Cambridge, UK

**Rodolfo Armas**
Consultant Ophthalmic Surgeon
Glaucoma Unit: Ophthalmology Department
University of Chile and Hospital del Salvador
Santiago, Chile

**Keith Bradshaw**
Vision Scientist
Department of Ophthalmology
Addenbrooke's Hospital NHS Trust
Cambridge, UK

**Arvind Chandna**
Consultant Ophthalmic Surgeon
Department of Ophthalmology
Alder Hey Children's Hospital
Liverpool, UK

**Stephen Charles**
Consultant Ophthalmic Surgeon
The Royal Eye Hospital
Manchester, UK

**John Elston**
Consultant Ophthalmic Surgeon
Oxford Eye Hospital
Oxford, UK

**Allen Foster**
Senior Lecturer
London School of Hygiene and Tropical Medicine
London, UK

**Clare Gilbert**
Clinical Lecturer
Department of Preventive Ophthalmology
Institute of Ophthalmology
London, UK

**Elizabeth M Graham**
Consultant Medical Ophthalmologist
The Medical Eye Unit
St Thomas' Hospital
London, UK

**Kevin Gregory-Evans**
Senior Lecturer & Consultant Ophthalmologist
Imperial College School of Medicine
Western Eye Hospital
London, UK

**Christopher M Harris**
Department of Ophthalmology
Hospital for Sick Children and Institute of Child
Health
University College London
London, UK

**Peter Hodgkins**
Consultant Ophthalmic Surgeon
Southampton Eye Unit
Southampton General Hospital
Southampton, UK

**David Hughes**
Consultant Ophthalmic Surgeon
Department of Ophthalmology
St Woolos Hospital
Newport, Gwent, UK

**Peng T Khaw**
Professor of Glaucoma and Wound Healing
Director, Paediatric Glaucoma Clinic and
Wound Healing Research Unit
Glaucoma Unit and Department of Pathology
Moorfields Eye Hospital and Institute of
Ophthalmology
London, UK

**Anthony T Moore**
Consultant Ophthalmic Surgeon
Addenbrooke's Hospital NHS Trust
Cambridge, UK
and
Moorfields Eye Hospital and Institute of
Ophthalmology
London, UK

**Andrew Narita**
Consultant Ophthalmologist
Royal Children's Hospital
Melbourne
Australia

**Carmel Noonan**
Consultant Ophthalmologist
Warrington Hospital NHS Trust
Warrington, Cheshire, UK

**Maria Papadopoulos**
Fellow
Moorfields Eye Hospital and Institute of
Ophthalmology
London, UK

**Jeremy Prydal**
Consultant Ophthalmic Surgeon
Department of Ophthalmology
Frederick Thorpe Administration
Leicester Royal Infirmary
Leicester, UK

**Nicola Ragge**
Locum Consultant Ophthalmologist
The Medical Eye Unit
St Thomas' Hospital
London, UK

**Geoffrey E Rose**
Consultant Ophthalmic Surgeon
Moorfields Eye Hospital and Institute of
Ophthalmology
London, UK

**Isabelle M Russell-Eggitt**
Consultant Ophthalmic Surgeon
Hospital for Sick Children
London, UK

**Rosalyn M Stanbury**
Specialist Registrar
The Medical Eye Unit
St Thomas' Hospital
London, UK

**Anthony Vivian**
Consultant Ophthalmic Surgeon
Department of Ophthalmology
West Suffolk Hospital
Bury St Edmunds, Suffolk, UK

**Antony Wells**
Fellow
Moorfields Eye Hospital and Institute of
Ophthalmology
London, UK

# Preface to the
# *Fundamentals of Clinical Ophthalmology* series

This book is part of a series of ophthalmic monographs, written for ophthalmologists in training and general ophthalmologists wishing to update their knowledge in specialised areas. The emphasis of each is to combine clinical experience with the current knowledge of the underlying disease processes.

Each monograph provides an up to date, very clinical and practical approach to the subject so that the reader can readily use the information in everyday clinical practice. There are excellent illustrations throughout each text in order to make it easier to relate the subject matter to the patient.

The inspiration for the series came from the growth in communication and training opportunities for ophthalmologists all over the world and a desire to provide clinical books that we can all use. This aim is well reflected in the international panels of contributors who have so generously contributed their time and expertise.

*Susan Lightman*

# Preface

Paediatric ophthalmology is now a well-established subspeciality within ophthalmology but is unique in that it encompasses such a broad range of eye and systemic disorders. It is the last bastion of the generalist in an era of increasing subspecialisation. It is impossible given the breadth of the subject to cover all aspects of paediatric ophthalmology in a short book. Rather, the aim has been to produce a concise, readable, well-illustrated account of the major disorders affecting the eye and visual pathways in childhood. A limited number of references to other more comprehensive texts or important original papers are given to allow the interested reader to pursue particular interests in more depth. The examination, investigation, and management of infants and young children is time consuming and very challenging; a quite different approach to that adopted in adults is required. I hope that the book will serve to highlight the specific needs of this young age group and to stimulate interest in this fascinating and rewarding area of ophthalmology.

I am grateful to the many people who have helped in the production of this book. Most of the illustrations have come from my own slide collection and I am grateful to Catherine Haslam, ophthalmic photographer, and her colleagues from the Medical Illustration Department at Addenbrooke's Hospital for their expertise and help. I am also grateful to the many colleagues, acknowledged in the text, who generously provided other slides and illustrations. I am also very grateful to the children and their parents who allowed their photographs to be reproduced. Linda Allars provided essential secretarial help and I am grateful to the staff of BMJ Books for their patience and guidance. Finally, I would like to thank Julia Moore for her editorial assistance, encouragement, and support during the production of this book.

*Anthony Moore*

# 1 Epidemiology of childhood blindness

CLARE GILBERT, ALLEN FOSTER

The word "epidemiology" comes from the Greek which means "diseases that visit the community", and is defined as the "quantitative measure of the distribution, determinants and control of diseases in populations". In this chapter, available data on the prevalence and magnitude of blindness in children will be presented, as well as data on the major causes. Possible measures for controlling blindness in children will be outlined.

"Childhood" is defined by UNICEF as an individual aged less than 16 years, and "blindness" as a corrected visual acuity (VA) in the better eye of less than 3/60, or a central visual field of less than 10° around the point of central fixation (the World Health Organization's categories of visual impairment). This definition immediately raises difficulties when applied to children as accurate measurement of VA and visual fields can be difficult in young children, and in those with additional handicap.

## Epidemiological parameters

### Sources of data

In industrialised countries information on the prevalence, incidence and causes of blindness in children can be obtained from registers of the blind (providing they are comprehensive, "live" registers), birth cohort studies, and surveillance systems. In developing countries data are not available from these sources, but children have been included in several surveys of whole populations. Incidence data are more difficult to obtain, requiring either very accurate registers of the blind, or very large follow-up studies.

## Prevalence, incidence and magnitude of childhood blindness

Prevalence data that are available are shown in Table 1.1 which show that the prevalence of blindness in children in developing countries is three to four times greater than in industrialised countries.[1] It has been estimated that there are approximately 1.5 million blind children in the world, the majority of whom live in developing countries (Table 1.2).[2,3]

Data from Scandinavian registers suggest that the incidence of visual impairment (i.e. visual acuity of <6/18), is approximately 8/100 000 children/year. There are no incidence data from developing countries but it has been estimated that 500 000 children become blind worldwide each year.[4] Many of the blinding conditions of childhood, particularly in developing countries, are associated with a high mortality rate, e.g. measles and vitamin A deficiency (VAD). In countries where VAD is a significant public health problem, it is thought that over 50% of children die within one to two years of becoming blind from this cause.

## Sources of data on the causes of blindness in children

In industrialised countries most data on the causes of blindness in children come from

Table 1.1   Prevalence of blindness and severe visual impairment in children by region and country

| Region/ Country | Year | Category of visual impairment | Prevalence (per 1000) | Age group (years) | Source of data |
|---|---|---|---|---|---|
| *Europe* | | | | | |
| England | 1985 | Variable | 0.10 | 0–4 | Registration |
| England | 1985 | Variable | 0.22 | 5–9 | Registration |
| England | 1985 | Variable | 0.23 | 10–14 | Registration |
| Scandanavia | 1992 | <3/60 | 0.15–0.41 | 0–15 | Registration |
| Iceland | 1980 | Variable | 0.36 | 0–14 | Survey |
| Eire | 1991 | <3/60 | 0.16 | 0–16 | Estimate |
| UK | 1988 | 3/60 | 0.34 | 10 | Cohort study |
| *Asia* | | | | | |
| Nepal | 1980 | <3/60 | 0.63 | 0–14 | Survey |
| Bangladesh rural | 1985 | Not stated | 0.64 | 0–5 | Survey |
| Bangladesh urban | 1985 | Not stated | 1.09 | 0–5 | Survey |
| China | 1992 | <6/18 | 0.94 | 0–13 | Survey |
| *Africa* | | | | | |
| Benin | 1991 | <3/60 | 0.60 | 0–15 | Survey |
| Morocco | 1994 | <3/60 | 0.30 | 0–15 | Survey |
| The Gambia | 1986 | <3/60 | 0.70 | 0–19 | Survey |
| Nigeria (Kaduna State) | 1994 | <3/60 | 1.0 | 5–14 | Survey |
| Malawi | 1983 | Functional definition | 1.10 | 0.5 | Survey |

registers of the blind. In developing countries some indication of the main causes can be obtained by examining children in schools for the blind, but these data are likely to be biased as only 5–10% of blind children are enrolled in special schools. Data from registers and from blind school studies will be biased if the causes of blindness in children included are different from the causes in children not registered or enrolled. In both situations this is likely; in industrialised countries children with multiple handicap may not be registered, and in developing countries children with additional handicap, those from isolated rural areas, and preschool age children are usually not catered for. The only way to obtain truly accurate data would be to identify and examine all the blind children in a representative sample selected at random from the population of interest. However, as childhood blindness is relatively rare, a very large sample of children would be needed.

## Classification of the causes of blindness in children

It is useful to be able to classify the causes of blindness in children using a descriptive classification (i.e. the principal site in the eye affected, e.g. cornea, lens), as well as an aetiological classification (i.e. the time of onset of the insult leading to blindness, e.g. during the intrauterine or perinatal periods).[5] Descriptive data are less

Table 1.2   Estimated prevalence and magnitude of childhood blindness, by region

| Region | Population aged 0–15 years (millions) | Blindness prevalence (per 1000) | Estimated number of blind children |
|---|---|---|---|
| Africa | 240 | 1.1 | 264 000 |
| Asia | 1200 | 0.9 | 1 080 000 |
| Latin America | 130 | 0.6 | 78 000 |
| Europe/USA/Japan | 240 | 0.3 | 72 000 |
| Total | | | 1 494 000 |

Table 1.3    Regional variation in the causes of blindness in children – descriptive classification

| Region | Number of studies | Cornea | Lens | Retina | Optic nerve | Glaucoma | Other* |
|---|---|---|---|---|---|---|---|
| Europe/USA | 10 | 0–1% | 4–15% | 21–40% | 9–44% | 0–3% | 21–47% |
| South America | 9 | 1–23% | 5–39% | 10–51% | 8–18% | 3–18% | 8–29% |
| Eastern Mediterranean region | 6 | 3–26% | 7–21% | 20–52% | 4–18% | 0–19% | 11–34% |
| Asia | 3 | 11–29% | 11–17% | 20–22% | 6–7% | 3–6% | 30–37% |
| Africa | 7 | 24–72% | 7–18% | 4–26% | 3–14% | 0–13% | 7–20% |

*Includes lesions of the whole globe such as microphthalmos, anophthalmos, and lesions of the higher visual pathways

useful for planning control measures but can be more readily obtained than information on the underlying cause, which is often not possible to determine even where there is expertise and facilities for investigation. Data from multiple sources (which have been reclassified using the system mentioned above) are summarised in Tables 1.3 and 1.4.

## Regional variation in the major causes of blindness in children

In industrialised countries genetic diseases and conditions occurring as a result of perinatal events are the major causes of blindness in children, acquired diseases being responsible for a small percentage. This is in contrast to developing countries where childhood conditions such as VAD and measles are major causes of blindness. In countries with developing economies, it appears that retinopathy of prematurity (ROP) is becoming an important cause of blindness.

## Changes in the major causes over time

As the major causes of blindness in children are strongly associated with levels of socio-economic development and healthcare provision, it is not surprising that the major causes change over time. For example, ROP accounted for almost half of causes in European countries and the USA during the 1950s, but now accounts for approximately 10%. In Saudi Arabia genetic causes have become more important as infectious diseases have been controlled.[6]

## Avoidable causes of blindness in children

The principles or prevention (which can be applied to any disease) are as follows:

- Primary prevention
  Prevention of the disease, e.g. immunisation. This reduces the incidence of the disease.

- Secondary prevention
  Treatment of the disease to prevent impairment, e.g. antibiotic treatment of infections. This reduces the incidence of impairment.

- Tertiary prevention
  Treatment of the impairment to restore function, e.g. surgery on a cataract blind patient; rehabilitation to prevent handicap. This reduces the prevalence of the impairment.

Table 1.4    Regional variation in the causes of blindness in children – aetiological classification

| Region | Number of studies | Hereditary | Intrauterine | Perinatal | Childhood | Unknown |
|---|---|---|---|---|---|---|
| Europe/USA | 5 | 30–50% | 1–11% | 11–33% | 5–19% | 0–40% |
| South America | 3 | 22–39% | 4–11% | 14–23% | 10–15% | 25–28% |
| Eastern Mediterranean region | 6 | 47–80% | 0–4% | 1–6% | 5–30% | 0–37% |
| Africa | 2 | 11–21% | 1–8% | 1–3% | 34–60% | 27–34% |
| Asia | 3 | 16–35% | 2–4% | 0–16% | 5–30% | 40–56% |

Conditions amenable to primary prevention include congenital rubella syndrome, VAD and measles. Blind school studies indicate that 28–32% of children are blind from entirely preventable causes in Eastern Europe, Africa, Asia and Latin America (Table 1.5). Conditions that can be treated to prevent blindness or to restore function are responsible for a further 14–17%. Overall, 42–54% of children in these four regions were blind or severely visually impaired from potentially avoidable causes.

## Genetic disease

In industrialised countries, genetic eye disease is an important cause of blindness in children, accounting for 16–51% of visual impairment. Aetiological data from developing and newly industrialising countries are more difficult to obtain due to lack of medical records, details of family history and facilities for investigation. In a high proportion of cases, it is not possible to determine the underlying causes. However, data from blind school studies suggest that genetic eye diseases assume greater relative importance in countries with higher levels of socio-economic development than in poorer countries, i.e. 11–32% in six African countries, 17–35% in four Asian countries and 22–39% in three Latin American countries. In most countries, auto-somal recessive diseases predominate (22–54%), and retinal dystrophies, such as retinitis pigmentosa and Leber's amaurosis, are the more common diseases (42–80%).[7]

In the eastern Mediterranean region, approximately two-thirds of blindness in children has been attributed to genetic causes, with 50–65% being due to an autosomal recessive disease. The high level of consanguineous marriage practised in the region (16–55% of all marriages) is probably an important factor as consanguinity is known to increase the risk of recessive diseases and multifactorial disorders.

The site and nature of the genetic abnormality have been determined for many genetic eye diseases, e.g. retinoblastoma is due to mutations of the RB1 gene on the long arm of chromosome 13 (13q14). It is being increasingly realised that the same clinical disease can occur as a result of mutations of different genes. For example, in

Table 1.5   Avoidable causes of blindness and severe visual impairment in children. Blind school studies where all data were collected using a standard method

|  | Eastern Europe (n = 275) | | Asia (n = 2235) | | Latin America (n = 830) | | Africa (n = 1407) | |
|---|---|---|---|---|---|---|---|---|
|  | n | per cent | n | per cent | n | per cent | n | per cent |
| *Preventable* | | | | | | | | |
| Measles/VAD/TEM | 0 | 0 | 470 | 21% | 9 | 1.1% | 310 | 22% |
| Ophthalmia neonatorum | 1 | 0.4 | 29 | 1.3% | 13 | 1.6% | 29 | 2.1% |
| Retinopathy of prematurity | 37 | 13.5 | 30 | 1.3% | 140 | 16.9% | 61 | 4.3% |
| Toxoplasmosis | 14 | 5.1 | 9 | 0.4% | 33 | 4% | 2 | 0.1% |
| Autosomal dominant | 2 | 0.7 | 62 | 2.8% | 38 | 4.6% | 59 | 4.2% |
| Rubella | 13 | 4.7 | 27 | 1.2% | 31 | 3.7% | 30 | 2.1% |
| Other | 10 | 3.6 | 86 | 3.8% | 20 | 2.4% | 35 | 2.5% |
| Subtotal: | 77 | 28.0 | 713 | 31.9% | 284 | 34.2% | 526 | 37.3% |
| *Treatable* | | | | | | | | |
| Cataract | 26 | 9.5 | 219 | 9.8% | 45 | 5.4% | 124 | 8.8% |
| Glaucoma | 13 | 4.7 | 76 | 3.4% | 75 | 9% | 79 | 5.6% |
| Other | 0 | 0 | 17 | 0.8% | 5 | 0.6% | 32 | 2.3% |
| Subtotal: | 39 | 14.2 | 312 | 14.0% | 125 | 15.1% | 235 | 16.7% |
| *Avoidable* | 116 | 42.2 | 1015 | 45.4% | 409 | 49.3% | 761 | 54.1% |

VAD = vitamin A deficiency.
TEM = (harmful) traditional eye medicines.

dominant retinitis pigmentosa, the majority of the genetic mutations identified have been found in the gene which encodes for rhodopsin, but mutations which encode for other proteins, such as peripherin, have also been identified.

## Strategies for the prevention of childhood blindness due to genetic diseases (Box 1.1)

Genetic counselling services, as part of tertiary eye care, or provided by a medical genetics department, should be available for affected families. A detailed family history, with examination and/or investigation of relevant family members to determine the mode of inheritance and to calculate the risks in subsequent pregnancies, are essential early steps in genetic counselling. There are techniques available to provide presymptomatic diagnosis, and to identify carriers of X-linked and recessive traits, giving prospective parents the information required to make informed decisions. Advances in molecular genetics also raise the possibility of future therapeutic interventions for affected individuals (e.g. gene therapy), or to prevent the condition through *in vitro* fertilisation. Germ line therapy may eventually be possible. In countries where

there are financial, religious or cultural constraints (e.g. where consanguineous marriage is practised) genetic counselling services need to provide options that are acceptable to the community.

## Intrauterine causes of blindness (Box 1.2)

Intrauterine causes of blindness in children occur as a result of the teratogenic effects of infections (e.g. rubella, toxoplasmosis and cytomegalovirus (CMV)), ionising radiation (e.g. $x$ rays), drugs (e.g. thalidomide, retinoic acid, and cocaine and alcohol abuse), maternal metabolic disturbances (e.g. diabetes) and environmental agents. The time of exposure is critical as different stages of organogenesis occur at different times during foetal development. Very early exposure (0–17 days) tends to cause death or complete recovery; exposure in the critical period (18–60 days) causes structural (and/or functional) abnormalities whereas exposure later in pregnancy (60 days or more) causes more general effects, i.e. growth and mental retardation, and functional changes.

Intrauterine causes are relatively rare in industrialised countries, but it appears that congenital ocular abnormalities (e.g. optic nerve hypoplasia) resulting from alcohol and drug abuse during pregnancy are increasing, particularly in deprived inner-city areas in the United States of America. Most industrialised countries have introduced rubella immunisation programmes, mainly measles, mumps & rubella (MMR) immunisation at one year of age. This has been very effective at preventing congenital rubella syndrome (CRS), which can cause cataract, glaucoma, microphthalmos and pigmentary retinopathy as well as other systemic abnormalities. There are few data on the importance of CRS as a cause of childhood blindness in developing countries, but a blind school study in Jamaica showed that 39% were blind from cataract, and CRS was implicated in almost half of these children. A recent study in India demonstrated that 26% of infants with congenital cataract had CRS.

---

**Box 1.1** *Strategies for prevention of childhood blindness due to genetic diseases*

| Level of prevention | Strategy |
|---|---|
| Primary | • Genetic counselling to allow informed choice about future pregnancies |
| | • *In vitro* fertilisation followed by pre-implantation diagnosis |
| | • (Germ line therapy) |
| Secondary | • Prenatal diagnosis, with termination of affected pregnancies |
| | • Early identification and treatment of genetic disease, e.g. congenital glaucoma |
| | • (Somatic cell therapy) |
| Tertiary | • Appropriate treatment, e.g. congenital cataract |

There are several different rubella immunisation strategies, e.g. immunisation of infants, or girls aged 12–14 years, or women of child-bearing age who are seronegative. In industrialised countries, immunisation of infants and seronegative women is the strategy most commonly used. In developing countries with low immunisation coverage rates, MMR immunisation alone should be avoided as this approach can lead to a higher proportion of women of child-bearing age who are seronegative and hence susceptible to infection during pregnancy. A preferred approach would be to immunise school girls, and women at marriage.

Toxoplasmosis is another unusual cause of blindness in children in industrialised countries, but is a significant cause in some Latin American countries.

---

**Box 1.2** *Strategies for prevention of childhood blindness due to intrauterine causes*

| Level of prevention | Strategy |
| --- | --- |
| Primary | • Health education to prevent the harmful effects of alcohol, drugs and *x*-rays during pregnancy; avoid cat litter during pregnancy; safe food preparation<br>• Rubella immunisation<br>• Screening programmes to identify women who develop toxoplasmosis during pregnancy, by detecting those who seroconvert, followed by intensive antibiotic treatment and follow up. This strategy has been adopted in France, but whether it is justified in other industrial countries is debatable, and is not feasible for financial and logistical reasons in developing countries |
| Secondary | • Early identification and treatment of affected infants, e.g. uveitis |
| Tertiary | • Appropriate treatment, e.g. of congenital cataract |

---

## Perinatal causes

The perinatal period is defined as from 28 weeks of gestation to 28 days following birth. Causes of blindness resulting from perinatal events includes ophthalmia neonatorum, lesions of the optic nerve and higher visual pathways, and retinopathy of prematurity.

### Ophthalmia neonatorum (Box 1.3)

Ophthalmia neonatorum (ON) is an exceptionally rare cause of blindness in children in industrialised countries, but is thought to be responsible for up to 5% of blindness in children in the poorer countries of the world. In Africa, up to 18% and 22% of women in antenatal clinics are infected with gonorrhoea and genital chlamydia respectively, and approximately 30% and 25–50% of infants exposed to *Neisseria gonorrhoea* and *Chlamydia trachomatis* develop neonatal conjunctivitis (Figure 1.1). The incidence of gonococcal conjunctivitis in European countries is 0.04–0.3/1000 live births compared with 40/1000 live births in Kenya and the Cameroon. The higher incidence of ON in African countries reflects the higher incidence of sexually transmitted diseases (STDs), which are often undetected and untreated, and lack of ocular prophylaxis in the newborn.

The treatment of gonorrhoea has been complicated by the emergence of drug-resistant strains, particularly to penicillin, tetracycline and

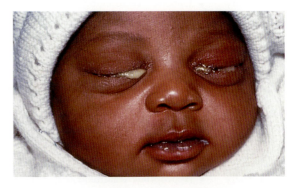

Figure 1.1 Nigerian baby with gonococcal ophthalmia neonatorum. (Courtesy of P S Lee)

some of the earlier cephalosporins. When drug resistance reduces the effectiveness of these drugs to less than 95% other antibiotics, such as third generation cephalosporins, are required.

---

**Box 1.3** *Strategies for the prevention of blindness due to ophthalmia neonatorum*

| Level of prevention | Strategy |
|---|---|
| Primary | • Prevention of STDs, by health education<br>• Identification and treatment of STDs in women of child-bearing age and during pregnancy. Transmission of HIV infection is higher if there is an associated STD and programmes for the control of STDs as a means of preventing HIV transmission in developing countries may have an impact on the incidence of ON in infants<br>• Ocular prophylaxis in the newborn, i.e. cleansing of the eyelids immediately after delivery of the head and before the eyes open, followed by instillation of an antiseptic (1% silver nitrate, or 2.5% aqueous povidone-iodine solution) or antibiotic (erythromycin or tetracycline ointment). This can be done by midwives, obstetricians and traditional birth attendants |
| Secondary | • Early identification of ON, with prompt and appropriate systemic and topical antibiotic treatment |
| Tertiary | • Optical iridectomy (or corneal grafting) to restore function. In most developing countries corneal grafting is not a realistic option as the risks of rejection are high, follow up often poor, and there may be lack of the following: corneal material, expertise and equipment to perform surgery, drugs to treat rejection |

---

## Lesions of the higher visual pathways

In the United Kingdom, 22% of newly registered children are blind from lesions of the higher visual pathways, and a further 20% from optic atrophy. Other European countries report 15–54% of children to be blind from CNS abnormalities (Box 1.4), attributed to a variety of factors including metabolic and genetic diseases, the effect of teratogens, intrapartum events associated with birth asphyxia, and postnatal events including tumours, trauma and meningitis. Up to 59% of children blind from CNS lesions have additional impairments, most commonly cerebral palsy (CP). Data from developing countries show a much lower proportion of children to be blind from CNS lesions, the majority of cases being due to postnatal events, e.g. meningitis, encephalitis, trauma, and tumours.

Hypoxia resulting from intrapartum events has been thought to be the underlying cause of both blindness and CP. However, there is a body of evidence which shows that indicators of birth asphyxia, such as low Apgar score, are poor predictors of neurological abnormality.[8] Other studies have shown that the incidence of CP in babies with normal birthweight has not declined despite improvements in obstetric care; the underlying cause of CP seems to be due to events occurring before birth which either cause cerebral damage, or which make the cerebrum more susceptible to damage from stresses during delivery. However, the same is probably not true of premature and low-birthweight babies, who are at risk of developing periventricular ischaemia and para- and intraventricular haemorrhage during the neonatal period, although the adverse effects of intrauterine events cannot be completely ruled out.

---

**Box 1.4** *Strategies for the prevention of blindness due to perinatal CNS factors*

| Level of prevention | Strategy |
|---|---|
| Primary | • Good antenatal care to prevent premature birth<br>• Good obstetric care<br>• Good intensive neonatal care |
| Secondary | • None possible |
| Tertiary | • None possible |

**Retinopathy of prematurity** (Box 1.5)

Retinopathy of prematurity (ROP) emerged as a cause of blindness in children in industrialised countries during the late 1940s and 1950s due to improvements in neonatal intensive care, including supplemental oxygen, and increased survival of preterm babies. During the 1950s, ROP was the single commonest cause of blindness in children in many industrialised countries (the "first epidemic"). Hyperoxia was identified as an important risk factor, and the use of oxygen was restricted in the mid-1950s which was followed by a reduction in the incidence of blindness from ROP, but a higher infant mortality rate. Oxygen was used more liberally in the 1960s, and blindness from ROP began to re-emerge. The introduction of increasingly sophisticated technology and accurate monitoring of blood oxygen levels (and other parameters) in the 1970s were probably the major factors responsible for reduction of blinding ROP observed during this period.

The major risk factors for ROP are prematurity (<32 weeks gestational age), low birthweight (<1500 g) and fluctuations in blood oxygen levels during the first few weeks after birth. More very low birthweight (VLBW; <1500 g) and extremely low-birthweight (ELBW; <1000 g) babies are surviving as neonatal services continue to improve. The population of babies at risk is therefore increasing, and there is some evidence that blindness from ROP is increasing again in some industrialised countries (the "second epidemic"). In industrialised countries, blindness from ROP is now largely restricted to infants in the ELBW group.

ROP has recently been described in infants in India, and data from blind school studies suggest that ROP may be becoming an important cause of blindness in Latin American countries, and in urban centres in newly industrialising countries.[9]

---

**Box 1.5** *Strategies for the prevention of blindness due to retinopathy of prematurity*

| Level of prevention | Strategy |
|---|---|
| Primary | • Good antenatal care to prevent premature birth<br>• Systemic steroids for women with impending premature delivery<br>• Good intensive neonatal care, with monitoring of oxygen levels and other biochemical parameters |
| Secondary | • Screening of infants less than 1500 g at birth and/or born at less than 32 weeks gestation to detect treatable disease, i.e. threshold disease (Stage III, "plus" disease affecting five or more continuous clock hours, or eight or more non-continuous clock hours). This should be done by ophthalmologists, using indirect ophthalmoscopy through a dilated pupil. Close cooperation with neonatologists is required<br>• Treatment of threshold disease with cryotherapy or laser photocoagulation |
| Tertiary | • Surgery for Stage V disease does not give good visual results |

---

## Childhood factors

Acquired diseases are unusual causes of blindness in children in industrialised countries, but are very important in poor countries. Worldwide, approximately 500 000 children are blind from corneal scarring, the majority caused by conditions occurring during childhood. The single commonest cause is vitamin A deficiency, which is often precipitated by measles infection, particularly in African children.

### Measles

Measles is a leading cause of child mortality in developing countries, accounting for an estimated 1.5 million deaths per year (10% of all childhood deaths). Overcrowding, which leads to a higher infecting dose of the virus, is thought to be the major reason for the severity of the condition, particularly in African children.[10]

Studies in Africa show that approximately 1–3% of children develop corneal ulceration following measles; in children with corneal ulceration, approximately a third give a history of recent measles, and up to 80% of children with corneal scarring give a history of measles.

The pathogenesis of corneal scarring following measles is complex and multifactorial and several mechanisms have been proposed. The measles virus can invade the cornea, giving rise to superficial ulceration which is usually self-limiting. Increased demand for and reduced intake of vitamin A, as well as loss in the urine and from the gut, can lead to acute vitamin A deficiency with corneal ulceration and keratomalacia. Measles infection reduces cell-mediated immunity, which encourages infection with herpes simplex virus (HSV) (Figure 1.2) keratitis.

Exposure keratitis in a very sick, dehydrated child can cause corneal ulceration, and secondary bacterial infection. Children with measles are often light sensitive, and in areas where measles is known to cause blindness, and where eye care services are not available or affordable, traditional remedies, which may be harmful, are often sought. Traditional medicines can cause corneal ulceration from secondary infection (e.g. *Gonococcus* if urine is used), thermal and chemical burns, and trauma (Figures 1.3 and 1.4).

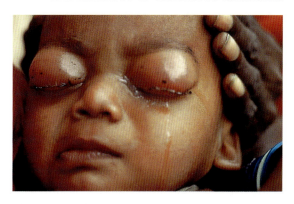

Figure 1.3    Child from Nepal whose mother rubbed oil mixed with soot onto the eyelids as a local remedy for conjunctivitis. (Courtesy of C Gilbert)

---

**Box 1.6** *Strategies for the prevention of blindness due to measles*

| Level of prevention | Strategy |
|---|---|
| Primary | • Measles immunisation<br>• Health education regarding the use of harmful traditional eye medicines |
| Secondary | • Appropriate treatment of corneal ulceration, i.e. high-dose vitamin A, antibiotics and antiviral agents |
| Tertiary | • Optical iridectomy (corneal grafting) |

---

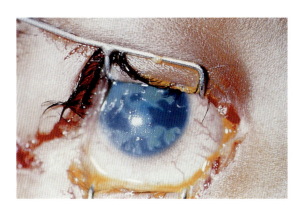

Figure 1.2    Tanzanian child with amoeboid herpetic corneal ulcer following measles infection. (Courtesy of A Foster)

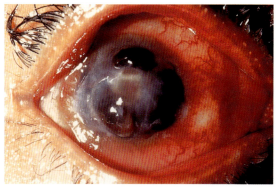

Figure 1.4 Corneal ulceration in a young Sierra Leonean who had used harmful traditional eye medicines to treat epidemic viral conjunctivitis. (Courtesy of C Gilbert)

Research is currently being undertaken to determine the most effective measles vaccine, and the best regimes (i.e. age at immunisation and vaccine titre), where measles is a leading cause of child mortality. In many developing countries, the Expanded Programme of Immunisation resulted in good coverage rates after it was first introduced. However, due to financial, logistical and political reasons, coverage in some African countries has fallen below the recommended level of 80%, and measles is becoming more common again.

## Vitamin A deficiency

Vitamin A is found as retinol in animal food sources, e.g. breast milk, cheese, fish, liver and eggs, and as carotenes and carotenoids in plant sources, e.g. yellow and red fruits (mango, papaya), dark green leafy vegetables and red palm oil. Vitamin A is necessary for cell differentiation and growth, particularly of epithelial tissues, and is an essential component of photoreceptor visual pigment. Vitamin A also plays a role in the immune system. Vitamin A is stored in the liver as retinal palmitate, and stores are usually sufficient for six months. It is released from the liver bound to retinol binding protein, which is transported to tissues bound to pre-albumin.

Vitamin A deficiency usually results from a combination of poor dietary intake, malabsorption and increased tissue demand. It is a condition of poverty, reflecting low levels of socio-economic development and education, and poor healthcare provision. Low dietary intake does not necessarily mean that affordable vitamin A rich foods are not available; inadequate breast feeding, traditional weaning and child-feeding practices and taboos are also important factors. Vitamin A deficiency is often associated with protein energy malnutrition and deficiency of other micronutrients. Severe diarrhoea is a cause of malabsorption, and measles leads to increased demand for vitamin A. Children born in communities where women of childbearing age have low vitamin A levels are

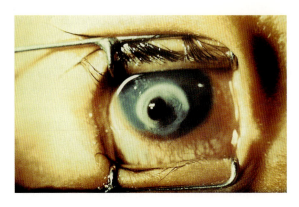

Figure 1.5    Peruvian child from a slum with a central penetrating corneal ulcer due to acute vitamin A deficiency. (Courtesy of L Gordillo Robles)

also more likely to be deficient. Children who are already vitamin A deficient with reduced liver stores can be precipitated into acute deficiency by measles or severe diarrhoea, resulting in corneal ulceration, keratomalacia and nutritional blindness (Figure 1.5).

In VAD, dedifferentiation of conjunctival and corneal epithelia leads to loss of goblet cells, squamous metaplasia and xerosis of the conjuctiva and cornea (xerophthalmia) (Figure 1.6). Bacterial action on deposits of keratin in the conjunctiva leads to accumulation of material which has a white, foamy, cottage cheese-like appearance. These accumulations, Bitot's spots (Figure 1.7), are usually located at the temporal limbus. Reduced photoreceptor rhodopsin causes night

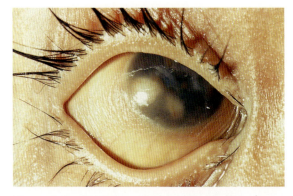

Figure 1.6    Child from Nepal with squamous metaplasia of the conjunctiva, and corneal xerosis and scarring due to vitamin A deficiency. (Courtesy of C Gilbert)

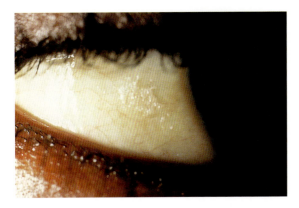

Figure 1.7 African child with a Bitot spot due to chronic vitamin A deficiency. (Courtesy of C Gilbert)

blindness and, occasionally in adults, fundus changes. Conjunctival xerosis and Bitot's spots are signs of long-standing VAD, found principally in children aged 3–8 years. Children most at risk of keratomalacia are those aged 6 months to 4 years, who may not have exhibited other features of xerophthalmia before the onset of corneal ulceration. Because not all children who are vitamin A deficient develop eye signs, it is important to be able to identify communities at risk, as children with xerophthalmia represent only the "tip of the iceberg" of those who are deficient in vitamin A in the community.

A simple, quick and cheap way of assessing the vitamin A status of a community is to determine the prevalence of the different grades of xerophthalmia, particularly of Bitot's spots, in children aged 0–6 years. The World Health Organization have suggested minimal prevalence criteria which indicate areas where there is a significant public health problem (Table 1.6).[11]

Table 1.6 Public health significance of xerophthalmia: minimal prevalence criteria

| Grade | Manifestation | Minimal prevalence (per 10 000 children) |
| --- | --- | --- |
| XN | Night blindness | 100 |
| X1B | Bitot's spots | 50 |
| X2,X3A,X3B | Corneal xerosis/ulcer | 5 |
| XS | Corneal scar | 10 |

**Box 1.7** *Strategies for the prevention of blindness due to vitamin A deficiency*

| Level of prevention | Strategy |
| --- | --- |
| Primary | • Health and nutrition education to improve the intake of vitamin A in children and women of child-bearing age, i.e. promotion of breast feeding; appropriate weaning foods; home gardening; instruction on the preparation and storage of vitamin A rich foods; food supplementation programmes<br>• Improved water supply and sanitation to prevent diarrhoea<br>• Education of women<br>• Child spacing and family planning programmes<br>• Vitamin A fortification of commonly consumed foods<br>• Measles immunisation programmes<br>• Vitamin A prophylaxis of individual children at risk, i.e. those with measles and severe diarrhoea from communities at risk<br>• Distribution of vitamin A to communities at risk, i.e. vitamin A (200 000 International Units for children aged 1–6 years and 100 000 International Units for children aged under 1 year) every 6 months. Distribution can be through existing healthcare facilities, in conjunction with immunisation programmes, or as a vertical programme |
| Secondary | • Vitamin A treatment for all children with signs of xeropthalmia, i.e. three doses given over two weeks |
| Tertiary | • Optical iridectomy (corneal grafting) |

## Conditions where the cause is often unknown

There is a significant proportion of blinding eye disease in childhood where the underlying cause cannot be determined with any degree of certainty. Data from the Nordic registers show that the underlying cause could not be determined in 32% of children, and data from developing countries show similar proportions (25–56%). This situation arises because many conditions have multiple possible causes, i.e. microphthalmos and cataract can be due to chromosomal and genetic abnormalities, or the effects of teratogens, and it is often not possible to determine the time of onset.

When the underlying cause is not known primary prevention is not possible, and prevention has to rely on strategies for early identification, appropriate treatment and follow up.

### Screening to detect treatable disease

The term "screening" should strictly be used to describe programmes which use a simple, non-invasive and inexpensive test to identify individuals with subclinical disease who can benefit from specific interventions. Screening programmes are usually targeted at high-risk groups. However, the term is often used loosely to describe methods of detecting disease, i.e. case finding.

Early identification of infants and children with ocular abnormalities and visual impairment is important. First, because early management of treatable conditions such as congenital cataract and glaucoma favourably influences the visual outcome, and second, because appropriate intervention can prevent or minimise the psychomotor developmental delay which often accompanies severe visual loss of early onset. To detect ocular abnormalities and visual impairment in children the following are recommended.

**Neonates** The eyes and adnexa of all newborn babies should be examined shortly after birth. Examinations are usually undertaken by paediatricians and neonatologists and clear guidelines need to be given on which cases to refer, and to whom the child should be referred. Children in families with genetic disease should be examined and investigated so that appropriate

interventions can be initiated early. Children who were premature, or who have certain systemic diseases where there is a high risk of eye disease (such as uveitis in Still's disease) should also be examined on a regular basis.

**Age two to three years** In countries with good primary healthcare systems, most children with major structural abnormalities and/or severe visual impairment have been identified by the age of two to three years either because parents or carers noticed a problem, or because the abnormality was detected by health workers during routine examinations. Accurate measurement of visual acuity in preschool age children is difficult and unreliable, leading to difficulties in the identification of children with unilateral or bilateral visual impairment due to less obvious structural abnormalities (such as retinal lesions, optic nerve disease). Screening of preschool age children, although desirable as early identification and treatment may favourably influence the outcome, raises several contentious issues, particularly concerning appropriate methods.

**Age three to four years** For children aged three to four years visual acuity measurement may be possible, but for younger children other methods are needed such as cycloplegic refraction, cover tests, tests of stereopsis, and photorefractive methods. In order not to miss true positive cases, and not to overload referral centres with false positives the screening test must have high levels of sensitivity and specificity. The issues of who should undertake the screening, and the cost effectiveness of preschool age screening programmes have not yet been resolved.

**Age five to six years** Most industrialised countries have vision screening programmes for five to six year-olds as part of a general assessment, providing a safety net to identify children with problems. In developing countries, vision screening of school children assumes greater importance and programmes, often undertaken by teachers, are being introduced in some developing countries, such as India.

## Overview of screening

The purpose of any screening programme is to detect disease early, using simple tests. Those who fail the screening test must be referred for confirmation of the diagnosis so that effective treatment can be instituted. The following all need to be considered:

- The seriousness and frequency of the disease in the population.
- The consequences of a delay in treatment.
- The risks and benefits of the screening procedure and the intervention.
- The feasibility and cost-effectiveness of the screening programme.

The following criteria should be fulfilled for screening programmes:

- The condition must be a significant health problem to the individual or community.
- The natural history of the condition must be known.
- A latent or preclinical phase must exist.
- An effective treatment must be available.
- The screening test should be simple, inexpensive, non-invasive and acceptable.
- The screening test must be valid, with reasonable levels of specificity and sensitivity.

- Full diagnostic and therapeutic services must be available.
- Early intervention must favourably influence the outcome.
- The screening programme should be cost effective.
- The screening programme should be continuous.

## References

1 Foster A, Gilbert C. Epidemiology of visual impairment in children. In: Taylor D, ed. *Paediatric Ophthalmology*, 2nd edn., chapter 1. Oxford: Blackwell Science, 1997.
2 Foster A, Gilbert C. Epidemiology of childhood blindness. *Eye* 1992; 6: 173–6.
3 Gilbert CE, Anderton L, Dandona L, Foster A. Prevalence of blindness and visual impairment in children – a review of available data. *Ophthal Epidemiol* 1999; 6: 73–81.
4 World Health Organization. *Prevention of Childhood Blindness*. Geneva: WHO, 1992.
5 Gilbert C, Foster A, Negrel D, Thylefors B. Childhood blindness: a new form for recording causes of visual loss in children. *WHO Bulletin* 1993; 71: 485–9.
6 Tabbara KF, Badr I. Changing pattern of childhood blindness in Saudi Arabia. *Br J Ophthalmol* 1985; 69: 312–15.
7 Gilbert C, Rahi J, Eckstein M, Foster A. Hereditary disease as a cause of childhood blindness: regional variation. *Ophthalm Genetics* 1995; 16: 1–10.
8 Paneth N. Birth and the origins of cerebral palsy. *New Engl J Med* 1986; 315: 124–6.
9 Gilbert C, Rahi J, Eckstein M, O'Sullivan J, Foster A. Retinopathy of prematurity in middle income countries. *Lancet* 1997; 350: 12–14.
10 Aaby P, Coovadia H, Bukh J, *et al*. Severe measles: a reappraisal of the role of nutrition, overcrowding and virus dose. *Med Hypotheses* 1985; 18: 93–112.
11 World Health Organization. *Vitamin A Deficiency and its Consequences: a field guide to detection and control*, 3rd edn. Geneva: WHO, 1994.

# 2 Paediatric eye examination

LOUISE ALLEN

While most infants and young children are referred with isolated ophthalmic problems that cause little or no long-term visual impairment, a minority will have serious ocular pathology which may be associated with other neurological or systemic abnormalities. Important aspects in the history of childhood eye disorders differ from those of interest in adult disease and, although older children may cooperate fully with a standard eye examination, special examination techniques are necessary in infants and toddlers. This chapter will describe the historical points and examination techniques which are of particular importance and use in the management of eye disease in young children.

## Ocular and visual screening services

The early identification of ocular and visual abnormalities optimises the results achieved by therapy and prompts early management of any associated systemic abnormality or psychomotor delay. Premature infants at risk of retinopathy of prematurity (ROP) are regularly screened for threshold disease by an ophthalmologist.[1] All other neonates are screened for congenital ocular abnormalities by medical staff prior to discharge from hospital. Routine checks of visual behaviour and eye development are repeated in the community at 6 weeks and 7–8 months of age. While many districts offer orthoptic and photographic refraction screening for preschool children, the service is expensive and the long-term advantages of the identification of strabismus and refractive error at this age continue to be debated.[2] In many health districts monocular visual acuity testing takes place at primary school entry and at 8 and 11 years of age, when colour vision is also screened.[3] It is doubtful if visual screening after the age of 6 years is worthwhile, as amblyopia detected at this age tends to respond poorly to treatment.

## History

Keep children under the age of 5 or 6 years amused with a toy or bottle during your discussion with their parents. Parental observations of the child's visual behaviour are usually correct and should be given due consideration. Older children may be able to describe their visual symptoms and care should be taken to establish a rapport with them and include them in the discussion. Children with congenitally poor vision or with acquired unilateral disease will often not complain of visual problems. Important questions at the initial clinic visit include:

- *What is the problem that has prompted the referral?*
    When was it first noticed and by whom?
    Have the parents themselves noticed the problem?
    Has there been any change since it was first identified?
    Have the parents noticed any other features, for example: photophobia, epiphora?

If the child has been referred for suspected strabismus:

How frequently is the deviation noticed by the parents?

Which eye converges/diverges or does it alternate?

Has the strabismus changed in frequency or laterality since it was first noticed?

Are there any precipitating factors, for example: fatigue, sunlight, close work?

Have the parents noticed a compensatory head posture?

- *Do the parents feel that there is a problem with the child's vision?*

Does the infant fixate and follow his/her parents' faces, show interest in his/her surroundings, smile or mimic the parents' facial expressions?

Does the infant tend to stare into bright lights or rub his/her eyes?

Have the parents noticed nystagmus?

Does the child tend to hold toys very close to his/her eyes while playing?

How does this child's visual development compare with that of his/her siblings?

Does the severity of visual impairment vary from day to day or in different lighting conditions?

- *Is the child otherwise healthy?*

Were there problems during the pregnancy, for example: maternal rash/fever, use of medication or drug abuse?

Was the child's birth premature?

Were there any medical problems in the perinatal period?

Is the infant thriving, do the parents, GP or paediatrician have any concerns?

Does the child have any other medical problems or use any medications?

Is the child reaching the expected developmental milestones; how does his/her development compare to his/her siblings at the same age?

How is the child doing at school?

- *Is there a family history of eye problems?*

Has anyone in the family had a squint, amblyopia or any serious eye problem?

Is there a family history of high refractive error?

Are the mother and father related?

Are there any other diseases which run through the family?

## Ophthalmic examination

### Initial observations

While talking with the parents, the child's general appearance, level of alertness, visual behaviour and motor development may be observed. A compensatory head posture may suggest an underlying ophthalmic cause, for example, nystagmus, visual field loss or ocular motility disturbance, or a musculoskeletal abnormality. Orbital asymmetry, abnormal lid position or gross strabismus may be noted. Physical and behavioural signs such as roving eye movements, eye poking (usually signifying bilateral retinal disease) or light gazing (a common feature of cortical visual loss) may suggest severe visual impairment.

### Visual development and acuity assessment

Although relatively well developed at birth, numerous anatomical changes occur in the eye and visual pathway postnatally which improve visual function. The first 6–8 weeks of life is an important period for normal visual development and unilateral or bilateral ocular pathology (such as dense cataract) left untreated by this time will permanently disrupt visual development.[4] The visual system retains its plasticity over the first decade of life and any ocular abnormality acquired during this period may also disrupt visual development, but the effect on vision reduces with increasing age. In general, the earlier the onset of the visual insult, the greater the resulting disruption of visual development.

15

## Infants/preverbal children

### Can this infant see?

Nystagmus may result from visual impairment due to ocular or anterior visual pathway disease but not cortical visual loss. An infant should be able to fix and follow faces within 2–3 weeks of birth.[5] A positive blink reflex to a burst of bright light, visually directed reaching and the ability of the infant to fixate and follow the examiner's face demonstrate that a basic level of vision is present. In the absence of nystagmus, the opto-kinetic drum may also confirm a visual response. When fixation can not be demonstrated, the spinning test may help the examiner differentiate between blindness and low levels of vision. The infant should be held at arm's length and rotated to provoke vestibulo-ocular nystagmus, the slow phase of which occurs towards the direction of the rotation (Figure 2.1). On stopping the rotation, the nystagmus should dampen quickly due to the fixation reflex. Absence of corrective saccades during rotation is a feature of ocular motor apraxia, while prolonged postrotational nystagmus suggests very poor visual function. Since all of these tests rely on the infant's motor responses, abnormal results require corroboration by electrophysiological tests.

### Quality of fixation

The ability of the young child to fixate and follow a small target is an important gross assessment of vision. Consistent objection from the child to having one eye occluded suggests that it has the better vision of the two. The ability of each eye to fixate a target centrally and steadily and to maintain this fixation through a blink gives a good indication of the quality of its vision. Eccentric fixation, where the child does not fixate with the fovea, is a sign of poor vision in that eye. The ability of a previously squinting eye to fixate a target centrally when the other eye is covered and maintain the fixation for several seconds when the cover is removed, indicates that the visual acuity in both eyes is similar; if the uncovered eye immediately moves to take over fixation, the tested eye must have poorer visual acuity. Fixation preference may be assessed in children without a manifest strabismus by creating an artificial vertical deviation with a 10 Dioptre prism held base down in front of one eye. If the visual acuity in the other eye is good, it will maintain fixation in the primary position but if its acuity is poor, the eye behind the prism will take up fixation, causing both eyes to move up.

### Forced choice preferential looking (FPL)

A popular way of quantifying infant vision, FPL is based on the natural tendency of an infant to prefer looking at a patterned stimulus rather than a plain one. Portable cards (Teller or Keeler cards) simultaneously present the infant with two targets, one with a square-wave grating with varying spatial frequency and the other of a homogeneous grey of matched mean luminance. The clinician, blinded to the location of the square-wave target, chooses the most likely location based on the observation of the infant's eye movements through a peep hole between the two targets. (Figure 2.2) An indication of the level of

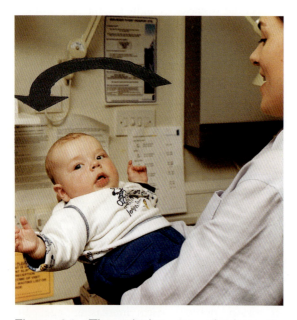

Figure 2.1 The spinning test stimulates the vestibulo-ocular reflex. The slow phase of the nystagmus occurs towards the direction of movement (shown by the arrow)

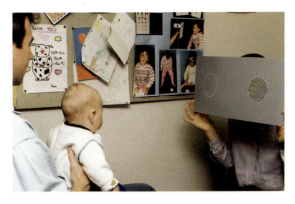

Figure 2.2 Forced choice preferential looking (FPL) measurement using Keeler acuity cards

the infant's spatial resolution is given when the eye movements indicate no preference between the targets. Although FPL may be inappropriate for infants with severe ocular motor defects, it may be assessed in the presence of horizontal nystagmus if the card is held vertically.

**Pattern visual evoked potential (PVEP)** (see Chapter 3)

The advantage of electrophysiological testing in assessing infant visual acuity is that no ocular motor response is required. A chequerboard pattern of varying size is used to stimulate the central retina and the occipital cortical response is measured with scalp electrodes. Meaningful results depend upon good fixation and correction of any refractive error. Neither PVEPs nor FPL measurements can be directly correlated with Snellen acuity and both underestimate the effect of strabismic amblyopia or macular disease. In the normal infant, PVEPs suggest the equivalent of 6/6 vision is achieved between 6 months and 1 year of life;[6] FPL measurements lag behind this (reaching 6/6 equivalent at 1–3 years of age),[7] probably due to the behavioural response required in its interpretation.[8] The "sweep visual evoked potential (VEP)", in which the frequency of grating is rapidly increased over a 10-second period, is faster to perform than the pattern reversal technique, potentially improving compliance with the procedure.[9]

## Verbal children

A variety of optotype tests are available for testing distance visual acuity in children (Figure 2.3):

- 1–2 years of age:     Cardiff acuity cards
- 2–3 years of age:     Kay pictures, matching optotypes (HOTV or Sheridan Gardiner)
- > 3 years of age:     Cambridge crowding cards, Snellen visual acuity chart, Stycar letters

Since isolated optotypes will overestimate vision in amblyopic eyes, crowding cards or full lines of Snellen characters should be used when amblyopia is suspected. Visual acuity with both eyes open and near visual acuity more accurately assess a child's functional visual impairment, especially if nystagmus is a feature of the condition. Near visual acuity charts include the reduced Snellen and Sheridan Gardiner tests read at 0.3 m or the Maclure test type (Figure 2.4).

## Visual field examination

The infant's visual field enlarges to reach normal adult values at 12–15 months of age.[10] While computerised perimetry, such as Humphrey field analysis, is useful in school-aged children, confrontation techniques are informative at any age. The child's attention should be drawn centrally using one toy, while another toy is introduced into their visual periphery. A child with normal visual fields will make a rapid head movement or fixation saccade to the target (Figure 2.5a,b). If the object is introduced into an area of relative field loss, the child may initially look past it before making a corrective eye movement to fixate it more accurately.[11] Hemianopic children may turn their heads towards an object in the non-seeing field and then rotate their eyes back to fixate the object of interest.[12] Older children will often cooperate with the confrontation techniques used in adults;

17

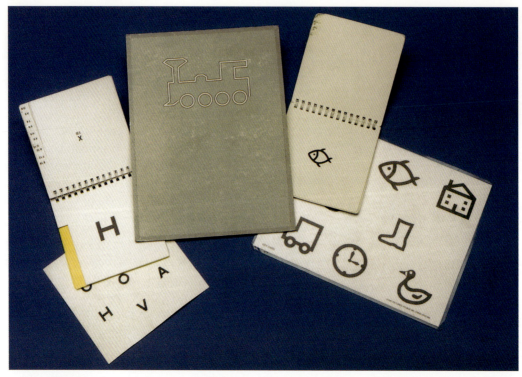

Figure 2.3   Visual acuity tests for preverbal children. From left to right: the Sheridan Gardiner test, Cardiff cards, Kay pictures

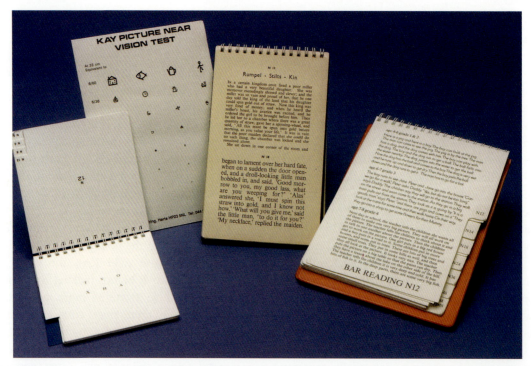

Figure 2.4   Near acuity tests. From left to right: the reduced Sheridan Gardiner test, the Kay picture near-vision test, the Moorfields reading test and Maclure bar-reading test

finger counting in the quadrants of the visual field is a particularly useful and quick method for identifying hemianopic field defects.

### Colour vision

Congenital colour vision abnormalities affect 6% of Caucasian males, the most common defect being deuteranomaly.[13] Colour vision assessment is an important diagnostic test both in children with decreased visual acuity and in the monitoring of progressive macular and optic nerve disorders. Although there are exceptions, the acquired optic nerve diseases tend to cause red–green colour defects, while acquired retinal diseases cause blue–yellow abnormalities in early disease. There are several colour vision tests available which are suitable for use with children (Figure 2.6a,b). Ishihara pseudoisochromatic plates screen for red–green colour defects only. Both the Hardy–Rand–Rittler (HRR) plates and the Mollon–Reffin test (in which the child is asked to identify a coloured chip placed randomly in a field of grey chips of varying luminosity) grade red–green and blue–yellow colour deficiencies and can be used for children as young as three.[14] The Farnsworth D15 test and City University plates are colour-matching tests which grade red–green and blue–yellow defects in older children.

### Ocular motility and tests of binocular vision

Nystagmus may have been noticed by the infant's parents. The frequency, amplitude and slow phase direction of the nystagmus, and the presence of an associated head posture should be noted. In general, the onset of nystagmus in the first month of life implies a benign cause such as congenital idiopathic motor nystagmus, while acquired nystagmus may indicate the presence of serious ocular or intracranial pathology.

Strabismus is a common referral diagnosis and the examination should be performed with certain goals in mind: to assess and measure the ocular deviation, to establish the cause for the deviation, to diagnose amblyopia and assess the binocular sensory status. While older children will be able to cooperate with a standard, full ocular motility examination, infants and young children often require special techniques, some of which are described below.

### Ocular alignment

Useful light reflex tests for infants include the Bruckner, Hirshberg and Krimsky tests. If an infant with strabismus fixates the light of a direct ophthalmoscope, the deviating eye will have a

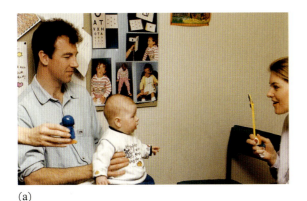

(a)

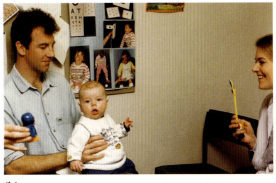

(b)

Figure 2.5   Visual field testing by confrontation. (a) The infant's attention is drawn towards the examiner while a toy target is introduced into the infant's peripheral field. (b) Once the infant is able to detect the target in his visual field, he will make a head movement to fixate it

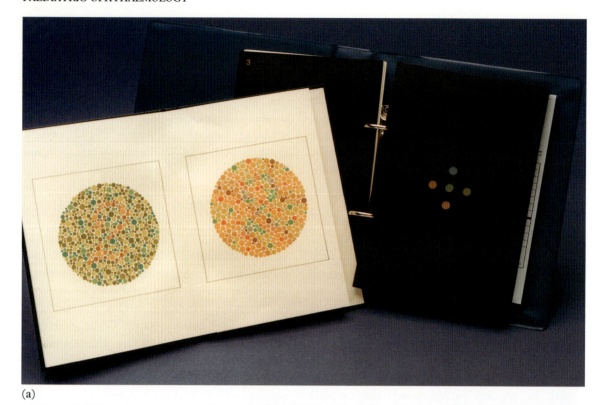

(a)

(b)

Figure 2.6   (a) Ishihara pseudoisochromatic plates and City University plates are commonly used for testing colour vision in older children. (b) Hardy–Rand–Rittler (HRR) plates and the Mollon–Reffin minimalist test are useful for the assessment of colour vision in children as young as 3 years of age

brighter red reflex than the fixating one (Bruckner test). If he/she then fixates the examiner's face while the torchlight is shone from a similar position, the corneal reflex will be eccentric in the non-fixing eye – the reflex will be displaced temporally in esotropia, nasally in exotropia and inferiorly in hypertropia. The angle of deviation may be estimated by the displacement of the light reflex (Hirshberg test) – displacement to the pupillary margin representing an angle of $15°$, to the mid-iris $30°$, and to the limbus $40°$, or measured using prisms (Krimsky test). In orthotropic children, the reflexes will both be slightly displaced nasally due to a physiological positive angle kappa.

The cover/uncover and alternate cover tests are difficult to perform on infants and younger children since they rely on good control of fixation. If a plastic cover is not tolerated, a thumb may act as an occluder while the examiner attempts to measure the ocular deviation at distance and at near (using an accommodative target) with a prism oriented with its apex pointing in the direction of the deviation.

## Eye movements

Cooperation time is limited in infants and toddlers, and observations have to be made quickly. A head posture may have already suggested a specific defect in motility. Versions are best assessed by encouraging the child to follow a target while a parent steadies its head. Voluntary abduction in infants with esotropia and crossfixation may be seen after patching one eye for a short period. The presence of supranuclear reflexes such as the vestibulo-ocular reflex and Bell's phenomenon may help in the exclusion of a paralytic or restrictive motility disorder. The vestibulo-ocular reflex is stimulated by the spinning test or the "doll's head" manoeuvre. Sixth nerve function can be assessed by studying abduction during rotation and abduction saccades. Similarly, optokinetic testing will demonstrate muscle weakness by the resulting slow and incomplete saccades in the field of action of the muscle in question. It may also demonstrate gaze abnormalities and saccade initiation failure (oculomotor apraxia).

## Assessment of binocular vision

The Lang and Frisby tests are frequently used for testing young children since they do not require the use of special glasses. Children over 5 years are usually tested with the Titmus fly and Randot stereopsis tests (Figure 2.7). Sensory fusion and anomalous retinal correspondence may be assessed in older children using the Worth four-dot test, Bagolini glasses or synoptophore. Motor fusion, as measured by prism fusional amplitudes, may be assessed from early childhood.

# Ocular examination

## Ocular adnexa

An initial examination should assess the child for dysmorphic features, head shape and size, symmetry and separation of the orbits and proptosis. Prominent epicanthic folds may cause pseudostrabismus. Ptosis is a common referral diagnosis and should be examined in the usual manner. Important features include the presence of a chin-up compensatory head posture, lid lag on downgaze characteristic of levator dystrophy, iris heterochromia caused by congenital Horner syndrome, jaw winking associated with Marcus Gunn ptosis (best observed when the infant feeds from a bottle) and assessment of the risk of amblyopia as indicated by the proximity of the lid to the visual axis. A pseudoptosis may occur with enophthalmos and in association with hypotropic eye (the ptosis disappears when the eye elevates to take up fixation).

## Pupil examination

Although the pupils are small and poorly reacting in the neonatal period, by the age of 3 months normal reactions should be present. Iris colour is permanent at $9-12$ months of age. Abnormalities in pupil shape and iris colour,

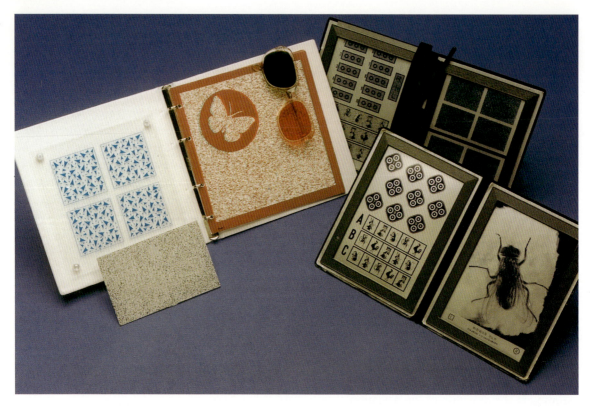

Figure 2.7    Tests for binocular vision and stereopsis. From left to right: the Frisby and Lang tests, the TNO test, the Randot and Titmus tests

such as colobomata, aniridia, iris heterochromia and leukocoria may be seen on torch inspection. Direct and consensual light reflexes and the presence of a relative afferent pupillary defect should be assessed, although maintaining distance fixation in young children during testing may prove challenging. A paradoxical pupil reaction is characterised by a brief pupillary constriction when the room lights are extinguished and may be a feature of congenital achromatopsia, congenital stationary night blindness or optic nerve hypoplasia. Anisocoria, if present, should be compared in light and dark environments and may require pharmacological confirmation of the cause.

### Slit-lamp examination

Slit-lamp examination allows visualisation of anterior segment abnormalities, identification of iris transillumination defects in albinism and determination of cataract type and position. Infants may be held prone by a parent, so that their forehead is touching the head band. Toddlers may reach the headrest by sitting on their parent's lap (Figure 2.8). Often there are only a few seconds of cooperation in which to examine the feature of interest, so the room should be completely darkened and the lamp made ready beforehand.

### Intraocular pressure (IOP) measurement

The IOP tends to be lower in children than adults; mean normal values are approximately 9.5 mmHg in neonates and rise to 14 mmHg by 5 years of age.[15] Measurement of IOP is ideally performed in the awake child since it may be influenced by anaesthetic agents and intubation.[16] Perkins tonometry under topical anaesthetic can be performed in most neonates, while Keeler Pulsair tonometry is helpful in young children. Goldmann tonometry may be tolerated by children as young as 5 or 6 years of age.

## Refraction

While older children may be able to cooperate with subjective refraction, cycloplegic refraction is necessary, at least initially, in all children. Cyclopentolate 1% (0.5% for infants under 3 months of age) is the most commonly used cycloplegic. It produces maximal cycloplegia 30–60 minutes after instillation and its effects last approximately 24 hours. Dose-related side-effects are rarely seen but include ataxia, cerebellar dysfunction and visual hallucinations. Prior instillation of proxymetacaine 0.5% can be useful in children who find the sting of cyclopentolate upsetting. Atropine 0.5% drops used three times a day for 3 days prior to refraction are useful for children with darkly pigmented irides. Parents should be warned to discontinue the drops if flushing, irritability and fever should occur.

Accurate refraction may be difficult in a tired and fractious child and, although some infants and toddlers may settle with a bottle, sometimes only the briefest of views is possible. In these cases, refraction with a +4 Dioptre lens will at least exclude myopia and high hypermetropia. For accurate measurements, refraction must be performed along the visual axis with the child fixating the light or examiner's face; a strabismic eye should be forced to fixate by occluding the other with a thumb or patch.

## Fundoscopy

Mydriasis may be augmented by the use of tropicamide 0.5% or 1%, or phenylephrine 2.5%. Fundoscopy should take place in a darkened room, with the infant cradled in the parent's arms and settled with a bottle. The indirect ophthalmoscope is used initially, with the examiner gently opening the baby's lids with his/her fingers. The lens should be held in position and the light quickly brought into view, providing a series of quick glimpses before lid squeezing and Bell's phenomenon develop. While a +20 Dioptre lens provides a useful overview of the fundus, a +28 Dioptre lens will provide a wider field of view, and a +14 Dioptre lens a better detail of the macula and optic nerve. Toddlers and young children are often the hardest group to coax into cooperating with the examination and may eventually require a short period of restraint in order to get a satisfactory view. Fortunately, older children are usually entertained by the appearance of the indirect ophthalmoscope and cooperate well with the procedure. Detailed examination of the macula and optic disc are possible using a +78 or +90 Dioptre lens at the slit-lamp in older children and by direct ophthalmoscopy – an especially useful technique in the detection of optic nerve hypoplasia – in infants.

## Examination under sedation and anaesthesia

Examination under sedation may be indicated if children will not tolerate vital aspects of the

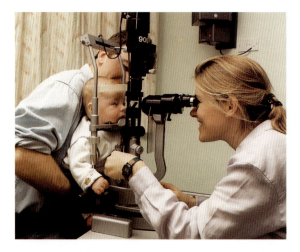

Figure 2.8 While toddlers may be able to reach the headrest while sitting on a parent's lap, infants should be held prone

ophthalmic examination, such as regular IOP measurements for congenital glaucoma. Most paediatric departments will have a protocol for children requiring examination under sedation and will provide paediatric support for the procedure. Chloral hydrate sedation will facilitate a full eye examination and IOP measurement. Ketamine, when used in subanaesthetic dosage, provides sedation and analgesia adequate for minor procedures such as suture removal. Administered by intramuscular or intravenous routes in theatre, it is also a useful initial agent if the case may proceed to major procedure on the results of the examination findings. If examination under general anaesthetic is necessary, the opportunity should be fully utilised to provide ophthalmic information, photographic records, phlebotomy, and contributions from other specialists involved in the child's care.

## Examination of family members

Examination of family members provides valuable information about the genetics of the condition – for example, by the detection of the maternal carrier state in X-linked ocular albinism – and may also indicate the likely visual prognosis in dominantly inherited conditions such as macular dystrophy and optic atrophy.

## Further investigations

Photographic records are useful for explaining the condition to family members and assessing changes in the appearance of the pathology over time and after surgery. Children with visual impairment often require electrodiagnostic and neuroradiological investigations before a specific diagnosis can be made. Since visual impairment in childhood results in psychomotor delay and congenital ocular abnormalities are often associated with other systemic problems, a paediatric specialist should be involved in the child's management.

## Services for visually impaired children

It is fortunately uncommon to have to tell parents that their child has severe visual impairment. The impact of this news often results in a tumult of emotions such as shock, fear, denial, anger, guilt, and sadness. Since the way in which the parents are told of their child's blindness may influence their ability to adapt to their loss, it is important to take the time to discuss the situation compassionately with the family in an appropriately private setting. Advice regarding the visual prognosis, stimulation of residual vision, education services and genetic counselling should be given, and parents should be informed about support groups and organisations such as LOOK and the RNIB (see Appendix). Contacting these groups often decreases the parents anxiety about the diagnosis and gives them something positive that they can do for their child. The local education authority should be informed soon after the diagnosis is made; a peripatetic teacher will be assigned to encourage the child's development and provide assistance with education. Many visually impaired children can be successfully integrated into local schools, while special schools may be more helpful for children with additional learning difficulties.

## Summary

The paediatric ophthalmic examination is tailored for the age of the child, the cooperation they are able to give, and towards identifying the eye disorders which occur in childhood. In many cases, the initial clinical examination alone will not provide a definitive diagnosis and further electrophysiological and radiological investigations are required. Establishing a good rapport with the child and his/her parents maximises the information gained during the examination and the support which can be given if the child's visual prognosis is poor. Although the paediatric eye examination is often approached with a sense of trepidation by many ophthalmologists more used to examining adult patients, some initial time spent establishing the child's and parents' trust together with a structured clinical approach will result in a detailed, complete and even enjoyable consultation.

## References

1 Report of a joint working party. *Retinopathy of Prematurity: Guidelines for Screening and Treatment.* London: Royal College of Ophthalmologists and British Association of Perinatal Medicine, 1995.

2 Stewart-Brown SL, Haslum MN. Partial sight and blindness in children of the 1970 birth cohort at 10 years of age. *J Epidemiol Community Health* 1988; **42**: 17–23.

3 Report of a joint working party. *Ophthalmic Services for Children.* London: Royal College of Ophthalmologists and the British Paediatric Association, 1994.

4 Vaegan, Taylor D. Critical period for deprivation amblyopia in children. *Trans Ophthalmol Soc UK* 1979; **99**: 432–9.

5 Willshaw HE. Traditional clinical methods of visual assessment in childhood. *Trans Ophthalmol Soc UK* 1985; **104**: 641–5.

6 Sokol S, Dobson V. Pattern reversal visually evoked potentials in infants. *Invest Ophthalmol Vis Sci* 1976; **15**: 58–62.

7 Mayer D, Dobson V. Visual acuity development in infants and young children as assessed by apparent preferential looking. *Vision Res* 1982; **22**: 1141–51.

8 Allen D, Bennett PJ, Banks MS. The effects of luminance on FPL and VEP acuity in human infants. *Vision Res* 1992; **32**: 2005–12.

9 Norcia A, Tyler C. Spatial frequency sweep VEP: visual acuity during the first year of life. *Vision Res* 1985; **25**: 1399–1408.

10 Mohn G, Van Hof-van Duin J. Development of the binocular and monocular visual fields of infants during the first year of life. *Clin Vis Sci* 1986; **1**: 51–64.

11 Good WV. Behaviors of visually impaired children. *Semin Ophthalmol* 1991; **6**: 158–60.

12 Zangemeister WH, Meienberg O, Stark L, Hoyt WF. Eye–head coordination of homonymous hemianopia. *J Neurol* 1982; **226**: 243–52.

13 Waardenberg PA, Franceschetti A, Klein D. *Genetics and Ophthalmology.* Thomas Springfield, Illinois: Thomas, 1963.

14 Mollon JD, Astell S, Reffin JP. A minimalist test of colour vision. In: Drum B, Moreland JD, Serra A, Eds. *Colour Vision Deficiencies.* Dordrecht: Kluwer, 1991.

15 Pensiero S, Da Pozzo S, Perissutti P, Cavallini GM, Guerra R. Normal IOP in children. *J Paediatr Ophthalmol Strabismus* 1992; **29**: 79–84.

16 Dear GD, Hammerton M, Hatch DJ, Taylor D. Anaesthesia and intra-ocular pressure in young children. *Anaesthesia* 1987; **42**: 259–65.

# 3 Electrophysiological investigations of infants and young children

KEITH BRADSHAW

Electrophysiological tests can be helpful in three ways. Firstly, for some clinical problems electrophysiology is essential to confirm the diagnosis (e.g. the flash electroretinogram in early onset retinal dystrophies). Secondly, they can provide important supplementary information about the likely degree of visual function, rather than provide data which influences the clinical diagnosis (e.g. the pattern visual evoked potential (VEP) may be used to estimate Snellen acuity). Thirdly, they can provide a degree of "comfort" that serious organic abnormality is not being missed (e.g. evidence of a VEP response in an apparently blind infant may provide positive support for a diagnosis of delayed visual maturation).

## Electrophysiological tests

There are four tests in routine use which allow the investigator to probe specific visual structures. The essential principles of each of these tests will be summarised here and the interested reader is referred to the book by Carr and Siegel[1] for a more detailed treatment. The books by Regan[2] and Heckenlively and Arden[3] are authoritative texts covering many aspects of human visual electrophysiology.

## The Electro-oculogram (EOG)

This term is used in two quite distinct ways. Firstly, it refers to procedures for measuring various characteristics of eye movements such as saccadic delay, velocity and duration (see Chapter 15). The second and more common use of the term refers to a specific procedure for measuring the electrical standing potential of the eye. This procedure has been used clinically for many years to assess the function of the retinal pigment epithelium (RPE).

The EOG test, sometimes also referred to as the Arden test, is a specific method for measuring the standing electrical potential of the eye. This standing potential is an electrical charge which develops across the RPE membrane and can be measured directly as a 60-mV potential difference between the front and the back of the eye, the back of the eye being negative relative to the front. The potential can be measured indirectly in patients by means of small disc electrodes placed on each side of the eye. If the eye is rotated alternately left and right through a fixed angle, the EOG signal will show up as a steady swing in voltage, going relatively negative as the eye rotates one way then relatively positive as the eye rotates the other way. The level of the standing potential changes during the course of dark and light adaptation. In the EOG test procedure, the signal is recorded in the way described at 1-minute intervals, first over a period of 15 minutes in total darkness and then over 15 minutes with the eyes exposed continuously to a fairly bright uniform light. During darkness, the signal amplitude falls reaching a trough at about 8 minutes, and then rises slowly in the light reaching a peak after about 8–10 minutes. The ratio of light peak to dark trough, called the Arden index, is about 2 : 1 in normal observers; a low Arden index indicates abnormal function of the RPE.

A clinical standard for the test procedure has now been published.[4] The test has only limited clinical value in paediatric ophthalmology, chiefly in the diagnosis of some retinal dystrophies such as Best's disease and some of the pattern dystrophies.

## Pattern electroretinogram (PERG)

This retinal signal, recorded directly from the eye by means of a small conductive foil or fibre electrode in contact with the sclera, is a response to pattern stimulation. The pattern is usually made up of black-and-white squares (checkerboard) or stripes (grating) and the PERG signal is evoked by the sudden reversal of contrast of each pattern element (black squares change to white and white to black). The response is very small and can only be measured by summating the response to about 200 pattern contrast reversals. In cooperative subjects, it takes only a few minutes to record the response but accurate refraction of the eye and careful fixation of the stimulus are essential and for these reasons the test is not possible in the youngest age groups. However, many older children cope perfectly well with the procedure. More detailed reviews can be found in Berninger and Arden.[5] Guidelines for recording the PERG in the clinic have been adopted and published by the International Society for Clinical Electrophysiology of Vision (ISCEV).[6]

When the rate of stimulation is relatively slow (say 2–4 contrast reversals per second) the PERG signal consists of two components, a positive-going response measuring 3–5 µV with a peak at about 50 ms and a negative-going potential measuring 4–6 µV with a peak at about 90 ms. An abundance of evidence from both clinical and experimental studies indicates that this response is generated in the inner retina, probably with a significant contribution from ganglion cells, with the central retina making the greatest contribution to response size under normal clinical test conditions. The PERG can therefore be used as a specific test of central retinal function and is very useful in the investigation of suspected macular dysfunction.[7] Moreover, because of the contribution of ganglion cells to the PERG response, the test can be used in conjunction with the VEP to assess both retinal and optic nerve function across the central field of vision, for example in suspected cases of hysterical amblyopia.

## Flash electroretinogram (flash ERG)

The flash ERG is the electrical response of the retina which is evoked by a diffuse flash of light. The ERG is essentially a wide-field response and so ERG stimulators are usually designed to present a uniform flash of light over a wide area (120° or more) so that all parts of the retina are stimulated equally well. This is best achieved by means of a dome, or Ganzfeld, stimulator which scatters the light from a small xenon flash lamp over the inner white surface of the sphere. The patient views the stimulus flash indirectly through a small viewing port.

Isolating the fundamental receptor mechanisms should be the starting point for any clinical ERG procedure. The rods and cones contribute their signals to the ERG in an independent way and the response of one system can be clearly separated from the other by relatively simple procedures that are based on well-established principles of photoreceptor physiology.[8] A rod-dominated signal can be obtained by presenting low-intensity flashes (below the activation threshold of cones) to the dark-adapted eye. Composite cone responses can be recorded by a variety of methods. One simple procedure involves suppression of rod activity by adaptation to a low-intensity white light. A bright flash of light presented against this background will then generate an ERG signal derived primarily from the cones. A white light flickering at 30 Hz will also elicit a cone response. A bright flash of light presented to the dark-adapted eye will elicit a maximal amplitude mixed rod–cone response. A standard for recording the clinical ERG has been adopted by ISCEV[9] and is revised every four years. More rigorous procedures for recording the ERG a-wave and for relating the response to the parameters of photo-transduction in photoreceptors have been described recently.[10-12] These procedures are essential in research studies of photoreceptor abnormality but are not required for routine clinical diagnosis at the present time.

In cooperative subjects the ERG is best recorded by means of an electrode in direct contact with the eye and the majority of older children will tolerate this recording procedure quite well. Younger children are unlikely to accept an electrode in contact with the eye without restraint or sedation and to avoid this the ERG can be recorded by means of a silver disc electrode placed on the skin just below the lower eyelid. There is loss of signal amplitude and an increase in the background noise with this procedure but all the standard rod and cone responses can be recorded with the Ganzfeld procedures described above. Ganzfeld stimulators cannot be used easily with children younger than 4 years old or with infants so an alternative procedure is to hold a small xenon flash lamp directly in front of the eyes. Infants only a few weeks old can be tested in this way. With disc electrodes on the skin and small hand-held stimulators, there is a sacrifice of technical rigour, but this procedure is capable of providing clinically useful information. It is also possible to obtain age-matched control data for each of these procedures, which is more difficult for protocols involving sedation and/or recording electrodes in contact with the eye.

The amplitude and latency of ERG components are measured carefully and compared with age-matched control data to determine whether rod and cone responses are abnormal. It is also possible to assess whether inner or outer retinal function is abnormal from our knowledge of which cells contribute to the various components of the ERG response. The photoreceptors make the most significant contribution to the early negative component (the a-wave) so a very low amplitude a-wave indicates primary photoreceptor abnormality. Cells in the inner nuclear layer appear to contribute more to the later positive-going component (the b-wave), so ERG responses with normal a-waves but depressed b-waves indicate inner retinal abnormality.

## The visual evoked potential (VEP)

This is the response recorded from one or more electrodes attached to the scalp at the back of the head over the occipital cortex. Responses at this site are low amplitude and "buried" in the background electroencephalograph (EEG) activity, so computer processing is essential for extraction of the VEP signal. Two types of stimuli are commonly used in clinical evoked potential investigations. The simplest is an unstructured, diffuse flash of light – usually a short-duration flash from a xenon lamp, as with the ERG. This stimulus has the advantage that the subject does not need to fixate carefully or pay attention and the response is unaffected by slight opacities of the media or uncorrected refractive errors. It has greatest value in assessing the visual pathway in infants and in older subjects where cooperation is limited. Clinical studies suggest that it is a rather robust response and it may be unaffected by quite severe lesions of the optic nerve (e.g. it may be normal in optic neuritis).

The more useful stimulus is a patterned field, usually a checkerboard as with pattern ERG studies. The pattern must be modulated or changed in some periodic manner in order to "drive" the visual system. There are two ways of doing this. One method is called pattern (or contrast) reversal because the elements of a continuously visible checkerboard are reversed in contrast periodically (e.g. twice per second). The second procedure is called pattern onset or pattern appearance because the checkerboard pattern "appears" (or replaces) a uniform grey field. The overall waveform morphology and the latency and amplitude of individual peaks depend on a variety of parameters including the mode of presentation (for the same pattern, reversal and appearance procedures generate markedly different responses), check size and field size. Each procedure has a particular role to play in investigation of visual pathway abnormalities in infants and children, which will be described later, and ISCEV has published a standard for clinical VEP testing.[13]

Visual acuity estimation is particularly important in young infants. Pattern-onset and pattern-reversal procedures have been investigated for this purpose. A further technique which is technically more complex but has the advantage of speed is the sweep visual evoked potential. This technique is based on the idea of recording the steady-state potential while sweeping rapidly through a range of pattern sizes up to and beyond the acuity limit. It is beyond the scope of this chapter to discuss in detail this difficult technical issue but an up-to-date and authoritative review is provided by Tyler.[14] At the present time, it is not certain which VEP procedure will give the best estimate of Snellen acuity, and none are immune to the practical difficulties inherent in testing the young infant.

## Clinical indications for electrophysiological tests

How can the ophthalmologist make best use of these tests? The best approach is to use them to test a specific structure (retina or optic nerves) and to answer a specific clinical question. When referring a patient for electrophysiology, the ophthalmologist should be clear what information is wanted from the test and should make requests as specific as possible – for example, "Is there ERG indication of a photoreceptor dystrophy?" or "Is there VEP evidence of albinism?". Each test can be quite lengthy and in infants and younger children, it may be possible to perform only one procedure per session.

Asking a specific clinical question will also help the electrophysiologist select the most appropriate test procedure. Here it is important to understand a distinction between the electrophysiological test itself and a particular test protocol. Each of the tests described can be implemented in a variety of ways and the particular method, or protocol, adopted will depend in part on the clinical question being asked. For example, if the likely diagnosis is retrobulbar neuritis, this could be confirmed by recording the pattern reversal VEP to a single pattern size from a single occipital electrode and taking careful measurement of response peak latency. However, if the ophthalmologist requires information about the level of useful pattern vision, a different test protocol would be required. Here, it would be essential to record the VEP in response to a wide range of check sizes, particularly sizes smaller than 12′ arc, and results would be evaluated on the basis of amplitude (not latency) relationships over the range of pattern sizes and by determining the smallest pattern giving a reliable response (i.e. determination of electrical threshold).

The success of the investigation depends very much on the cooperation and, in the case of the VEP, the level of alertness of the infant. Development of test protocols appropriate for specific age groups and clinical problem, and careful patient handling are crucial in ensuring that technically satisfactory recordings are obtained. However, it must be accepted that even for a single test procedure, it may not always be possible to obtain all the information required at the first visit. But with patience and persistence it is usually possible to obtain all necessary data, either completely at a second visit or cumulatively over several visits.

## Assessing retinal function

### Assessing the young infant

Flash ERGs are indicated in infants presenting at a few months of age with nystagmus, especially if there are other associated signs (e.g. photophobia) or fundal abnormality, and in infants with other organic disease and apparently symmetrical visual loss where retinal abnormality may be suspected (e.g. in metabolic disorders).

Figure 3.1 shows the flash ERGs of three infants recorded by means of silver disc electrodes on the skin below each eye. A small, handheld strobe lamp was used to stimulate the eyes. Recordings on the left are for a normal 1-year old. The lowest trace is an isolated rod response which has only a positive-going (upward) b-wave and the next response is a mixed rod–cone response to a maximal intensity white flash which has both a negative (downward) a-wave followed by a b-wave. Cone responses are shown in the upper three traces.

**Case 1** A one-year-old female who presented with nystagmus and apparently poor vision was referred for investigation. She was otherwise healthy with normal development. There was a family history of retinitis pigmentosa. The ERG is shown in the centre panel of Figure 3.1. There was no measurable cone response to any of the three stimuli and no mixed rod–cone response to the brightest flash. The absence of an a-wave indicates photoreceptor degeneration. These results confirmed severe, extensive abnormality of both rod

and cone photoreceptors and supported a diagnosis of infantile-onset rod–cone dystrophy. In this case, the ERG confirmed the clinical diagnosis.

**Case 2** A one-year-old girl presented with dysmorphic features, hypotonia, feeding problems and possible seizures. She appeared to have poor vision but fundal examination was normal. At the time of referral for ERG studies, she was under investigation for a possible peroxisomal disorder. Responses are shown in the right panel of Figure 3.1. There was only minimal cone response to 30-Hz flicker and no convincing response to red flash (light adapted white flash not obtained). Very low amplitude, subnormal rod–cone and rod responses were obtained in the dark (lower two traces). These results indicated severe, extensive abnormality of both rods and cones indicating that she had a retinal dystrophy in addition to her other systemic abnormalities.

## Assessing retinal function in young children

Older, more cooperative children can be tested with better ERG procedures incorporating diffuse field stimulators and proper control of dark and light adaptation of the eye, though often

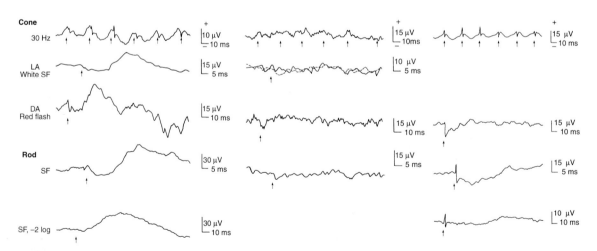

Figure 3.1 ERGs recorded by means of silver disc electrode on the skin below each eye. Small handheld strobe stimulator. Left panel: Normal 1-year old. Centre panel: Leber's amaurosis. Case 1. Right panel: Peroxisomal disorder, Case 2. Both were 1-year-old females with severe extensive photoreceptor abnormality. All ERG responses could not be recorded in the patients for technical reasons. The arrows indicate the time of the stimulus flash

disc electrodes on the skin must be used instead of foil electrodes in contact with the sclera. Some children tested in this age group may have an infantile-onset retinal dystrophy which has not yet been diagnosed accurately whilst others may have developed symptoms after a period of normal visual development. Most retinal dystrophies affect both rods and cones, but in some dystrophies only one type of photoreceptor is affected and it is important for correct diagnosis and genetic counselling to determine which photoreceptors are abnormal (see Chapter 10).

The left panel of Figure 3.2 shows recordings obtained in a normal 11-year old. The lower two traces show isolated rod responses (b-wave only present at these low light intensities) and the next two higher traces are mixed rod–cone (mainly rod) responses which show both an a-wave and a b-wave, the amplitude of the response increasing with increasing intensity.

The upper traces are isolated cone responses to three different stimuli.

**Case 3** A 10-year-old boy presented with deteriorating vision. His visual acuity was reduced to 6/60 in each eye and he had no measurable colour vision on testing with the Ishihara plates. His visual fields were reduced to 30°. On examination he showed a subtle bull's eye maculopathy but there was no evidence of peripheral retinal changes. The ERG responses are shown in the right panel of Figure 3.2. Only poorly defined, very small cone responses are evident to 30-Hz flicker and white flash and there is no measurable response to red flash. Rod and rod–cone responses are clearly present but amplitudes are subnormal when compared with age-matched controls. These results indicated extensive rather than localised photoreceptor abnormality and suggested a diagnosis of cone–rod dystrophy rather than a macular dystrophy.

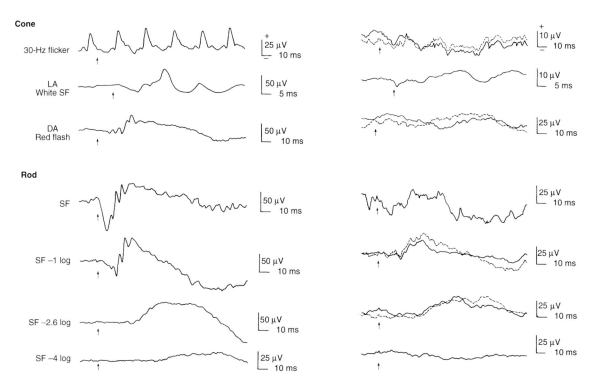

Figure 3.2    ERGs recorded by means of silver disc electrodes on the skin below each eye. Full-field Ganzfeld stimulation. Left panel: Normal 11-year-old male. Right panel: Cone–rod dystrophy. Case 3. 10-year-old male with extensive abnormality of both rod and cone function. Note the different amplitude calibrations for two panels. The arrows indicate the time of the stimulus flash

Some retinal dystrophies affect only the cone system. Two forms, rod monochromatism and blue cone monochromatism are present from birth but the diagnosis may be missed early in life (see Chapter 10). The ERG is especially useful in these conditions as there may be no detectable fundal abnormality. Typical ERG findings are shown in Figure 3.3.

**Case 4** This 6-year-old boy presented with reduced vision and photophobia which had been present from early infancy. Visual acuity was reduced to 6/36 in each eye and there was poor colour vision. Fundus examination was normal. The ERG (centre panel of Figure 3.3) show normal rod responses. However, there was no measurable response to any of the three cone specific stimuli (note that with a red flash it is only components occurring within the first 50 ms after the flash that are cone specific, the later positive component resulting from rod activity). These results show extensive cone photoreceptor abnormality confirming the clinical diagnosis of a cone dystrophy.

**Case 5** This girl was aged 4 years at the time of her first ERG. She presented initially at age 4 months with apparently poor vision, photophobia, and nystagmus. When examined at age 4 years acuity was 6/60, she was significantly long sighted and had fine, rapid pendular nystagmus. Fundus examination was very difficult but no definite abnormalities were seen. She coped well with ERG procedures and normal rod responses were obtained (lower two traces of Figure 3.3, right panel). Mixed rod–cone responses were slightly reduced in amplitude but she did sometimes avert her eyes to these brighter stimuli and the attenuation was therefore regarded as artefactual. As with Case 4 there was no measurable response to a red flash or to a 30 Hz flicker, but possibly a very low amplitude response to a white flash on a rod-suppressing background. Based on the age of onset, associated clinical signs and severity of the cone ERG abnormality, a diagnosis of rod monochromatism was made.

It is important to distinguish between retinal dystrophies which affect the photoreceptors (which in many cases will be progressive) and those disorders that affect postreceptoral structures (which may be non-progressive). Abnormalities of the inner retina give rise to distinct abnormalities of the ERG which are illustrated in Figure 3.4.

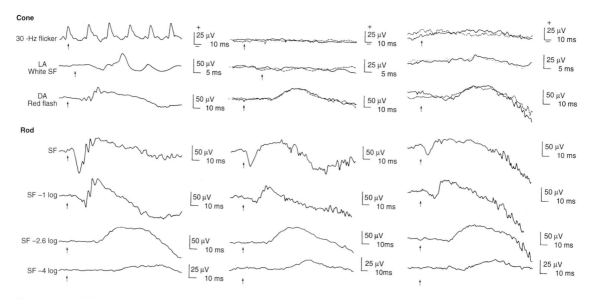

Figure 3.3 ERGs recorded as described for Figure 3.2. Left panel: Normal 10-year-old male. Centre panel: Cone dystrophy, Case 4. Right panel: Rod monochromatism, Case 5. Both patient ERGs show normal rod responses but no measurable cone response

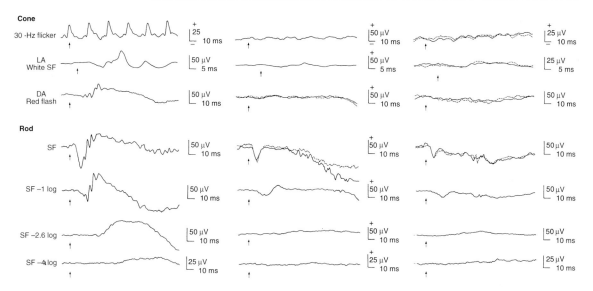

Figure 3.4   ERGs recorded as described for Figure 3.2. Left panel: Normal 10-year-old male. Centre panel: XLRS, Case 6. Right panel: CSNB, Case 7. Both patient ERGs show slightly low a-waves (photoreceptor response) but severely reduced amplitude or absent b-waves and oscillatory potentials indicating extensive abnormality of inner retina

**Case 6**  This 10-year-old boy first presented age 3 years with hypermetropia and a convergent squint for which he subsequently had surgery. The vision was reduced in each eye and he was thought to have bilateral amblyopia. At age 9 years his acuity was 6/12 right eye and 6/18 left eye. Fundoscopy revealed bilateral cystic changes of both maculae. There was a shallow peripheral schisis with large inner leaf break in the left eye. The ERG responses are shown in the centre panel of Figure 3.4. There was no measurable b-wave to the two lowest intensity stimuli suggesting rod photoreceptor abnormality. However, brighter stimuli evoked well-defined, normal amplitude or only slightly low amplitude a-waves. Normal a-waves but subnormal b-waves were also recorded to cone-specific stimuli, making a diagnosis of a photoreceptor dystrophy unlikely. The ERG abnormality was clearly specific to the b-wave, therefore indicating an inner retinal disorder. Based on the clinical appearance and ERG abnormality a diagnosis of X-linked retinoschisis (XLRS) was made. The ERG is very important when XLRS is suspected as the disorder shows variable clinical expression and retinal changes may be subtle. Moreover, foveal schisis is not confined to XLRS (e.g. it may be a feature of Goldmann–Favre syndrome), but the ERG features help to differentiate this disorder (see Chapter 10).

**Case 7**  This male infant presented initially at age 7 weeks apparently blind but with a normal fundus and a normal pupil reaction. A computed tomography (CT) scan of the head was normal. Vision improved and at age 17 weeks variable vertical nystagmus was noted. Flash VEPs at this time were normal. One year later he was noted to have moderate myopia and persistent nystagmus. He was very difficult to test but a single bright flash ERG showed a normal a-wave but reduced amplitude b-wave indicating that there was an inner retinal dystrophy. Full ERG responses, shown in the right panel of Figure 3.4, were eventually obtained when he was 6 years old. Normal or near-normal a-waves were recorded to all stimuli, but b-waves were absent or at a very reduced amplitude. The bright flash ERG (condition SF in Figure 3.4) showed the typical "negative-wave" appearance of inner retinal abnormality. A diagnosis of congenital stationary night blindness (CSNB) was made. The fundus appearance is normal in CSNB so the ERG is essential to confirm this diagnosis (see Chapter 10).

## Assessing optic nerve and primary visual cortex function

While the VEP can provide information which directly aids correct clinical diagnosis, the main value of this response is in providing objective evidence of intact visual pathways and possibly the level of useful pattern vision.

### Assessing infant vision

The VEP test is indicated when visual behaviour is poorer than expected for the age of the infant and when there is no nystagmus or other ocular abnormality to account for the poor vision. The flash VEP is the easiest response to obtain in this age group.[15] Very little cooperation is needed from the infant but the eyes should be open and the child must be awake and preferably alert because behavioural state can affect the response. Careful comparison with age-matched control subjects is absolutely essential because waveform morphology alters dramatically with age. There is only a single, long-latency positive component in the response of very young infants. Peak latency shortens during the first 8 weeks and then waveform morphology changes so that by about 16 weeks a complex series of negative and positive deflections is seen in the response. By 1 year of age the response is similar to that of an adult. The presence of a flash VEP

response will provide evidence of intact visual pathways and waveform morphology can be used as a rather coarse index of visual maturation.

**Case 8** Flash VEPs in the left panel of Figure 3.5 are for a normal infant at 3 and 6 months of age. Recordings on the right are from an infant who was apparently blind on initial presentation at 12 weeks. The child had a normal delivery, there were no neonatal problems and the eye examination was normal. Flash VEPs recorded at this visit (top-right trace, Figure 3.6) showed clear evidence of a response with a waveform (single positive component) appropriate for the age but with peak latencies which were prolonged and outside normal confidence limits for the age group. Although abnormal, the presence of a response confirmed intact visual pathways and helped to reassure the referring ophthalmologist who suspected a diagnosis of delayed visual maturation. When re-examined at age 6 months, the child was much more visually alert and was following light and toys well. Preferential looking indicated acuity of 6/130. The flash VEP showed improvement with shortening of peak latencies but the waveform did not have the more complex features appropriate for the age

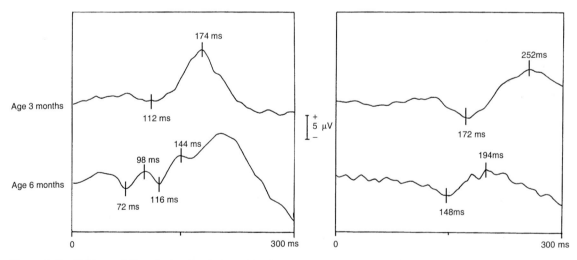

**Figure 3.5** VEPs to diffuse flash stimulation of both eyes together and recorded by means of a single silver disc electrode on the scalp 3 cm above the inion. Left panel: Normal male. Right panel: Delayed visual maturation. Case 8, an apparently blind infant presenting at age 3 months. A response was present at this time and showed some maturational improvement (shortening of peak latencies) when recorded again at age 6 months. However, the response remained abnormal when compared with age-matched controls

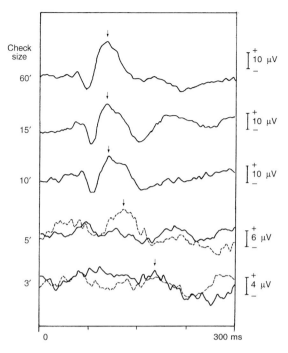

Figure 3.6   Pattern-reversal VEPs. Functional visual loss. Recording procedure as described for Figure 3.5. Size of check pattern shown to left of each trace. Case 9, a 12-year-old boy with a volunteered acuity of 3/60. The arrows indicate the normal P100 component which can be recorded down to 3′ arc check pattern size. The broken line traces are repeat recordings shown to confirm the presence of normal low-amplitude response to the two smallest pattern sizes. Note the size of the amplitude calibration bars

(compared with the normal 6-month old shown on the left) and was classified as abnormal.

The pattern VEP can also be used in this age group. A single size of check pattern can be used to give an indication as to whether the infant has any pattern vision, or a wide range of pattern stimuli can be used in an attempt to estimate acuity level.[13,14]

**Assessing young children**

Pattern VEPs are a more sensitive indicator of visual function and can be used with greater ease in older children as a means of assessing the level of pattern vision, especially in cases of visual loss with no obvious clinical cause.

**Case 9** A 12-year-old boy had been found to have reduced vision at a routine eye check one year earlier. His acuity was recorded at 3/60 in each eye. He had poor colour vision and constricted fields. There was no history of night blindness. The eye examination was normal. Pattern reversal VEPs are shown in Figure 3.6. This response is dominated by a positive component with a latency of about 100 ms. called the P100 (indicated by the arrow). Recordings show a normal latency and amplitude P100 to a 60′, 15′ and 10′ check and a response could be monitored down to 3′ check patterns. These responses were indistinguishable from normal recordings and suggested an acuity level much better than 3/60. Based on the normal eye examination, normal VEP and normal flash ERG (not shown), a diagnosis of functional visual loss was made.

Particular abnormal features of the pattern VEP can be a signature indicating specific types of abnormality of the visual pathways, which may aid accurate diagnosis in a few rare neuro-ophthalmological conditions. In demyelination, pattern-reversal response amplitude may be normal or near normal but peak latency is always prolonged. However, unlike adult forms of the disease, peak latency often recovers to normal over time. Conversely, in optic atrophy peak latencies may be normal but amplitudes are reduced, especially to smaller check patterns.

The pattern VEP can be very helpful in the diagnosis of albinism (see Chapter 16). Pattern-onset stimulation (not reversal) must be used with a relatively large check pattern and recordings must be obtained from three occipital electrodes as shown in Figure 3.7. The upper traces are normal-onset responses from the right and left eyes to a 60′ check pattern. The response is largest at the mid-occipital electrode and decreases symmetrically about the midline. Computer subtraction of the response recorded over the right occipital region from that recorded over the left occipital region give a interhemispheric "difference" signal as shown in the right panel of Figure 3.7. Stimulation of the right and left eye give similar derived responses. Recordings are

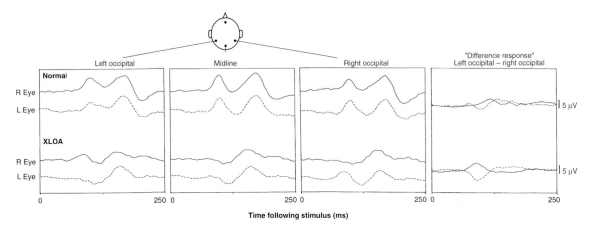

Figure 3.7   Pattern-onset VEPs. 60′ check pattern. Three recording electrodes positioned as shown on the diagram. Each eye was tested separately. Upper traces of each panel are for a normal male and the lower traces are for an age-matched male with a clinical diagnosis of X-linked ocular albinism (XLOA). The extreme right panel shows the response computed by the subtraction of the right occipital response from the left occipital response to give an interhemispheric "difference" signal. For the normal subject, the "difference" signal is similar for right- and left-eye stimulation, but for the XLOA, the signal for the right eye is opposite in polarity to that for the left eye, indicating misrouting of optic nerve fibres

quite different in albinos as shown in the lower traces of Figure 3.7. Firstly, the response is abnormal at the midline. Secondly, the response is asymmetrical about the midline, the normal "M"-shaped waveform being recorded over the hemisphere contralateral to the stimulated eye. Thirdly, the computed "difference" signal has the same latency but opposite polarity when stimulating the left eye compared with the right eye. This type of abnormality appears to be specific to albinism[16] and is presumed to be a consequence of the abnormal crossing of optic nerve fibres at the chiasm. Albinism may sometimes be easy to diagnose on clinical grounds, but not all clinical features are present in every affected individual and in some patients there may be doubt about the diagnosis. However, abnormal crossing of optic nerve fibres is believed to be a characteristic feature of all albinos, and therefore the VEP asymmetry may be a reliable signature of the condition when clinical signs are equivocal.

## Summary

In summary, several electrophysiological tests are available to aid clinical diagnosis. Each test is adapted and implemented in a manner most appropriate to the age of the patient and the clinical question being asked. Each provides a means of measuring visual performance at a specific level of visual processing. Each has a place in the evaluation of visual loss in childhood. They should be used appropriately within the context of the overall clinical assessment and with specific clinical questions in mind.

## References

1  Carr RE, Siegel IW. *Electrodiagnostic Testing of the Visual system*. Philadelphia: FW Davis, 1990.
2  Regan D. *Human Brain Electrophysiology* Amsterdam: Elsevier, 1989.
3  Heckenlively JR, Arden GB. *Principles and Practice of Clinical Electrophysiology of Vision*. St Louis: Mosby Year Book, 1991.
4  Marmor MF, Zrenner E. Standard for clinical electro-oculography. *Doc Ophthalmol* 1993; **85**: 115–25.
5  Berninger T, Arden GB. The pattern electroretinogram. *Eye* 1988; **2**(suppl): 257–83.
6  Marmor MF, Holder GE, Porciatti V, *et al.* Guidelines for basic pattern electroretinography. *Doc Ophthalmol* 1995/6; **91**: 291–8.
7  Arden GB, Carter RM, Macfarlan A. Pattern and Ganzfeld electroretinograms in macular disease. *Br J Ophthalmol* 1984; **68**: 878–84.
8  Gouras P. Electroretinography: some basic principles. *Invest Ophthalmol* 1970; **9**: 557–69.
9  Marmor MF, Zrenner E. Standard for clinical electroretinography (1994 update). *Doc Ophthalmol* 1995; **89**: 199–210.

10 Hood DC, Birch DG. Assessing abnormal rod photo-receptor activity with the a-wave of the ERG: applications and methods. *Doc Ophthalmol* 1997; **92**(4): 253–67.

11 Smith NP, Lamb TD. The a-wave of the human electroretinogram recorded with a minimally invasive technique. *Vision Res* 1997; **37**: 2943–52.

12 Friedburg C, Thomas RM, Lamb TD. A 4-flash protocol improves the *in vivo* recording of the complete time-course of the rod response measured using the ERG. *Invest Ophthalmol* 1999; **40**: S17.

13 Harding GFA, Odom JV, Spileers W, Spekreijse H. Standard for visual evoked potentials. *Vision Res* 1996; **36**: 3567–72.

14 Tyler CW. Visual acuity estimation in infants by visual evoked cortical potentials. In: Heckenlively JR and Arden GB eds. *Principles and Practice of Clinical Electrophysiology of Vision*. St Louis: Mosby Year Book, 1991.

15 Apkarian P. VEP assessment of visual function in paediatric neuro-ophthalmology. In: Albert DM and Jacobiec FA, eds. *Principles and Practice of Ophthalmology*. Philadelphia: WB Saunders, 1994.

16 Apkarian P, Reits D, Spekreijse H, Van Dorp D. A decisive electrophysiological test for human albinism. *Electroenceph Clin Neurophys* 1983; **55**: 513–31.

# 4 Normal and abnormal visual development

ARVIND CHANDNA, CARMEL NOONAN

Visual development, both normal and abnormal, has fascinated generations of philosophers and scientists. Empirical questions regarding early vision were being asked in the 17th century but the singular experiments of Torston Weisel and David Hubel in the middle of this century provided a fascinating insight into normal and abnormal visual development. With a model of monocular visual deprivation in cats and monkeys, they observed changes in the primary visual cortex in the form of anatomical shifts in cortical ocular dominance towards the non-deprived eye and the lack of physiological responses from the cells driven by the deprived eye. These changes were profound if they occurred during the early period of life providing evidence of a critical or sensitive period. In addition, these changes were to a large extent reversible if deprivation was reversed within the critical period giving rise to the concept of plasticity. These observations served as a catalyst for exploration of visual function in the early years and aid clinicians in the understanding and treatment of visual defects in childhood.

A normal visual system allows us to see with a combination of motor and sensory visual subsystems in perfect harmony. A peripheral object of interest is perceived triggering an eye movement in order to bring the image of the object on the fovea from where appropriate signals are sent for component analysis in the visual cortex for contrast, colour, form, motion, orientation and depth in relation to itself and its background.

The oculomotor system steadies the eyes and stabilises the image on the fovea with small eye movements which permit the object to be perceived continuously. This simplistic explanation of the functioning of a mature visual system is prefaced by a complex period of pre- and postnatal development.

For centuries, arguments have ranged between an innate visual system preprogrammed to develop and a learned visual system which is influenced by postnatal visual experience. The truth, as always, lies in a combination of these nativist and empiricist theories of visual development. Both concepts need to be explored with the underlying belief that normal, and abnormal, visual development progresses on a visual system that is preprogrammed to respond sensitively to visual experience in the early years of childhood.

Our present understanding of visual development is based on clinical observation, psychophysical threshold estimates, electrophysiological recordings, neurophysiological and detailed neuro-anatomical studies in animals and, recently, human infants. Recent attention has focused on the molecular level with advances in determining the role of chemical mediators, opening up new areas of research and treatment options.

This chapter explores the body of research that has emerged over the last thirty years and attempts to link basic research findings to clinical aspects of disordered visual development. Wherever possible, human visual development is explored but if human investigations are lacking, monkey and cat visual development is presented. A correction factor for comparing monkey and human visual development is accepted at 4 : 1.

## Normal visual development

Common with all sensory systems, an orderly development takes place in the visual system. The prenatal period lays down the visual system template dominated by cell generation and the establishment of connections between the retina, lateral geniculate nucleus (LGN), visual cortex and associated areas. The onset of electrical activity just before birth initiates the process of refinement of the template for the development of different visual functions. The postnatal period is characterised by the onset of visual experience which completes the process of normal visual development.

## Visual development under genetic/molecular control

Little is known regarding cell generation with the human visual system. In studies on macaque monkey, retinal cells are generated at embryonic day 30 (E30), LGN cells at E36 and cortical cells at E40. Retinal cells are generated initially near the future foveal area and later in the peripheral area. All human foveal cells are generated by 14 weeks of gestation.

The cell layer at the fovea is the thickest with a single layer of primitive rods and cones. Human foveal pit formation begins at 24–28 weeks gestation by a progressive lateral migration of the ganglion cells and Mueller cells, with only a single layer of ganglion cells being present at birth in the human infant.[1] Within the central retina the parafoveal area (1.5 mm from fovea) is the area of the highest rod density (rod ring). It shows mature rod photoreceptors at birth. Parafoveal photoreceptor (rods and cones) maturity is in advance of foveal cone maturity. This indicates that early neonatal acuity may be dependent on parafoveal photoreceptor function until foveal cone vision takes over.

Although appearances of the human foveal pit are adult like by 15 months of postnatal age, further changes in foveal cone population and morphology occur until approximately 13 years of age. Relative to adult cone density, foveal cones population increases from 17% at birth, to 52% at 45 months of age with adult cone density values (208 000 cones mm$^2$) at 13 years of age. The increase in length (thin, tapered) of the cones improves the efficiency of light capture (funnelling of light); the increase in density contributes to the improvement in spatial resolution (Figure 4.1a,b).

For peripheral retinal development there is a six-fold increase in area before birth, while the central retina remains stable. This leads to a decrease in density of the photoreceptors, the rods decreasing to a third and the cones to half their original density. Rods outnumber cones in density in the mid-peripheral retina and are the principal photoreceptors in the far periphery.

Cells within the visual cortex arise below the future layer VI and are termed "subplate cells". Cells from layer VI migrate upwards to the superficial layers in a radial fashion to form the characteristic six layers (I to VI) and organise themselves in an anatomical columnar fashion which later have important physiological implications. Some cells migrate in a lateral direction making short range connections and others migrate longer distances (long range) connecting cells and columns with similar physiological properties. These long and short-range connections are implicated in contour integration. This visual function has been found impaired by amblyopia.[2] Treatment of amblyopia with occlusion therapy results in an improvement in contour integration on a separate time course relative to improvement in high contrast letter (Snellen) acuity.

Cell generation in the retina, LGN and the visual cortex is accompanied by the establishment of connections via axonal afferents between these visual stations. The migration of axons from the ganglion cell layer, the crossing

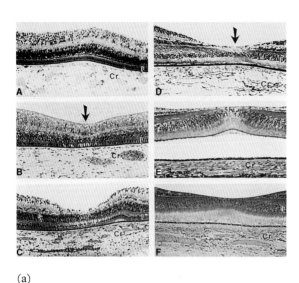

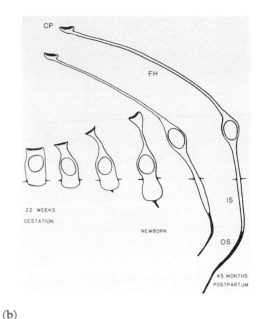

(a)                                                       (b)

Figure 4.1 (a) The maturation of the human fovea. Cr = choroid; P = outer nuclear layer. A: 22-week foetus lacking foveal depression. B: 24–26-week foetus with the beginning of a foveal depression. C: 5-day postbirth with foveal depression. D: 15-month-old; fovea well demarcated containing only cone photoreceptors. E: 45-month-old foveal cone layer thicker with an external fovea. F: 72-year-old adult fovea. Note a progressive thinning of retinal ganglion cell layer and inner nuclear layer from (A) to (D) and complete absence in (D). (Reprinted courtesy of Hendrickson AE, Yuodelis C. The morphological development of the human fovea. *Ophthalmology* 1994; **91** (6): 603–12) (b) Schematic drawing for development of human cones. Left to right at 22, 24, 26 and 34–36 weeks of gestation; newborn; 15 and 45 months postpartum. The inner segment (IS) develops before and the outer segment (OS) develops after birth. The fibre of Henle (FH) and cone pedicle (CP) are present before birth. Considerable elongation and thinning occurs in the foveal cone especially at postnatal ages.[1] (Reprinted courtesy of Hendrickson AE, Yuodelis C. The morphological development of the human fovea. *Ophthalmology* 1994; **91** (6): 603–12

over of the nasal half of the fibres in the optic chiasm, the initial coarse topographic localisation in the lateral geniculate and visual cortex, are also under genetic and molecular control. Evidence for this control is seen in misrouting of axons at the optic chiasm in albinism where most of the fibres cross over giving rise to characteristic abnormalities detected by specific visual evoked potential recordings.

### Onset of electrical activity

The next step in development is the onset of electrical activity. The purpose of this stage is to strengthen appropriate connections and eliminate inappropriate projections. Increased activity

in the postsynaptic cell provides feedback signals to potentiate the synaptic process. Conversely, low levels of activity will lead to activation of a similar feedback process which in this event leads to a depression of activity. Such activity occurring over a prolonged period of time will lead to potentiation for some afferents (long-term potentiation; LTP) and depression of activity at some afferents long term depression (LTD). Recent work investigating patterned electrical activity within retinal ganglion cells explains aggregation of afferents with like properties and segregation of right eye, left eye and binocular inputs at the LGN and visual cortex. Electrical activity within retinal ganglion cells originates at a point and spreads across as a wave

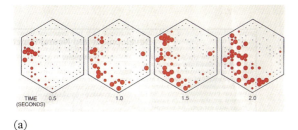

(a)

(b)

Figure 4.2 Patterned electrical activity in retinal ganglion cells (see text for details). (Reproduced with permission from Schatz CJ. The developing brain. *Sci American* 1992; **267**: 34–41)

over a discrete area of the retina. Waves occur in succession in the same eye but no two waves are superimposed in the same eye (Figure 4.2a,b). This local aggregation suggests that neighbouring retinal cells with similar physiological properties (see receptive fields, discussed later) fire in local synchrony. This local synchrony led the investigator Carla Shatz to suggest "cells that fire together wire together".[3]

Such patterned electrical activity is for the most part uncorrelated for retinal areas between the two eyes leading to potentiation of synaptic connections from one and depression of synaptic connections from the other eye leading to segregation of eye-specific layers in the LGN and primitive ocular dominance columns in the visual cortex. At some point in time synchronous firing from corresponding retinal areas of the two eyes leads to binocular potentiation of neurones leading to binocularly driven cells. Though LGN segregation may occur with such patterned electrical activity alone, refinement of ocular dominance columns and cells sensitive to disparity (stereopsis) require visual experience in addition

to electrical activity. Development dependent on electrical activity alone is dominant from prebirth until 3 weeks post birth (12 weeks in the human) with visual experience development becoming dominant between 3–6 weeks (12–24 weeks) for the evolution of stereopsis.

## Two distinct pathways

Even in the early stages of onset of electrical activity, there is evidence of two distinct pathways originating at the retinal ganglion cells. Retinal ganglion cells serving fine detail and colour (P cells) project to the four dorsal small cell layers (parvocellular layers) and retinal ganglion cells dealing with movement (M cells) to the two ventral large cell layers (magnocellular layers) of the LGN and thence to the layer IV of the primary visual cortex. Here we need to consider the complexity of layer IV to understand the two distinct pathways. Layer IV is subdivided into IVA, IVB, IVC-alpha, and IVC-beta. The magnocellular pathway terminates in IVC-alpha which projects to IVB. The afferents from the parvocellular layers of the LGN terminate in IVC-beta and IVA. Layer IV projects to layers II and III which in turn project to layer V. Layer VI receives afferents from layers II, III and V. Layer V and VI in turn send projections back to superior colliculus and LGN, respectively.

## Receptive fields

Further development under the influence of visual experience leads to refinement of properties such as disparity detection, orientation and in addition aggregation of cells and neuronal connections with similar properties termed "receptive fields". A receptive field defines the physiological behaviour of a cell or a population of cells. A group of cells responding in a similar manner (for example, to a specific degree of orientation) are wired together in the visual system.

At a basic level these receptive fields have a simple substructure of a centre which may respond to a stimulus by increasing (on-centre) or decreasing (off-centre) its rate of firing (electrical activity) and a surround which will behave in an opposing (inhibitory or excitatory) manner to the centre. Receptive field properties of centre-surround; on-off are true for the retinal ganglion cells and the LGN but adopt far more complex properties in the visual cortex. Receptive fields in the cortex have been defined on the basis of orientation specificity, direction of preferred movement and disparity. Receptive field size also varies, being small for fine detail (at the fovea) and larger for coarser detail (retinal periphery). The study of the development of receptive fields has led to our understanding of different visual functions.

## Chemical mediators and neuromodulatory transmitters

Much attention has now focused on chemical mediators that control the morphological development and neuromodulatory transmitters which modify the actions of the chemical mediators. Electrical activity causes release of chemical mediators which lead to receptor-mediated opening of ionic channels in the postsynaptic cell membrane with influx of chemical mediators into the cell. Intracellular secondary messengers are activated leading to formation of new cellular components.

The neurotransmitter dopamine is involved in several visual functions, one being a neurotransmitter in the retina where it controls the circular receptor field characteristics of the retinal cells. In photopic luminance levels, dopamine is released, horizontal cells uncouple, creating smaller receptive fields. In the dark, dopamine release is inhibited by gamma-aminobutyric acid (GABA) and therefore horizontal cells become coupled creating larger receptor fields with reduced inhibition. The release of dopamine in the retina has been found to be a graded response (i.e. more light, more dopamine). Coupling and uncoupling appear dependent on inner plexiform cells which provide a feedback loop between horizontal cell receptive fields. It is thought that the control of the horizontal cell receptor fields in turn influences the ganglion cell receptor fields.

In animal models of amblyopia, it has been shown that there is reduced retinal dopamine and that receptive fields are larger. In addition, retinal dopamine is thought to participate in the pathway linking visual experience and postnatal axial eye growth.

The myopia associated with form deprivation has been prevented by administration of dopamine-related agents. Since dopamine is reduced in the retina of chicks and monkeys with deprivation amblyopia, it is conceivable that there are also changes in the dopaminergic system occurring in humans with strabismic or anisometropic amblyopia.[4]

Modulatory neurotransmitters such as acetylcholine, adrenaline, dopamine and serotonin appear to influence the visual cortex via modulatory pathways from other sites within the cerebral cortex. They are found in abundance during the critical periods and decline to lower levels or disappear during later periods.[5]

In studies on kittens, intracortical 6-hydroxydopamine (6-OHDA) administered during the critical period disrupts plasticity by interfering with both cholinergic and adrenergic transmission, raising the possibility that acetylcholine and noradrenaline facilitate synaptic modifications in the cortex by a common molecular mechanism. Glutamate is a synaptic transmitter within the visual cortex acting on three types of receptors on the post-synaptic cell: N-methyl-D-aspartate (NMDA), AMP-kainate and the metabotropic receptors. Of these, the NMDA receptor appears to be the most important.

The exact role of individual neurotransmitters in controlling cortical plasticity is not known, but the correlation with the time frame of the critical period provides an explanation for the success of amblyopia treatment if carried out during the critical period and decreasing success when detected and treated beyond the period of plasticity.

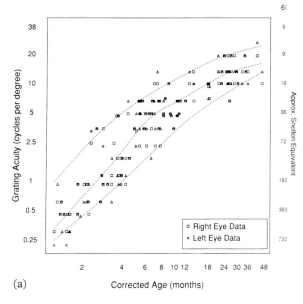

(a)

Figure 4.3   (a) The development of grating acuity from 4 weeks to 48 months of corrected age derived by the forced-choice preferential-looking method using a staircase paradigm. The central curve represents the median with 5% (lower) and 95% curves representing acuity values for 90% of the tested population. Acuity develops rapidly for the first 6 months of life followed by a further slower increase with adult acuity values in the region of 30 cycles/degree just achieved at 4 years of age.[6] (b) (i and ii) Acuity development for right and left eyes over the first year of life for a representative group of four normal infants superimposed on the overall acuity norms from (a). Each infant has a somewhat different developmental course within the acuity norms. Importantly for clinical practice, each individual child does not have a difference of more than a half octave between their right and left eyes at any given age. For all children tested, acuity values between children at any age may vary by as much as two octaves but for each child the acuity difference between eyes was never more than a half octave.[5]

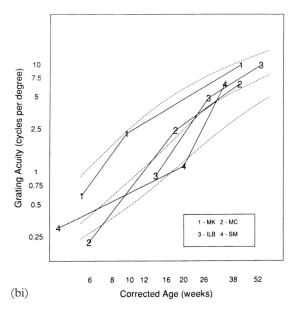

(bi)

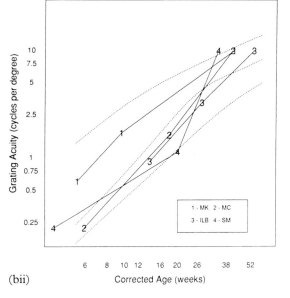

(bii)

## Correlation with developing visual functions

Visual acuity to high contrast gratings develops rapidly for the first 6 months of life from 1 cycle/degree to approximately 25 cycles/degree and slowly thereafter reaching adult acuity levels of 30–40 cycles/degree by about 5 years of age (Figure 4.3a,bi,bii). This is largely explained by the changes occurring in the cone photoreceptors. Limitations of infant acuity cannot be explained entirely by the immaturity of the retina which accounts for approximately 40–55% of the difference between neonatal and adult acuity. Further improvement is dependent on the refinement of connections between retina, LGN and visual cortex.

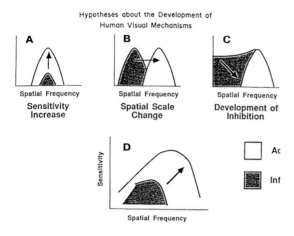

Figure 4.4 Hypothesis regarding development of spatial mechanisms in the human infant. Infant functions are shown in grey and adult in white with arrows indicating direction of change. (A) Increase in sensitivity due to an increase in efficiency of the cones. (B) A change towards higher spatial frequencies due to increased density of cones at the fovea. (C) Low-frequency fall off probably due to development of lateral inhibition in the receptive field centre-surround. (D) Overall increase in contrast sensitivity function from infant to adult.[7] (Reprinted from Wilson HR. Development of spatiotemporal mechanisms in infant vision. *Vision Res* 1988; 5: 611–28, with kind permission from Elsevier Science Ltd, The Boulevard, Longford Lane, Kidlington, OX5 IGB)

Contrast sensitivity function in the infant is characterised by a low overall contrast sensitivity curve, a fall off at the low and a cut off at high spatial frequencies (Figure 4.4). Overall contrast sensitivity improves due to an increase in efficiency of the cones and contrast at high spatial frequencies due to increased density of cones at the fovea. The low frequency fall off is probably related to the development of lateral inhibition in the receptive field centre-surround.[7]

Orientation specificity and direction of motion selectivity develop due to physiological changes in the responsiveness of cortical cells. This occurs in parallel with changes occurring in LGN and retina. Though these responses are present at birth they mature over the first 6 months of life in conjunction with refinement of the orientation columns in the visual cortex.

The development of stereopsis separates visual development into two distinct phases. The prestereoptic phase (where infants do not show a preference for visual stimuli with disparity) extends for the first three months when there is a considerable degree of overlap between right and left eye driven cells in layer IV. The post stereoptic phase, where infants show a preference for stimuli with disparity, starts at three months of age coinciding with improvement in spatial temporal frequency discrimination (acuity and contrast sensitivity), segregation of right and left eye inputs in layer IV and more importantly convergence of right and left eye signals on cells in layers other than layer IV.[8] These binocularly driven disparity cells are now further subdivided into cells for crossed versus uncrossed disparity and near versus far stereopsis.

In summary, genetic influences lay down the template. The onset of electrical activity, release of chemical mediators, neuromodulatory transmitters and visual experience refine the system with development of visual functions. Each developing visual function has a different time course and is dependent on the development of other visual functions. Therefore for each visual function there is not only an independent critical period of development but also an interdependence of critical periods between visual functions.

If affected, visual functions may be regained with appropriate treatment, indicating plasticity[9] within the visual system. The plastic period may extend beyond the critical period especially when the visual function that is affected has undergone some normal development during the critical period. In addition, critical periods can be modified or delayed in onset as is seen in dark rearing of animals and then subsequently exposing them to normal visual experience. This will be discussed in the next section.

## Abnormal visual development

Most of what we know regarding normal visual development has been derived from the experimental study of abnormal visual development. Strabismus, refractive errors and media opacities presenting in early childhood lead to abnormal visual development. Strabismus is commonly associated with refractive error; cataracts may initially lead to monocular visual deprivation and later to strabismus.

Clinical manifestations of disordered visual development are seen as amblyopia, suppression and loss of binocularity. Amblyopia manifests as loss of acuity and patients complain of muddled vision. Suppression is commonly seen in strabismus where the absence of diplopia provides indirect evidence of vision being switched off in the non-fixing eye. Loss of binocularity is evidenced as inability to perceive depth on standard clinical tests. Animal studies using deprivation paradigms and clinical observations of visual function deficits in children have helped in our understanding of the changes that occur in the abnormal visual system.

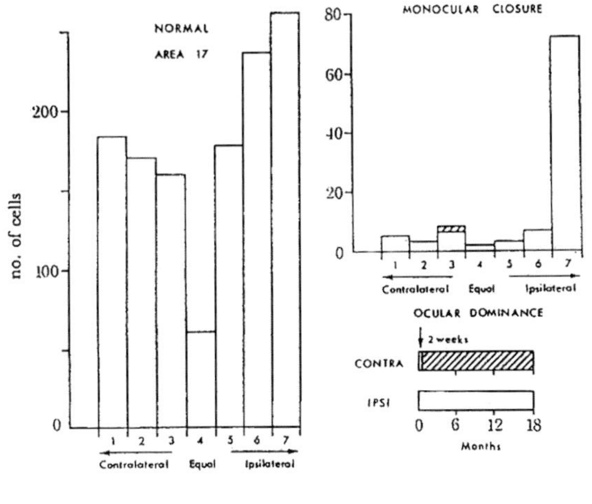


Figure 4.5 Histogram of cell responses in area 17 of the visual cortex in normal and monocularly deprived monkeys. The normal histogram is characterised by an equal population of cells being driven by either eye (group 1 and 7) or by both eyes (group 4) and others sharing an input (groups 2,3; 5,6). With monocular visual deprivation with eye closure (contralateral eye) from two weeks to 18 months the distribution changes to most cells being driven by the open eye and very few cells being driven by the previously closed eye.[10]

## Monocular deprivation

The paradigm of monocular deprivation[10] has been studied intensively in kittens and monkeys. Following monocular visual deprivation, the deprived eye is opened and recordings made from the LGN and visual cortex. The eye on examination is entirely normal; the LGN cells show normal though slowed physiological responses and anatomically the layers receiving input from the deprived eye are thin in cross-section (Figure 4.5).

Cells in the visual cortex responding to stimulation of the deprived eye showed abnormal responses. Only a few cells responded to stimulation of the deprived eye and their responses were slowed and did not show orientation tuning. These changes are specific to the time of onset and duration of deprivation. Early onset followed by prolonged duration leads to profound effects, whereas late onset with short durations leads to less severe deficits. These experiments gave rise to the concept of a critical period where sensitivity to modified visual input is dependent on timing. The critical period is species specific. Monkeys have an earlier onset critical period which lasts longer compared to cats. Within the same species different visual functions such as acuity, contrast sensitivity, motion and stereopsis have different critical periods. Human acuity develops from birth over an approximately five-year span whereas stereopsis develops with an onset at approximately three months and reaches adult levels by six months of age. Despite separate critical periods, developing visual functions are highly interdependent. Contrast sensitivity function at higher frequencies is dependent on acuity development.

## Eye reversal

For the clinician the next series of experiments provided the principles of therapy, on which occlusion of the good eye for amblyopia is based. Following early monocular deprivation, simply opening the deprived eye does not lead to recovery of visual function. However, if deprivation is now reversed (eye reversal) visual function recovers in the previously deprived eye. Recovery is dependent on eye reversal occurring for an appropriate duration during the critical period. However, all visual functions do not recover and this may be due to different critical periods for different visual functions. Contrast sensitivity function may remain abnormal despite good recovery of acuity in the previously amblyopic eye. This is borne out by abnormal cortical physiological recordings and anatomy despite successful eye reversal.

### Strabismus

Subsequent experiments which induced strabismus (e.g. cutting the medial rectus muscle) revealed findings different from that of monocular deprivation. Here, cortical cells are arranged in ocular dominance columns which respond either to the left or the right eye with only a few binocularly driven cells. In normal dominance columns the majority of cells are innervated from both eyes with each cell showing a preference for one or the other eye. Thus alternating strabismus will enable either eye to develop monocular abilities but binocularity will not develop. This is mirrored in the clinical observation of equal acuity in a large-angle alternating early-onset esotropia which may not recover binocularity despite good alignment following surgery. In an ideal situation, surgery before the critical period of development of binocularity may restore binocularity. In practical terms, this would imply surgery between three and six months of age. There is some evidence that this is the case though incontrovertible evidence favouring early surgical alignment is still awaited through appropriately controlled prospective studies.

Suppression of the non-viewing eye is a well accepted clinical finding in childhood strabismus without diplopia. In the model described above with equal dominance from either eye, suppression is difficult to explain and this model may serve those rare cases where diplopia is present or manifests after intensive occlusion therapy. A shift of ocular dominance towards the preferred eye with suppression of the non-preferred eye (strabismus with a fixation preference) is possible to postulate by taking this model one step further. Long-term potentiation of electrical activity at binocular cortical synapses strengthening input from the preferred eye will lead to a weakening of the input from the non-preferred eye (competition) leading to suppression and if continued long enough decrease in acuity or amblyopia in that eye. Recent evidence regarding patterned neural activity originating in retinal ganglion cells also helps in understanding this shift in ocular dominance.

### Binocular deprivation

The nature-versus-nurture question was answered in another series of experiments. Binocular deprivation was achieved by either bilateral lid closure allowing some light and motion to be perceived or complete deprivation by rearing kittens and monkeys in the dark.

Unlike monocular deprivation where the cells are driven largely by the non-deprived eye, in binocular deprivation there are equal proportions of cells being driven by either eye and some binocularly driven cells. This picture is similar to a newborn normal animal giving rise to the presence of an innate influence on visual development. However, though the majority of cells respond to visual stimuli there are no orientation or direction-specific cells, the receptive fields of the monocularly driven cells are immature with inappropriate on–off properties and responses are slow. This is reflected in clinical measurements of decreased spatial resolution (acuity) and contrast sensitivity. This is despite a normal photoreceptor mosaic and normal responsiveness at the LGN neurones.

NMDA receptor activity at the geniculocortical synapses is initiated by exposure to light-dependent sensory activity and closely follows the course of the critical period. This activity is not seen in dark-reared animals but on subsequent exposure to light proceeds normally. Thus dark rearing delays the onset and time course of the critical period. Initial experiments manipulating the critical period have shown plasticity in the visual system in dark-reared animals at 12–20 weeks of age whereas light-reared animals at this age do not demonstrate plasticity of their visual system. In clinical terms such alternations in the critical period with pharmacological or sensory means may help in treatment.

The study of abnormal visual development goes some way in answering the nature-versus-nurture question. Patterned visual activity (nurture) is essential for normal development at the geniculocortical synapse whereas for the earlier synapses at the retina and LGN there appears to be an innate influence (nature) guiding it towards normal development.

The anatomical changes and abnormal physiological responses seen in abnormal visual development are different with different paradigms of deprivation. The clinician treating the consequences of disordered visual development needs to tailor treatment accordingly. Attempts are being made to investigate treatment options for amblyopia and suppression and are discussed in the next section.

## Clinical aspects of abnormal visual development

Traditionally, amblyopia has been classified according to the clinical abnormality found on examination:

- strabismic amblyopia when there is an obvious constant deviation of one eye;

- anisometropic amblyopia in the presence of an asymmetrical refractive error;

- ametropic amblyopia in the presence of bilateral high refractive errors preventing well-defined focused images;

- meridional amblyopia in the presence of an astigmatic error;

- deprivation amblyopia in the presence of an identifiable obstruction to vision such as cataract, corneal opacity or ptosis.

More than one amblyogenic factor (strabismus with anisometropia) may combine to give a "mixed" type of amblyopia. This classification does not examine the underlying differences in the amblyopia based on sensory (acuity, contrast sensitivity) and motor (fixation, smooth pursuit, saccades) abnormalities which has been the subject of recent investigations.[11]

## Sensorial adaptations to strabismus and amblyopia

### Suppression

Suppression is a protective adaptive mechanism to prevent diplopia and confusion. This is best exemplified in strabismus where suppression can be mapped to the area of visual field in the deviating eye which overlaps a similar area in the fixing eye. Clinically, in an esotropic deviation this would be seen in central areas (termed "central suppression"). Like amblyopia, it is seen only in abnormal visual development while the visual system is immature, whereas in the mature visual system of adults adaptation to suppression is not possible and diplopia results. Diplopia is also seen when treatment for strabismus results in positioning the deviating eye into a non-suppressed area as in overcorrection of exotropia. The development of suppression is usually a barrier to development of fusion and stereopsis.

### Anomalous correspondence

Clinically this is incorrectly described as anomalous (or abnormal) retinal correspondence (ARC). The correspondence is throughout the visual system and not just retinal. This is an uncommon sensorial adaptation to a strabismic deviation. Normal visual development will lead to corresponding areas (receptive fields) between the two eyes linked together in the entire visual system relaying corresponding visual images of the visual scene which, when fused and seen in depth, are characteristics of normal binocularity.

In the presence of an early-onset constant strabismus, the foveal corresponding area in the fixing eye may develop a correspondence with a peripheral extrafoveal area on the retina in the deviating eye (such correspondence may be seen for all other areas). This anomalous correspondence creates a form of binocular cooperation during early visual development even resulting in the ability to fuse and occasionally achieve subnormal stereopsis.

## Relationship between amblyopia, suppression and anomalous correspondence

The relationship between amblyopia and suppression remains unclear though clinical experience indicates an interdependent relationship. The precise cause and effect relationship between these two sensorial adaptations to abnormal visual development remains unknown. It is possible that asymmetrical binocular visual inputs lead to a "switching off" of the eye with the weaker input and is clinically termed "suppression" which in turn leads to reduced visual acuity in the affected eye which manifests as amblyopia.

Amblyopia remains a monocular event diagnosed on the basis of reduction in monocular visual acuity (except for the uncommon bilateral amblyopia). Suppression is seen under binocular viewing circumstances diagnosed on the basis of absence of diplopia or a fixation preference of the dominant eye. Amblyopia remains a fixed entity with reduced visual acuity at all times and at all distances whereas suppression is more of a dynamic event. There is some improvement in acuity for near vision in amblyopia. The cause remains unclear, though it may be due to linear magnification. Children with intermittent exotropia may show suppression at times when the deviation is manifest in contrast to perfect binocularity when the deviation is latent and this is true for intermittence at various distances of

fixation or state of alertness (or tiredness).

Anomalous correspondence may coexist with suppression as is seen in cases of small-angle esotropia (microtropia) where an extrafoveal area in the deviating eye corresponds with the foveal area in the fixing eye with a small suppression area associated with the foveal area. Both may coexist with mild degrees of amblyopia. In addition, anomalous correspondence may exist with normal correspondence but this may be due to testing conditions.

## Treatment of amblyopia

Amblyopia (blunted sight) is defined as diminished acuity in one or both eyes without any discernible ocular abnormality ("functional amblyopia") though deprivation amblyopia may be due to a visible abnormality such as a cataract or an upper-lid ptosis. In clinical terms, amblyopia is usually assessed with high-contrast letter acuity though there are other abnormalities as evidenced by abnormal contrast sensitivity. In children unable to cooperate with recognition acuity tests, amblyopia is managed by tests of fixation pattern and preferential-looking behaviour.

At present there is increasing controversy over screening for amblyopia, efficacy of treatment and even whether treatment is worthwhile from a quality-of-life aspect. These questions have led to sufficient concern among clinicians, stimulating ongoing clinical research to prove the efficacy of treatment of amblyopia. A recent retrospective meta-analysis of studies comparing the results of patching as a treatment for amblyopia concluded that successful treatment was related to the age and the depth of visual loss at presentation. These conclusions supported the value of early detection and treatment of all types of amblyopia.[12] The type of amblyopia (e.g. strabismic, anisometropic), though significant in one group of studies, was not found to be significant in another comparable group and the final answer for this question remains to be resolved.

## Methods of treatment

In this section we discuss traditional treatment options and examine new treatment options for the future.

## Occlusion

The mainstay of amblyopia treatment continues to be occlusion of the better eye. This is achieved by depriving the dominant eye of light and formed visual stimuli encouraging improvement of acuity in the amblyopic eye. Therapy may be full- or part-time occlusion. Empirical occlusion schedules have been developed though evidence-based practice on type of occlusion is still lacking.

Full-time occlusion of the preferred eye is the most effective method for treating strabismic amblyopia. Improvement also is likely to be more rapid when occlusion is worn full-time (Figure 4.6a,b). Alternating monocular full-time occlusion is practised by patching on a weekly schedule with more days of occlusion of the dominant eye. It has the advantage of preventing occlusion amblyopia and recent evidence suggests prevention of abnormal binocular interaction.

Refractive correction alone may be sufficient to correct amblyopia in anisometropic amblyopia. If the visual acuity fails to improve, occlusion therapy is added. This group of patients has a good prognosis, despite late presentation.

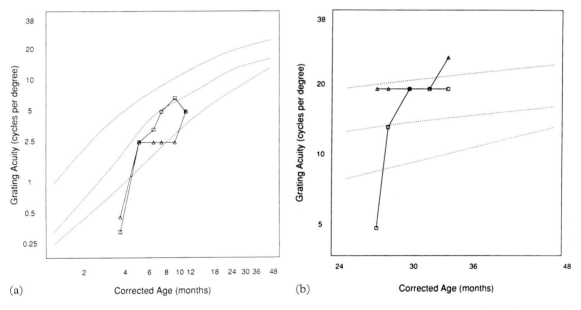

(a)    (b)

Figure 4.6   Development of grating visual acuity in children with ocular pathology superimposed on acuity norms from Figure 4.3(a). Acuity values were obtained without knowledge of clinical diagnosis or management unless obvious to the tester. Acuity values for right eye represented with a square and left eye with a triangle. (a) Acuity values well below the 5% curve for both eyes at presentation in an infant with bilateral cataracts. Surgery and contact lens correction at 6 months of age leads to an improvement in acuity. Loss of contact lens left eye leads to a decrease in acuity value recorded. Successful contact lens wear leads to a rapid improvement in acuity over the next 4 months reaching the lower norm spread at 12 months of age. (Chandna A. Evaluation of Preferential Looking in Clinical Practice. MD Thesis. University of Bristol). (b) An older child presenting at 26 months of age with right-eye acuity well below norm for that age and an interocular acuity difference (IAD) of 2.0 octaves (normal IAD = ± 0.5 octave). Correction of refractive error (anisohypermetropia) and occlusion therapy for a constant right esotropia leads to an improvement in right-eye acuity and a decreasing IAD over the 9 months with an insignificant IAD at the end of therapy.[6] (Chandna A. Evaluation of Preferential Looking in Clinical Practice. MD Thesis. University of Bristol)

However patients with myopic or myopic/mixed astigmatism have poorer visual outcomes.

Patients with ocular abnormalities, e.g. optic nerve hypoplasia, may also have amblyopia. Full-time occlusion has produced good results in this group of patients.[13] These children, following completion of their primary treatment, need maintenance treatment until visual maturity to retain vision is achieved.

Deprivation amblyopia appears to have severe effects on visual development and the cause (e.g. congenital cataract) needs to be treated early and vigorous occlusion therapy needs to be instituted for any improvement to occur.

## Penalisation

Penalisation of the non-amblyopic eye leading to defocus, may be useful in patients who are non-compliant with occlusion or have latent nystagmus. Pharmacological penalisation with topical atropine will blur the vision in the non-amblyopic eye. Optical penalisation involves the use of lenses to blur the visual acuity of the better eye. This is achieved by adding a strong convex lens (or a strong concave lens) to the better eye. The aim of these methods is to give the amblyopic eye better distance and near vision. When used in isolation the results are generally disappointing but improve if both modalities are used simultaneously. Published retrospective studies have indicated the need for larger prospective randomised comparative treatment trials comparing occlusion and penalisation therapies.[14,15] While optical penalisation has the advantage of ease of application, it is costly and atropine may have toxic and allergic effects. Monitoring visual acuity in the normal eye to rule out reversal of amblyopia is difficult, as children may not be able to co-operate with a pinhole visual acuity during treatment.

## Regression

Following successful treatment of amblyopia, visual acuity may regress in amblyopic eyes presenting with dense amblyopia and affected by mixed strasbismic-anisometropic amblyopia. Approximately 40% of children with a pre-treatment vision between 6/60 and 6/18 and a diagnosis of pure strabismic or anisometropic amblyopia will lose 0.65 of a Snellen line and 60% of children with a pre-treatment vision of less than 6/60 and a diagnosis of strabismic-anisometropic amblyopia will lose on average 2 Snellen lines.[16] However, regression to pre-treatment levels is rare, indicating a net benefit of treatment.

## Compliance

Compliance with occlusion treatment is a signficant problem in treatment of amblyopia. Poor visual acuity in the amblyopic eye, discomfort with the adhesive patch, parental lack of understanding and social stigma are some of the factors resulting in poor compliance. Nucci et al. (1992) reported an 18% incidence of non-compliance overall with higher incidences in the younger age group (1 to 2 year olds) and children with dense amblyopia at presentation.[17] In a recent study by Simons and Preslan (1999) of the 18 children with amblyopia who failed to comply with prescribed treatment (spectacles, occlusion), 17 did not show an improvement and the amblyopia worsened in seven children,[18] indicating the benefits of treatment and the importance of compliance. Compliance needs to be addressed with informed counselling of parents and older children, record books and a system of rewards for the younger child.

## Other methods

The use of graded filters (Baengerter filters) to degrade acuity in the dominant eye has successfully reversed amblyopia and equalised fixation pattern, though long-term studies are lacking. The use of occlusive contact lenses is to be discouraged since complications of extended wear soft contact lenses in the paediatric population are well known and put the dominant eye at significant risk of severe visual deficit and blindness.

## Delayed visual maturation (DVM) (see Chapter 18)

An ill-understood phenomenon in visual development is seen in infants who in the first two to three months of life appear not to see and over the next four to six months show a remarkable improvement in vision. Extensive observational and investigative studies have led to a classification of DVM.[19] In isolated DVM, the eye is visibly normal but the visual evoked potential may be abnormal and there may be delayed developmental milestones. Subsequent visual development is rapid and complete. DVM may be associated with ocular disease especially when associated with nystagmus. Here vision is much worse than one would expect and subsequent development is slower than in isolated DVM and usually not complete. DVM may be associated with systemic disease (infantile spasms, hydrocephalus) resulting in subnormal mentation, in addition to the poor vision.[20] The aetiology of the delayed visual development is unclear.

## Looking to the future

The association between amblyopia and neurotransmitters is strongly supported by extensive literature showing the involvement of catecholamines, GABA, glutamate, acetylcholine and serotonin in visual plasticity. Recent experimental studies have concentrated on the use of neurotransmitters/neuromodulators in an attempt to prolong the plastic period of the visual system, with initial encouraging results.

Recent studies have also looked at the effect of levodopa[21] with or without occlusion on visual acuity in children, both during and beyond the plasticity period. Results have shown a one-line improvement in visual acuity following a single dose of levodopa and in longitudinal studies an improvement that remained stable over a five-month follow-up period. As the improvement

was also seen in older children, levodopa, particularly in combination with occlusion therapy may offer hope to amblyopic teenagers and adults. A more limited study on the use of citicoline and the effect of its use in amblyopia, found an improvement in visual acuity in both the good and the amblyopic eye. These results pave the way for further studies and provide new hope for future management of amblyopia.

## References

1 Hendrickson AE, Yuodelis C. The morphological development of the human fovea. *Ophthalmology* 1984; **91**: 603–12.
2 Polat U, Sagi D, Norcia AM. Abnormal long-range spatial interactions in amblyopia. *Vision Res* 1997; **37**: 737–44.
3 Schatz CJ. The developing brain. *Sci American* 1992; **267**: 34–41.
4 Stone RA, Lin T, Laties M, Iuvone PM. Retinal dopamine and form-deprivation myopia. *Proc Natl Acad Sci USA* 1989; **86**: 704–6.
5 Bear MF, Singer W. Modulation of visual cortical plasticity by acetylcholine and noradrenaline. *Nature* 1986; **320**: 172–6.
6 Chandna A. Evaluation of Preferential Looking for Clinical Practice. MD Thesis. Bristol: University of Bristol, 1993.
7 Wilson HR. Development of spatiotemporal mechanisms in infant vision. *Vision Res* 1988; **5**: 611–28.
8 Thorn F, Gwiazda J, Cruz AAV, *et al.* The development of eye alignment, convergence, and sensory binocularity in young infants. *Invest Ophthalmol Vis Sci* 1994; **35**: 544–53.
9 Sillito AM. Plasticity in the visual cortex. *Nature* 1983; **303**: 477–8.
10 Hubel DH, Wiesel TN, LeVay S. Plasticity of ocular dominance columns in monkey striate cortex. *Trans Roy Soc Lond* 1977; **278**: 377–409.
11 McKee SP. The classification of amblyopia on the basis of visual and oculomotor performance. *Trans Am Ophthalmol Soc* 1992; **90**: 123–48.
12 Flynn JT, Woodruff G, Thompson JR *et al.* The therapy of amblyopia: an analysis comparing the results of amblyopia therapy utilising two pooled data sets. *Trans Am Ophthalmol Soc* 1999; **97**: 373–90.
13 Bradford GM, Kutschke PJ, Scott WE. Results of amblyopia therapy in eyes with structural abnormalities. *Ophthalmology* 1992; **99**: 1616–21.
14 Repka MX, Ray JM. The efficacy of optical and pharmacological penalisation. *Ophthalmology* 1993; **100**: 769–74; discussion 774–7.
15 Simons K, Gotzler KC, Vitale S. Penalisation versus part-time occlusion and binocular outcome in treatment of strabismic amblyopia. *Ophthalmology* 1997; **104**; 2156–60.
16 Levertovsky S, Oliver M, Gottesman N, Shimshoni M. Factors affecting long term results of successfully treated amblyopia: initial visual acuity and type of amblyopia. *Br J Ophthalmol* 1995; **79**: 225–8.

17 Nucci P, Alfarano R, Piantanida A, Brancato R. Compliance in antiamblyopia occlusion therapy. *Acta Ophthalmol (Copenh)* 1992; **70**: 128–31.

18 Simons K, Preslan M. Natural history of amblyopia untreated owing to lack of compliance. *Br J Ophthalmol* 1999; **83**: 582–7.

19 Fielder AR, Russell-Eggit IR, Dodd KL, Mellor DH. Delayed visual maturation. *Trans Ophthalmol Soc* 1988; **104**: 653061.

20 Chen TC, Weinberg MH, Catalano, RA *et al.* Development of object vision in infants with permanent cortical visual impairment. *Am J Ophthalmol* 1992; **114**: 575–8.

21 Leguire LE, Walson PD, Rogers GL, *et al.* Longitudinal study of levodopa/carbidopa for childhood amblyopia. *J Pediatr Ophthalmol Strabismus* 1993; **30**: 354–60.

# 5 Developmental disorders of the globe

KEVIN GREGORY-EVANS

Developmental abnormalities of the eye occur either in isolation or as part of a multisystem syndrome. These ocular abnormalities are usually bilateral but can be asymmetrical. Such disorders are almost always clinically apparent from birth (congenital) and are essentially non-progressive although the consequences of these abnormalities can result in further damage to the eye, e.g. glaucomatous optic nerve damage in aniridia and nanophthalmos. All such developmental disorders occur as a result of disordered maturation of foetal ocular tissue. They are usually associated with one of three pathologic processes: retardation of growth, aberrant growth or failure of fusion of the foetal cleft.

## Aetiologic influences

A wide range of endogenous and exogenous factors have been causally linked to developmental abnormalities of the eye but in many cases the underlying aetiology is unclear. Of these the most important factor is genetic. Developmental eye abnormalities may occur in association with chromosomal abnormalities or be caused by autosomal or sex-linked genetic mutations. Ocular malformations are very frequently associated with systemic abnormalities, limb and auricular/facial abnormalities being the most common associations.

The developing eye is a complex organ comprised of embryonic tissue derived from ectoderm, endoderm, and mesoderm. A great many genetic influences therefore come into play. A

wealth of literature exists on the genetic control of ocular development in animals. Correlation of this work with human ocular development is however still at an early stage. To date, the most important gene found to be involved in the control of human eye development has been Pax6.[1] The central importance of Pax6 is illustrated by the fact that the gene is conserved throughout the animal kingdom.[2] Pax6 is one of a number of paired-box genes encoding nuclear transcription factors, and was initially associated with disease in the mouse and rat Small eye (Sey) mutant. Subsequently, Pax6 mutations have been associated with a number of developmental abnormalities of the anterior segment of the human eye (see below). Another member of this group of genes that has been implicated in human disease is Pax3. This gene has been associated with Waardenberg syndrome[3] type I and III, a dominantly inherited audito-pigmentary syndrome, characterised by sensorineural hearing loss, facial dysmorphism and abnormal pigmentation of the eyes, hair and skin. In addition to these features, type III cases exhibit limb hypoplasia and contractures. Some (20%) of cases of Waardenberg syndrome type II (deafness and ocular hypopigmentation) have been associated with mutations of microphthalmia-associated transcription factor (MITF) the human homologue of a recessive mouse microphthalmia gene. Mutations of Pax2 have been found to cause a rare syndrome of optic nerve coloboma and renal abnormalities.[4] An autosomal recessive microphthalmos locus has recently been identified on chromosome 14q32.[5]

No disease gene has yet been identified at this locus.

Other genes involved in ocular development and disease in animal models include Chx10,[6] Rx,[7] Dlx1,[2] GH6,[2] Msx12 and CrX.[8] A number of other genes have been specifically associated with lens development and cataract. These include genes encoding cytoskeletal proteins (e.g. Vim), structural proteins such as the crystallin genes (Cryg) and membrane proteins (e.g. Mip). The relevance of this work to human disease awaits full assessment.

A large number of environmental influences are also known to predispose to ocular maldevelopment. Intrauterine exposure to radiation and infection, including rubella, varicella, and toxoplasmosis (see Chapter 10) are important causative associations. A large number of teratogens, including thalidomide, cocaine and alcohol, have also been implicated. Retinoic acid is a potent teratogen thought to interfere with neural crest cell migration during development. Maternal use has been associated with a "retinoid syndrome" in which affected children may show cleft lip and palate, thymic hypoplasia, congenital heart disease and spina bifida. Ocular associations include microphthalmos, Goldenhar syndrome, and optic nerve anomalies.[9]

## Developmental disorders of the whole globe

### Anophthalmos

Anophthalmos is a rare condition diagnosed when there is absence of the globe or when it is replaced by a tiny cystic remnant (Figure 5.1). Microphthalmos, in an adult, is diagnosed when the globe diameter is less than 21 mm (less than 19 mm diameter in a one year-old child). In Europe, it has been estimated that the overall prevalence of eye malformations is approximately 3.7/10 000 newborns. The most frequent is anophthalmia/microphthalmia (2.1/10 000), followed by congenital cataract (0.6/10 000) and ocular coloboma (0.5/10 000).[10]

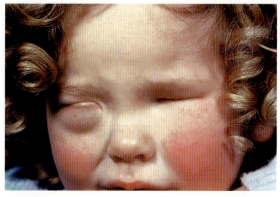

(a)

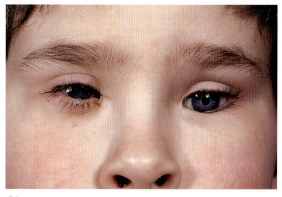

(b)

Figure 5.1    (a) Young child with bilateral anophthalmos associated on right side with an orbital cyst. (b) Same child after excision of cyst and fitting of orbital prosthesis

Anophthalmos/microphthalmos results from either complete failure or early arrest of optic vesicle budding. Anophthalmos is frequently bilateral but is usually asymmetric. Most cases are sporadic and idiopathic, although the condition has been seen to segregate in a few families. Chemicals (e.g. LSD), radiation and other environmental exposures early in foetal development have also been implicated in its aetiology. Extreme microphthalmos can usually be differentiated from anophthalmos on clinical examination, but if there is doubt the microphthalmic globe can be imaged using ultrasound, computed tomography (CT) or magnetic resonance imaging (MRI) scanning.

Infants born with anophthalmos should be referred to a paediatrician or geneticist with an interest in dysmorphology so that any other congenital malformations can be excluded and accurate genetic counselling given. The parents need to be given advice about bringing up a visually impaired child and the support services available; referral to the peripatetic teacher for the visually impaired should be made at an early stage. The anophthalmic orbits are managed by inserting gradually enlarging conformers to stimulate growth and a final orbital prosthesis fitted once a reasonable orbital size has been achieved (Figure 5.1b).

## Microphthalmos

Microphthalmos may be simple (in isolation) or complex (associated with other ocular abnormalities). The smaller the eye or the more severe the complex type abnormalities, the more severe the visual deficit. Isolated microphthalmos is usually idiopathic but autosomal dominant, recessive and X-linked pedigrees have been described.

Complex microphthalmos involves association with uveal abnormalities (colobomatous microphthalmos), anterior segment dysgenesis (e.g. Peters' anomaly) cataract or retinal diseases such as retinopathy of prematurity and Norrie disease. Systemic syndromes are common associations with microphthalmos. Mental retardation and chromosomal abnormalities are notably seen with microphthalmos. Other associations include facial defects, cleft palate, dental abnormalities (oculodentodigital syndrome), brain abnormalities such as microcephaly (GOMBO syndrome), dermal aplasia (MIDAS syndrome) and albinism (Cross syndrome). Occasionally microphthalmos is seen in association with a rapidly expanding orbital cyst which communicates with the microphthalmic eye (Figure 5.1a). This is a feature of Delleman syndrome when microphthalmos and orbital cyst are seen in association with skin tags, hydrocephalus and mental retardation. Cryptophthalmos syndrome is microphthalmos seen in association with varying degrees of lid skin fusion to the globe.

## Nanophthalmos

Nanophthalmos is a rare condition characterised by a small hypermetropic eye with microcornea, often complicated by angle closure glaucoma. Scleral thickening is seen due to abnormal collagen and fibronectin deposition. Intraocular surgery in nanophthalmic eyes is often complicated by severe uveal effusion and serous retinal detachment which can be treated by vortex vein decompression.

## Cyclopia and synophthalmos

Complete (cyclopia) or partial (synophthalmos) fusion of the two eyes occurs very rarely and is almost always associated with severe central nervous system and other malformations mostly incompatible with life.

# Developmental disorders of the anterior segment

Anterior segment maldevelopment affects the cornea, trabecular meshwork, and iris.[11] Lenticular opacities are a common association. Those that affect the iridocorneal angle are often associated with early-onset glaucoma (buphthalmos).

## Primary corneal abnormalities (see Chapter 6)

### Megalocornea

Megalocornea is a rare congenital abnormality diagnosed if the corneal diameter is >13 mm in the first two years of life in the absence of raised intraocular pressure. The condition is always bilateral and symmetrical; endothelial cell density and corneal thickness are normal. Most commonly, megalocornea occurs as a simple X-linked isolated corneal disorder but can be seen in association with uveal pigment dispersion, miosis, and cataract. Systemic associations include mental retardation, albinism, ichthyosis, and hyperglycinanaemia. Megalocornea is also seen in a number of syndromes including

Marfan syndrome, Aarskog syndrome (X-linked) and Crouzon syndrome.

**Cornea plana**

Cornea plana is a rare, bilateral and congenital flattening of the cornea with hypermetropia. The condition is usually seen in association with microphthalmos, sclerocornea or uveal coloboma. These secondary associations are seen particularly in the autosomal recessive form of the disease. The autosomal recessive cornea plana disease gene (CNA2) has been mapped to chromosome 12q. Autosomal dominant pedigrees of more mild disease not associated with other ocular or systemic manifestations are also known.

**Corneal dermoids**

Corneal dermoids are idiopathic (usually), solid, white, choristomas composed of connective tissue, pilosebaceous material, keratinised epithelium and occasionally lipid. Central corneal dermoids are very rare, either inherited as an X-linked trait or as part of a syndrome. Epibulbar dermoids (Figures 5.2 and 5.3) are a common finding in Goldenhar syndrome. Sclerocornea is another congenital abnormality resulting in white opacification ("scleralisation") of the peripheral cornea. Congenital glaucoma is a common association and sclerocornea can be associated with mental retardation and facial abnormalities.

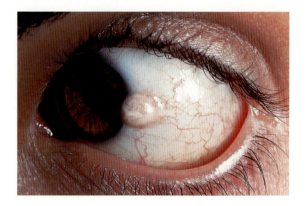

Figure 5.3    Limbal dermoid left eye

**Peters' anomaly**

Peters' anomaly (Figure 5.4) is another well recognised condition associated with opacification of the cornea. Histologically there is absence of central corneal endothelium with abnormal stromal lamellae and excessive amounts of fibronectin. The lens may be adherent to the central cornea. This anomaly is frequently bilateral and symmetrical and may be found in isolation; accompanied by other ocular malformations such as glaucoma, cataract, microphthalmos and iris dysgenesis; or associated with systemic diseases such as heart defects,

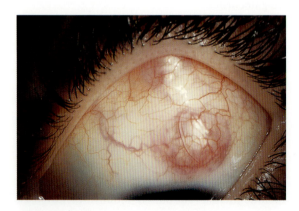

Figure 5.2    Epibulbar dermoid adjacent to superior limbus

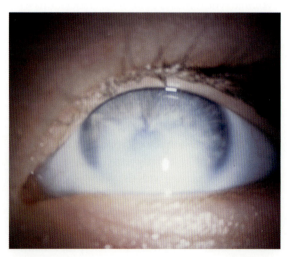

Figure 5.4    Corneal opacity with underlying iridocorneal adhesions in child with Peters' anomaly

mid-line CNS abnormalities or genitourinary disease. Peters' anomaly plus is a distinct entity consisting of bilateral (in 80% of cases) corneal opacities with short stature, cleft lip/palate, abnormal ears and developmental delay. Peters' anomaly may be seen in association with the foetal alcohol syndrome, ring chromosome 21, chromosome 11 deletion and with Pax6 mutations.[12]

## Abnormalities of the iridocorneal angle
(see Chapter 8)

A range of iridocorneal angle dysgenesis defects occurs. The commonest is posterior embryotoxon. This is visible clinically as a prominent white line demarcating Schwalbe's ring. Posterior embryotoxon is frequently seen in isolation (often with little consequence) but is also seen in Alagille syndrome and in association with ocular albinism. In Axenfeld's anomaly posterior embryotoxon is associated with adhesions between the peripheral iris and Schwalbe's ring indicating that there is more extensive iridocorneal dysgenesis. Axenfeld's anomaly may be complicated by glaucoma which is of a variable age of onset.

## Iris maldevelopment

Rieger anomaly[13] is a phenotypically variable, primary iris abnormality. Varying degrees of iris hypoplasia, polycoria and ectropion uveae are seen with posterior embryotoxon and iridotrabecular bridges. Glaucoma is evident in over 60% of cases and corneal and lens opacities are common. Systemic features (Rieger syndrome-autosomal dominant) include maxillary hypoplasia, dental abnormalities, inguinal hernias and hypospadias. Genomic localisations for causative mutations include chromosomes 6, 4q25 and 13.

Complete or almost complete hypoplasia of the iris is seen in aniridia (Figure 5.5).[13,14] Iris abnormalities are often associated with corneal opacity, cataract, lens dislocation, ciliary hypoplasia, foveal hypoplasia (Figure 5.6) and optic nerve

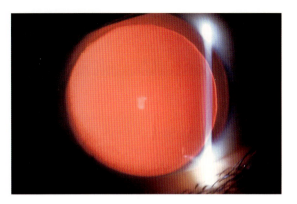

Figure 5.5    Aniridia with small rim of iris nasally

hypoplasia. Glaucoma is a common complication. Aniridia has a population frequency of 1 : 60 000 to 1 : 100 000.[14] In the majority of individuals with aniridia there is a family history consistent with autosomal dominant inheritance. Isolated cases represent new autosomal dominant mutations. Sporadic aniridia may be associated with Wilms' tumour and genitourinary abnormalities (WAGR syndrome). Chromosome analysis of such patients shows deletions of chromosome 11p which encompass the PAX6 locus and the adjacent Wilms' tumour gene. Isolated aniridia is associated with mutation of PAX6.[13,14]

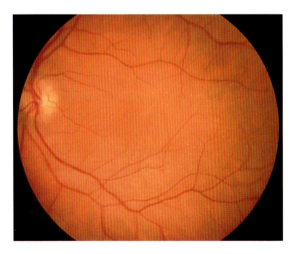

Figure 5.6    Left fundus of same patient as Figure 5.5 showing foveal hypoplasia

# Developmental disorders of the posterior segment

## Congenital vitreous anomalies (see Chapter 10)

At the nine-week stage of ocular development, primitive, vascularised vitreous is replaced by secondary, avascular tissue. Aberrations of this process are relatively common. A persistent hyaloid artery can be identified in 3% of children. Mostly these regress with time, but remnants often persist at the optic nerve head (Bergmeister papilla) or posterior lens capsule (Mittendorf dot). More severe abnormalities of vitreous maturation are seen in persistent hyperplastic primary vitreous. Most cases are unilateral and idiopathic although affected families have been described. Histopathologically, a thick, vascular retrolental mass is found. Clinically this often presents as a uniocular leucocoria. The condition is progressive and tractional retinal detachment (seen on ultrasound assessment), anterior chamber shallowing and glaucoma precede ocular phthisis.

## Norrie disease (see Chapter 10)

Norrie disease[15] is an X-linked recessive condition resulting in bilateral retrolental masses, vitreous haemorrhage and tractional retinal detachment.

Phthisis bulbi is common. Affected males are blind at birth or in early infancy. The Norrie disease gene (*NDP*) has been mapped to chromosome Xp11.3. Its specific function is unknown but the NDP protein does share homology with proteins known to be involved in cell adhesion, extracellular proteins such as mucins and growth factors such as transforming growth factor and nerve growth factor. The NDP protein may play a role in neural differentiation and in establishing neuronal connections in the developing eye. The gene is expressed in a number of tissues and systemic abnormalities such as sensorineural deafness, growth retardation, and hypertelorism are found. Behavioural abnormalities have been attributed to contiguous gene abnormalities, since in this subgroup of Norrie disease sufferers, Xp11.3 microdeletions have been found.

## Primary chorioretinal abnormalities

### Colobomatous abnormalities

Abnormal closure of the developing optic vesicle can lead to colobomatous abnormalities of the choroid and retina (Figure 5.7). These most commonly occur in the inferionasal retina and are associated with static superiotemporal field defects. These abnormalities can be unilateral or bilateral. Chorioretinal colobomas are associated with a significant risk of rhegmatogenous retinal detachment. Retinal tears can develop in the thinned retina overlying the colobomatous defect. Lens colobomas may also be associated with giant retinal tears. Chorioretinal colobomas are commonly seen in association with iris and optic nerve colobomas and affected eyes are often microphthalmic (Figure 5.8a,b). Colobomatous abnormalities are usually seen as isolated ocular abnormalities but may be found in a large number of systemic syndromes and are a common finding in children with chromosomal abnormalities.

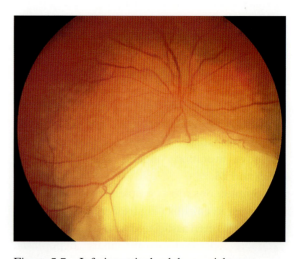

Figure 5.7   Inferior retinal coloboma right eye

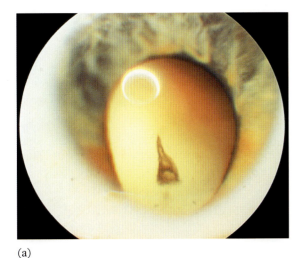

(a)

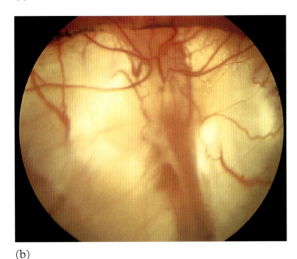

(b)

Figure 5.8   Right iris coloboma (a) and associated extensive optic disc and retinal coloboma (b)

## North Carolina macular dystrophy

Colobomatous-like chorioretinal defects are occasionally seen outside the inferionasal quadrant. Congenital toxoplasmosis is a common cause. North Carolina macular dystrophy is a rare, non-progressive, autosomal dominant condition that can present with bilateral congenital chorioretinal defects at the macula.[16] There is wide variation in phenotype with mild cases presenting with minimal retinal pigment epithelial abnormalities at the macula. The peripheral retina is normal and visual acuity is usually better than 6/24 even in severe cases. The North

Carolina macular dystrophy gene has been mapped to chromosome 6q.

## Congenital hypertrophy of the retinal pigment epithelium (CHRPE)

Congenital hypertrophy of the retinal pigment epithelium (CHRPE) is a well-recognised fundus abnormality often found incidentally. The lesions appear as isolated brown or black lesions in the mid-peripheral retina (Figure 5.9). Visual field defects corresponding to the site of the lesion can be elucidated on detailed perimetry and reflect photoreceptor atrophy overlying the lesion. Isolated cases are usually sporadic. Multiple, bilateral CHRPE lesions may be associated with autosomal dominant adenomatous polyposis coli. Clumps of small patches of retinal pigment epithelium (RPE) hyperpigmentation are called "bear tracks" and are innocuous. Clumps of depigmented retinal pigment epithelium have also been described (polar bear tracks).

## Aicardi syndrome

Aicardi syndrome[17] is a very rare X-linked dominant condition, lethal *in utero* in males. Affected females often appear normal at birth but soon develop infantile spasms and numerous

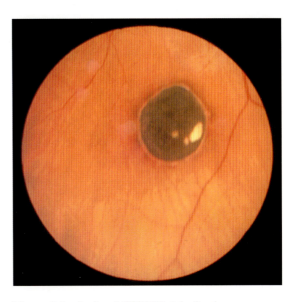

Figure 5.9   Isolated CHRPE right fundus

other neurological deficits. Characteristic, well-demarcated, large lacunae of chorioretinal hypopigmentation are evident on ophthalmoscopy (Figure 5.10). Optic nerve head abnormalities and microphthalmos are also commonly seen in affected females.

## Developmental anomalies of the optic nerve (see Chapter 18)

A diverse range of congenital abnormalities of the optic nerve head are known. Although congenital pigmentation of the disc itself is rare, pigmentation around the optic disc is very common. Myelinated nerve fibres around the disc are also common and represent abnormal extension of optic nerve fibre myelination beyond the cribiform plate. Visual field defects are often found corresponding to the area of myelination. This congenital abnormality is occasionally associated with unilateral high myopia and amblyopia (Figure 5.11).

### Optic nerve hypoplasia

Optic nerve hypoplasia[18] is an uncommon bilateral condition which in the more extreme

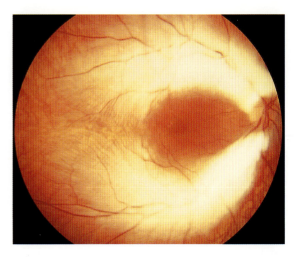

Figure 5.11 Right fundus of child with unilateral high myopia, myelinated nerve fibres and anisometropic amblyopia

cases presents with nystagmus and severe visual impairment in early infancy. Less severe and unilateral cases often present with static visual field defects or strabismus. A complete ring of bare sclera around the optic nerve head is a useful diagnostic feature in such mild cases, whereas severe cases are usually obvious on examination.

Optic nerve hypoplasia is usually seen as an isolated finding but may be seen in association with absence of the septum pellucidum (De Morsier syndrome), pituitary stalk abnormalities and endocrine disturbance, particularly growth hormone deficiency. All children with optic nerve hypoplasia should therefore be monitored regularly by a paediatrician or paediatric endocrinologist. Neuroradiologic imaging is only necessary if there are other congenital abnormalities or if there is concern about other neurological abnormalities. Optic nerve hypoplasia has also been reported in association with foetal alcohol syndrome and with maternal use of cocaine, LSD and certain antiepileptic drugs during pregnancy. It has also been reported to be more frequent in infants born to mothers with diabetes.

Familial cases are described but, apart from an association with autosomal dominant

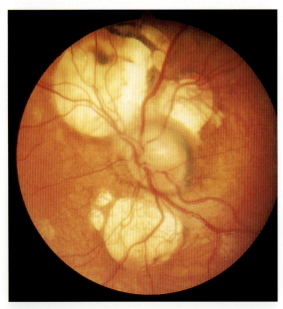

Figure 5.10 Fundus appearance in Aicairdi syndrome, (Courtesy of Dr R Buncic)

aniridia, no clear genetic abnormality has been associated.

Complete aplasia of the optic nerve is very rare and is usually associated with other severe ocular abnormalities, such as microphthalmos and abnormalities of the central nervous system.

## Optic nerve head coloboma

Optic nerve head coloboma can be an isolated finding or seen with colobomas of the iris, ciliary body, and choroid. Colobomas are relatively common and present either as an incidental finding on routine eye examinations or with non-progressive visual field defects. When seen in isolation, most cases are sporadic although autosomal dominant inheritance with variable expressivity and rarely autosomal recessive inheritance has been described. Systemic associations are known. Mutations of the *PAX2* gene on chromosome 10q24–q25 have been associated with optic disc coloboma and kidney abnormalities.[4] Coloboma may also be seen in chromosomal syndromes such as trisomy 13 and be amongst the consequences of teratogens such as thalidomide, retinoic acid, and alcohol.

Optic disc pits may be mild cases of optic nerve head coloboma. These usually present in adulthood as cases of central serous retinopathy or in cases where glaucomatous disc cupping is suspected. Pits are small herniations of neuroectodermal tissue into the nerve substance. They usually occur temporally near the disc margin. Morning glory syndrome is an extreme example of optic nerve head coloboma. The optic nerve head is displaced backward within a staphalomatous pocket and covered with varying degrees of glial tissue. Characteristically, retinal vessels radiate like the spokes of a wheel from the centre of the anomalous disc. Affected eyes have poor vision from birth. It is usually an isolated, idiopathic finding but associations with central nervous system abnormalities are described.

Tractional retinal detachments have been reported in affected eyes.

## References

1 Hanson I, Van Heyningen V. *Pax6* – more than meets the eye. *Trends Genetics* 1995; **11**: 268–72.
2 Graw J. Genetic aspects of embryonic eye development in vertebrates. *Develop Genetics* 1996; **18**: 181–97.
3 Tassabehji M, Newton VE, Liu X–Z, *et al.* The mutational spectrum in Waardenberg syndrome. *Human Molec Genetics* 1995; **4**: 2131–7.
4 Schimmenti LA, Cunliffe HE, McNoe LA, *et al.* Further delineation of renal-coloboma syndrome in patients with extreme variability of phenotype and identical *Pax2* mutations AU:JN: *Am J Human Genetics* 1997; **60**: 869–78.
5 Bessant DAR, Khaliq S, Hameed A, *et al.* A locus for autosomal recessive congenital microphthalmia maps to chromosome 14q32. *Am J Human Genetics* 1998; **62**: 1113–16.
6 Maas R. Keeping an eye on eye development. *Nature Genetics* 1996; **12**: 346–7.
7 Mathers PH, Grinberg A, Mahon KA, Jamrich J. The *Rx* homeobox gene is essential for vertebrate eye development. *Nature* 1997; **387**: 603–7.
8 Freund CL, Gregory-Evans CY, Furukawa T, *et al.* Cone-rod dystrophy due to mutations in a novel photoreceptor-specific homeobox gene (*CRX*) essential for maintenance of the photoreceptor. *Cell* 1997; **91**: 543–53.
9 Evans K, Hickey-Dwyer MU. Bifid anterior segment with maternal hypervitaminosis A. *Br J Ophthalmol* 1991; **11**: 691–2.
10 Bermejo E, Martinez-Frias ML. Congenital eye malformations: clinical epidemiological analysis of 1 124 654 consecutive births in Spain. *Am J Med Genetics* 1998; **75**: 497–504.
11 Elston J. Developmental abnormalities of the anterior segment. In: Taylor DSI, ed. *Paediatric Ophthalmology*, 2nd edn, Vol 23. London: Blackwell, 1997: 252–65.
12 Hanson IM, Fletcher J, Jordan T *et al.* Mutations at the *PAX6* locus are found in heterogeneous anterior segment malformations including Peters' anomaly. *Nature Genetics* 1994; **6**: 168–73.
13 Churchill A, Booth A. Genetics of aniridia and anterior segment dysgenesis. *Br J Ophthalmol* 1996; **80**: 669–73.
14 Hanson I, Jordan T, van Heyningen V. Aniridia. In: Wright AF, Jay B, Eds *Molecular Genetics of Inherited Eye Disorders*, Vol 19. Harwood Academic Press, 1994: 445–67.
15 Black G, Redmond RM. The molecular biology of Norrie's disease. *Eye* 1994; **8**: 491–6.
16 Moore A, Evans K. Inherited macular dystrophies. In: Taylor DSI, ed. *Paediatric Ophthalmology*, 2nd edn, Vol 23. London: Blackwell, 1997: 599–613.
17 Barth P. The Aicardi–Goutiere's syndrome. *Molec Chem Neuropathol* 1996; **27**: 47–9.
18 Hoyt CS, Good WV. Do we really understand the difference between optic-nerve hypoplasia and atrophy? *Eye* 1992; **6**: 201–4.

# 6 Disorders of the conjunctiva and cornea

JEREMY PRYDAL

The cornea and conjunctiva are susceptible to a wide range of disorders in childhood. Broadly, the abnormalities may be congenital, often associated with other developmental abnormalities of the eye, or acquired. Infections are common and are an important cause of visual impairment in the developing world. Trachoma, although rare in industrialised countries, is a common cause of morbidity worldwide. Immunological disorders range from the mild discomfort of seasonal allergy to part of potentially fatal systemic disease. A wide variety of genetic disorders also affects the cornea, often resulting in deposition of abnormal material in the corneal stroma or instability of the surface epithelium. The cornea is also affected in a wide variety of inherited metabolic disorders which present in childhood.

## Bacterial conjunctivitis

Bacterial conjunctivitis is common in children. It can be categorised into three groups by its time course: hyperacute, acute and chronic. Characteristics of each are given in Table 6.1.

## Aetiology

Skin and mucous membranes become colonised by commensal organisms within days of birth. The normal flora of the external eye consists mainly of *Staphylococcus epidermidis* and *Staph. diphtheroides* which inhibit invasion by other organisms but may occasionally be pathogenic themselves, often for unknown reasons.

Staphylococci produce a range of biologically active substances including coagulases, hyaluronidases, lipases, proteases, nucleases, fibrolysin, and several toxins. This accounts for the different manifestations of infection: blepharitis, keratitis, marginal ulceration, phlyctenulosis as well as conjunctivitis. *Staph. aureus* is a common cause of acute and chronic conjunctivitis.

Some strains of *Streptococcus pneumoniae*, commensals in the upper respiratory tract, cause conjunctivitis. Beta-haemolytic streptococci cause more severe disease often with membrane formation. *Haemophilus* species are a common cause in children under two years of age. The infection may spread to give a preseptal cellulitis.

Table 6.1  Bacterial conjunctivitis

| Hyperacute | Acute | Chronic |
| --- | --- | --- |
| Abrupt onset with progression over a few hours | Onset over one or two days | Poorly defined onset |
| Copious purulent discharge | Irritation and tearing of one eye, spreading to other within two days | Duration of longer than one month |
| Chemosis | Duration less than one month | Less severe symptoms and signs |
| Lid oedema | Moderate mucopurulent discharge | |
| Cornea often involved | Diffuse bulbar and tarsal hyperaemia | |
| | Intense papillary reaction | |
| | Possible mild punctate epithelial keratitis | |

*Neisseria gonorrhoeae* and *N. meningitidis* are always considered pathogenic when isolated from the eye. They cause a severe hyperacute conjunctivitis which can progress to involve and even perforate the cornea. Meningococcal conjunctivitis may be associated with septicaemia. Infection by *Corynebacterium diphtheriae* is rare but serious, causing an acute membranous conjunctivitis with scarring and symblepharon.

## Management

Treatment in mild disease is with a topical broad-spectrum antibiotic, such as chloramphenicol. In severe cases, or if there has been an inadequate response, Gram stain and culture on blood and chocolate agar is used to exclude gonococcal, meningococcal, and other serious infections. If antibiotic treatment has already been started it should be discontinued for 24 hours before samples are taken for culture. The choice of antibiotic is then based on the results of laboratory tests. Sensitivity of common pathogens are given in the Table 6.2.[1] Treatment of *Neisseria* infections is discussed in the section on neonatal conjunctivitis.

## Chlamydial conjunctivitis

*Chlamydia* are neither bacteria nor viruses. Like bacteria they have both RNA and DNA, as well as a discrete cell wall, but like viruses they can only replicate within host cells. The species *Chlamydia trachomatis* is responsible for the human ocular infections, trachoma, inclusion conjunctivitis and ophthalmia neonatorum. *Chlamydia* attach to conjunctival epithelial cells and induce them to become phagocytic. Once inside they divide to form clusters of particles seen on Giemsa staining as "inclusion bodies" around the nucleus. These are released to infect other cells.

## Trachoma (see Chapter 1)

In parts of Africa, Asia and India trachoma is endemic. In rural areas with poor sanitation, little water and crowded living conditions, nearly all children are infected by two years of age. Transfer is by direct contact within the family and indirectly by flies. Flies are also responsible for epidemics of bacterial superinfection. Repeated reinfections by *Chlamydia* and bacteria continue until much of the eye surface is replaced by scar tissue. This limits the infective phase of the disease and by the age of 15 there is little active infection. However, by this time there is often visual impairment from repeated bacterial keratitis, pannus, cicatricial entropion, and trichiasis.[2]

An important clinical sign of chlamydial disease is that it primarily affects the superior

Table 6.2    Sensitivity to antibiotics (modified from Smolin G and Thoft RA. *The Cornea*[1])

| Bacterium | Ch | Ci | Of | Ge | Me | Ne | Pe | Fu | Va | Po |
|-----------|----|----|----|----|----|----|----|----|----|----|
| *Staphylococcus epidermidis* | ± | + | + | + | + | ± | ± | + | + | − |
| *Staphylococcus aureus* | ± | + | + | + | + | ± | ± | + | + | − |
| MRSA | | + | + | + | − | | − | | + | − |
| *Streptococcus* sp. | + | + | ± | − | + | − | + | | + | − |
| *Streptococcus pneumoniae* | + | + | + | − | + | − | + | | + | − |
| *Clostridium* sp. | ± | − | ± | − | | − | + | | + | − |
| *Neisseria gonorrhoeae* | + | + | + | ± | ± | + | ± | | − | − |
| *Neisseria meningitidis* | + | + | + | ± | | + | + | | − | − |
| *Escherichia coli* | − | + | + | + | − | + | − | | − | + |
| *Moraxella* sp. | | + | + | ± | + | | + | | − | + |
| *Haemophilus influenzae* | + | + | + | ± | + | + | ± | | − | + |
| *Pseudomonas aeruginosa* | − | + | + | + | − | ± | − | | | + |

MRSA = methicillin-resistant *Staphylococcus aurens* + = sensitive; − = resistant; ± = variable sensitivity
Ch = chloramphenicol; Ci = ciprofloxacin; Of = ofloxacin; Ge = gentamicin; Me = methicillin; Ne = neomycin; Pe = penicillin G; Fu = fucidin; Va = vancomycin; Po = polymixin B

tarsal conjunctiva and upper limbus. MacCallan,[3] in 1908, proposed a classification of the disease into four sequential stages:

### Stage I: Incipient trachoma
The first signs of infection are follicles and papillary hypertrophy on the superior tarsus. There may be a mild punctate keratitis and fine superior pannus.

### Stage II: Established trachoma
IIA. Follicular hypertrophy
Active inflammation results in maturation of follicles which become "grain-like" in appearance (Figure 6.1). Follicles form at the limbus and subepithelial infiltrates in superior cornea.
IIB. Papillary hypertrophy
In stage IIB, papillae undergo further hypertrophy, obscuring follicles. Pannus grows down from the superior limbus.

### Stage III: Cicatrising trachoma
Follicles on the tarsal conjunctiva and at the limbus become necrotic, and are replaced by scar tissue (Figure 6.2). At the limbus the process leaves small depressions which become covered with transparent epithelium, Herbert's pits, a diagnostic sign of the disease. Under the lid, scars may join to form lines (Artl's lines). There is gross pannus and contraction of scar tissue begins to cause cicatricial entropion (Figure 6.3).

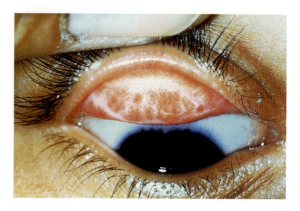

Figure 6.2 Subtarsal scarring due to trachoma. (Courtesy of WHO)

### Stage IV: Healed trachoma
Inflammation resolves once much of the eye surface has been replaced by scar tissue; there are no follicles or papillae and the disease is no longer infectious. Contraction of the tarsal conjunctiva causes entropion with trichiasis abrading the cornea. Scarring of conjunctiva obstructs lacrimal ducts and replaces goblet cells resulting in tear deficiency. The dry abraded corneal surface develops persistent epithelial defects and ulcers. At this stage there is profound loss of vision.

The World Health Organization have proposed a simpler grading system[4] (Table 6.3).

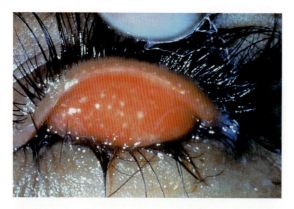

Figure 6.1 Superior tarsal conjunctiva in active trachoma showing follicular hypertrophy. (Courtesy of WHO)

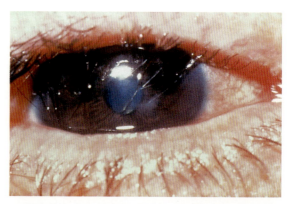

Figure 6.3 Cicatricial upper lid entropion with trichiasis due to trachoma. (Courtesy of WHO)

## Other chlamydial conjunctivitis

Inclusion conjunctivitis usually results from inoculation of organisms into the eye from genital infection and is therefore rare in children, except in neonates acquiring the disease during birth. Inclusion conjunctivitis presents after about 5 days' incubation with a unilateral purulent discharge and marked follicular response. Corneal changes are mild with epithelial keratitis and micropannus. Unlike trachoma, it resolves without scarring.

### Laboratory diagnosis

Giemsa staining to show cytoplasmic inclusion bodies used to be the standard method of diagnosis, but has now been replaced by more sensitive and specific immunofluorescence techniques. Antibodies against different strains can be used to serotype the organism. Methods using the polymerase chain reaction (PCR) have been developed but are not in routine use.

*Chlamydia* are usually cultured on McCoy cells, an irradiated monolayer of tissue cultured human fibroblasts. They can also be grown in the yolk sac of embryonated hens' eggs.

### Treatment

Systemic treatment is required to produce sufficiently high blood levels of antibiotic to eradicate the organism. Topical therapy can have a pronounced effect, but this is short lived and unnecessary with systemic treatment. After the age of 12, tetracycline is the standard choice (1 g/day for one month). In younger children, binding to calcium leaves deposits in growing bone and teeth and may cause hypoplasia. In this age group, and in nursing mothers, erythromycin is used (less than 2 years 250 mg/day, 2–8 years 500 mg/day, older than 8 years 1 g/day). Treatment of trachoma in endemic areas is not aimed at eradicating the infection. Periodic topical treatment reduces the severity of sight-threatening threatening complications. Surgery may be required for lid abnormalities.

## Viral conjunctivitis

### Adenovirus conjunctivitis

Adenovirus is remarkably hardy. It can survive in a dry state for more than two months, and is resistant to both alcohol and ether. The virus only infects humans, usually in epidemic outbreaks. Spread may be by direct droplet transmission, or via soap, towels, and other shared items.[5] Of the 47 known serotypes and subgroups, type D is usually responsible for eye infections. There are three clinical presentations.

- *Epidemic keratoconjunctivitis*
  The infection presents suddenly after a one-week incubation with irritation, soreness and foreign-body sensation which soon spreads to involve the other eye. It may be associated with an influenza-like illness. The eye is red with lid swelling, conjunctival oedema, and both papillae and follicles on the tarsal conjunctiva. Early in the disease, virus replication in corneal epithelial cells causes a diffuse punctate keratitis. This occurs in nearly all cases. Over the next few days these coalesce to form small raised islands of grey infiltrate. Immune responses clear the virus, but leave

Table 6.3  Simplified grading of trachoma

| TF | Trachomatous inflammation – follicular | The presence of five or more follicles in the upper tarsal conjunctiva; inflammation |
|---|---|---|
| TI | Trachomatous inflammation – intense | Pronounced inflammatory thickening of the tarsal conjunctiva that obscures more than half of the normal deep tarsal vessels |
| TS | Trachomatous scarring | The presence of scarring in the tarsal conjunctiva |
| TT | Trachomatous trichiasis | At least one eyelash abrading the eye |
| CO | Corneal opacity | Easily visible corneal opacity over the pupil |

infiltrates under healed epithelium, often with reduced visual acuity (Figure 6.4). Untreated, they may persist for years. Dendritic-like epithelial lesions, disciform keratitis, anterior uveitis and glaucoma are rare.

- *Pharyngeal conjunctival fever*
  Acute follicular conjunctivitis with pharyngitis and fever is a common form of the disease in children. It is milder than epidemic kerato-conjunctivitis with little corneal involvement. Subepithelial infiltrates are rare.

- *Non-specific follicular conjunctivitis*
  Non-specific follicular conjunctivitis is a mild infection seen in children. It does not require treatment.

### Diagnosis

Laboratory investigations are not usually required. Giemsa staining of conjunctival epithelial scrapes show intranuclear inclusion bodies (chlamydial inclusion bodies are in the cytoplasm). Culture, fluorescent antibody tests and the PCR are rarely used unless there is doubt about the diagnosis.

### Treatment

Topical non-steroidal anti-inflammatory agents and tear substitutes may relieve some of the discomfort. Antibiotics to prevent secondary bacterial infection are often used, but are probably unnecessary. Keratitis with reduced acuity should be treated with intensive topical steroids. Specific antiviral agents have not yet been developed.

### Herpes simplex

Until the age of six months, babies are partially protected by maternal antibodies. This does not prevent herpetic infection in the newborn, but reduces the severity of disease. Infection after the age of six months is common, but in 95% it is asymptomatic. There may be an acute follicular conjunctivitis, pre-auricular lymphadenopathy and skin vesicles (Figure 6.5). The corneal disease is different from that seen in adults because the child has not developed a specific immune response. It is limited to epithelium with diffuse punctate keratitis. Dendritic lesions if present are small. Hypersensitivity reactions causing stromal disease are unusual.[6] Treatment is with topical acyclovir.

### Measles

Ocular infection is associated with the systemic disease. Usually there is only a follicular conjunctivitis and other manifestations (extraocular muscle paralysis, chorioretinitis, optic atrophy, encephalitis) are rare. In developing countries, corneal ulceration with scarring and

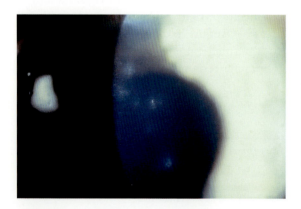

Figure 6.4 Subepithelial infiltrates in adenovirus keratitis

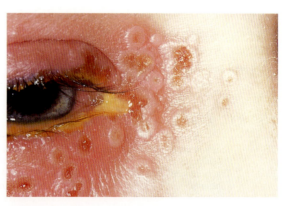

Figure 6.5 Primary herpes simplex infection in a young child showing multiple skin lesions

even perforation may occur, particularly in children with vitamin A deficiency (see Chapter 1).

## Other viral infections

Mumps may be associated with a superficial punctate keratitis and lacrimal gland involvement, but they resolve without treatment. Acute acquired rubella, unlike congenital disease, is a mild and self-limiting follicular conjunctivitis and superficial keratitis. Molluscum contagiosum causes a round raised skin lesion with umbilicated centre (Figure 6.6). If near the eye, antigens shed from the lesion cause a follicular conjunctivitis sometimes with keratitis. The lid lesion often goes unnoticed resulting in a chronic unilateral follicular conjunctivitis. Curettage or excision leads to resolution of the conjunctivitis.

## Ophthalmia neonatorum

Ophthalmia neonatorum is defined as any conjunctivitis occurring within the first month of life. It usually results from exposure to microorganisms during passage through the birth canal and varies from mild conjunctival hyperaemia to severe keratitis occasionally with perforation of the cornea. The time of onset gives

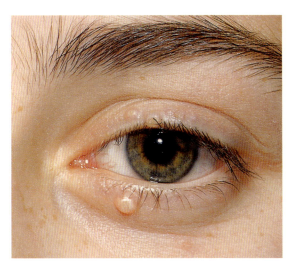

Figure 6.6   Umbilicated skin lesion of molluscum contagiosum. (Courtesy of Mr MG Kerr Muir)

some indication of the causative agent: toxic conjunctivitis usually presents within the first few days, bacterial infections within the first week, herpes simplex by the second week, and *Chlamydia* by the third week.[7] However, several other factors are relevant, including premature rupture of the maternal membranes, prolonged labour, and any prophylactic treatment used. A definitive diagnosis cannot be made from clinical examination alone. Laboratory tests should be performed in all cases.

## Gonoccocal infection

*Neisseria gonorrhoeae* attaches to mucosal surfaces by its capsule and is one of the few organisms that can penetrate intact corneal epithelium. The capsule also makes the organism relatively resistant to phagocytosis. It has become a less common cause of neonatal conjunctivitis in industrialised countries, initially because of routine prophylaxis with silver nitrate and more recently with the reduced prevalence of maternal infection. It remains common in developing countries[8] (see Chapter 1).

### Clinical features

Inflammation begins 2–4 days after birth rapidly progressing to a copious purulent discharge with intense conjunctival hyperaemia, chemosis and lid swelling. Membranes or pseudomembranes may form. Corneal ulceration may lead to perforation and widespread dissemination of infection.

### Diagnosis

Treatment may be started on clinical suspicion, but laboratory diagnosis is essential. Gram-negative diplococci are seen on Gram stain, usually on the surface of epithelial cells or within polymorphonuclear leucocytes. Epithelial scrapes are therefore more likely to give a positive result than examination of the purulent discharge. The organism can be grown on chocolate agar at high humidity with 5–10% carbon dioxide, but enriched agars with antibiotics to prevent growth of other organisms are now in common use.

**Treatment**

Resistance to penicillin is common and treatment should be with a third-generation cephalosporin, such as ceftriaxone 25–50 mg/kg, intravenously for 7 days with frequent ocular irrigation and penicillin drops.[8] Parents will also require treatment.

**Other bacteria**

Staphylococci, streptococci, enterococci, species of *Haemophilus* and *Pseudomonas* can cause ophthalmia neonatorum.[7] *Haemophilus* species are important as infection may be associated with preseptal cellulitis and meningitis, and *Pseudomonas* because it can cause endophthalmitis and septicaemia.

*Chlamydia*

This is now the most common cause of neonatal conjunctivitis in industrialised countries,[7,8] with up to 13% of women suffering from genital chlamydial disease.

**Clinical features**

After 5–14 days' incubation there is a mild mucopurulent papillary conjunctivitis (follicles cannot form until 6–8 weeks of age). The disease rapidly becomes bilateral with lid swelling, some chemosis and a fine epithelial keratitis. Pannus and stromal involvement with haze and peripheral infiltrates is rare. Ocular disease may be a manifestation of more widespread infection and pneumonitis occurs in 10–20% of cases.

**Diagnosis**

Traditional techniques for identification of chlamydial infection are Giemsa staining of conjunctival epithelial scrapes for intracytoplasmic inclusion bodies and McCoy cell culture. These have been replaced by more specific and sensitive tests using immunofluorescent antibodies or enzyme-linked immunosorbent assay (ELISA) techniques.

**Treatment**

Unlike adults, topical treatment is sufficient for local eye disease, but as there may be other sites of infection, systemic therapy is preferred: oral erythromycin syrup 50 mg/kg daily in four divided doses for 2–3 weeks in addition to topical erythromycin ointment.[8]

**Herpes simplex**

Herpes simplex is a rare cause of ophthalmia neonatorum, acquired from the mother and thus the type 2 virus. There may be vesicles on the lid, and fluid from them can be used to confirm the diagnosis by culture on cultured human fibroblasts. Herpetic conjunctivitis may be complicated by keratitis. Treatment is with systemic acyclovir.

**Other causes**

Silver nitrate used for prophylaxis against *Gonococcus* can itself cause a transient toxic reaction.[8] If suspected, no treatment is required and the child should be re-evaluated in 24 hours. Conjunctivitis may be secondary to congenital nasolacrimal duct obstruction, causing a mild unilateral mucopurulent discharge with reflux on massaging the lacrimal sac. The most common bacteria are *Haemophilus* species and *Strep. pneumoniae*. Treatment is with sac massage and antibiotics if necessary. Spontaneous resolution of the obstruction occurs in the majority of infants but if still present at 12 months of age requires mechanical probing (see Chapter 13).

# Immunological disorders

## Vernal keratoconjunctivitis

Vernal keratoconjunctivitis is a chronic fluctuating disease of children who often have other atopic problems. It causes intense itching with giant papillae on the superior tarsal conjunctiva, limbal disease and a characteristic keratopathy. Treatment can be difficult, but the disease is eventually self limiting.[9] In 90% of cases there are other allergic diseases: asthma, eczema, hay fever, as well as a family history of such conditions. It usually starts before the age of 10 and lasts 5–10 years.

### Clinical features

Intense itching, foreign-body sensation and photophobia are characteristic in this condition. The absence of itching makes a diagnosis of vernal keratoconjunctivitis unlikely.[9] Papillae coalesce to form giant papillae or "cobblestones" in the superior tarsal conjunctiva. They are flat topped, have a fibrovascular core and may cover the entire tarsal surface (Figure 6.7). Lid thickening can cause ptosis and deprivation amblyopia. There is a milky coating over the papillae and abundant stringy mucous discharge. Limbal involvement is commoner in dark-skinned people with single or multiple pale gelatinous nodules. Tranta's dots are collections of degenerate epithelial cells and eosinophils, usually limited to the superior limbus (Figure 6.8). They come and go, lasting less than a week.

Corneal involvement starts with a superficial punctate keratitis usually across the superior mid-periphery of the cornea. The necrotic epithelium can coalesce to form a vernal ulcer, a shallow horizontally oval epithelial defect in the superior third of cornea. These are also known as

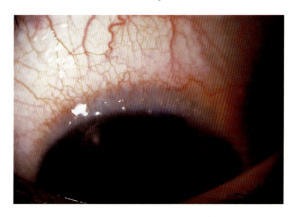

Figure 6.8  Vernal keratoconjunctivitis with Tranta's dots at the limbus

"shield" ulcers as mucus and fibrin form a plaque which inhibits healing. Pannus is rare.

### Differential diagnosis

A diagnosis can usually be made the from the history and examination. The physical signs are similar in giant papillary conjunctivitis, but here there is a source of mechanical irritation such as a suture, contact lens, or foreign body. The signs are different from those of seasonal allergic conjunctivitis in which the papillae are small, mainly on the lower tarsal conjunctiva, with no corneal changes.

### Treatment

It is not usually possible to completely eliminate symptoms. The aim is to achieve a background level of control using topical mast cell-stabilising agents and treat exacerbations with short courses of topical steroids. Sodium cromoglycate (4%) inhibits the release of inflammatory mediators from mast cells and should be used continually four times a day until the disease has burnt out. Side effects are rare. Lodoxamide and nedocromil are newer drugs with a similar action and might be more effective in relieving symptoms.[10] The mucolytic agent acetylcysteine (up to 10%) reduces the quantity and nature of mucus discharge. Neither topical or oral antihistamines are of benefit. Steroids are effective, but their use must be kept to a

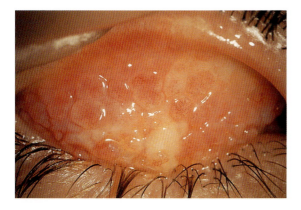

Figure 6.7  Cobblestone appearance of upper tarsus in child with vernal conjunctivitis. (Courtesy of Mr MG Kerr Muir)

minimum because of the risks of glaucoma and cataract formation. Exacerbations should be controlled with dexamethasone (0.1%) or prednisolone (1%) drops every hour for several days, rapidly reducing the frequency after one to two weeks. It is the high dose of steroids that controls inflammation and makes it possible to discontinue them after a short course. This regime results in fewer side effects than long-term low-dose therapy. Corneal ulceration is also treated with intensive topical steroids. Surgical removal of the plaque may be necessary to enable healing.

## Erythema multiforme

Erythema multiforme is an acute self-limiting, but potentially fatal disease, triggered by infection or drugs with blistering of skin and mucous membranes. It usually occurs in healthy individuals less than 30 years of age and is more common in men. There are three variants. Erythema multiforme minor is defined as disease with one or no sites of mucous membrane involvement. In erythema multiforme major (Stevens–Johnson syndrome[11]) there are two or more sites, one of which is usually the conjunctiva. The most severe form is toxic epidermal necrolysis in which there is extensive necrosis of the epidermis.

### Precipitating factors

Almost any drug can precipitate erythema multiforme; the more common are sulphonamides (including acetazolamide), penicillins, salicylates, phenylbutazone and phenytoin. Infection may be the precipitating factor, including herpes simplex, *Mycoplasma pneumoniae*, psittacosis, coxsackie virus and echovirus. BCG, polio and vaccinia vaccines may also be responsible. In many cases a trigger cannot be identified.[12]

### Clinical features

Malaise, fever, cough, headache and arthralgia precede the onset of skin and mucosal lesions. The skin lesions (maculae, papules, vesicles, and wheals) occur in crops, usually symmetrically distributed and affecting mainly the limbs including the palms and soles. Bullae scar after bursting. Haemorrhage into a vesicle results in "target" lesions, which have a red centre, pale surrounding zone and an outer red ring (Figure 6.9a). The mucosa of the mouth is commonly affected, leaving patients unable to eat or drink. Half of all patients suffer ocular disease and a third of these are left with permanently impaired vision. In the acute phase, there is a severe cicatrising conjunctivitis with swelling and ulceration of the eyelids (Figure 6.9b). Secondary infection is common. Late complications include symblepharon, ankyloblepharon, cicatricial entropion, trichiasis, corneal exposure, corneal keratinisation, and vascularisation. Stevens–Johnson syndrome may recur, but recurrent eye disease is

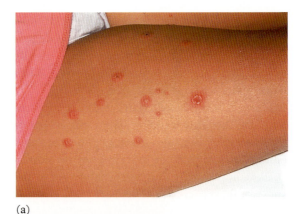

(a)

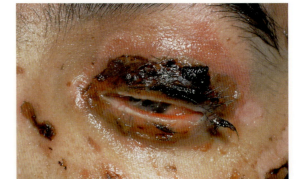

(b)

Figure 6.9    Typical target lesions on forearm (a) with associated lid and conjunctival involvement (b) in erythema multiforme

rare. Some patients, particularly those with severe mouth and throat lesions, are susceptible to overwhelming respiratory infection.

### Pathogenesis

There is a necrotising vasculitis with perivascular lymphocyte and macrophage infiltrate, circulating immune complexes and deposition of $C_3$, IgM, and IgG in blood vessel walls. The disease is associated with HLA-Bw44, the dominant subgroup of B12.

### Treatment

If a precipitating infection can be identified it should be treated, and all non-essential drugs stopped. Intravenous fluids and antibiotics may be required. Systemic high-dose corticosteroids are sometimes given although their use is controversial. If recurrent disease is preceded by herpes simplex infection, long-term low-dose acyclovir is indicated. There is no evidence that topical ocular steroids influence the severity of long-term complications, but they are usually used in the acute phase of the disease. Appropriate topical antibiotics should be given for secondary bacterial infection. Daily separation of adhesions does not usually stop permanent symblepharon formation. Large bandage contact lenses may be more effective. After the acute phase, the aim is to protect the cornea from tear deficiencies and eyelid abnormalities. Mucous membrane grafts may be required to reconstruct the fornices.

### Epidermolysis bullosa

Epidermolysis bullosa is a group of conditions in which there is a tendency for the skin to blister after minimal trauma. It may be acquired, autosomal dominant or autosomal recessive. In mild forms blisters heal without scarring, but at its worst patients may be disabled by progressive formation of limb contractures due to scar formation. The fingers can become completely encased in a keratinous shell and the bones resorb. Corneal epithelial cysts migrate to the surface causing transient defects and pain. Other findings include symblepharon, cicatricial entropion, trichiasis, blepharitis, and scarring of lacrimal punctae.[13] Treatment is supportive with artificial tears and correction of lid problems as required.

### Phlyctenulosis

This inflammatory disorder is a result of cell-mediated hypersensitivity to local bacterial antigens. It mainly affects children and young adults. Tuberculosis used to be the most common associated infection, but in industrialised countries it is now staphylococcal lid disease.[14] There may be single or multiple phlyctens which ulcerate and heal within two weeks. Conjunctival lesions are relatively asymptomatic, but corneal ones heal with stromal scarring and vascularisation. Topical steroids are usually effective although corneal disease associated with staphlycoccal infections can be resistant to treatment, recur and cause substantial visual loss. Treatment of blepharitic lid disease is important.

Table 6.4 Epithelial dystrophies

| Dystrophy | Synonyms | Inheritance | Age of onset | Appearance | Recurrent erosions | Pathology | Treatment | Graft | Visual acuity |
|---|---|---|---|---|---|---|---|---|---|
| Meesmann dystrophy | Juvenile hereditary epithelial dystrophy | Autosomal dominant | < 10 years | Intracellular vesicles | Rare | Thickened epithelium, intracytoplasmic vesicles | None required | No | Good |
| Cogan's dystrophy | Epithelial basement membrane dystrophy, Map–dot–fingerprint | May be dominant, usually sporadic | > 30 years | Map, dot and fingerprint opacities | Some | Thickened basement membrane and microcysts | For recurrent erosions | No | Good |
| Reis–Bücklers' dystrophy | Bowman's layer dystrophy | Autosomal dominant | <10 years | Subepithelial opacities, irregular surface | Frequent | Vacuoles in basal epithelium, absent or abnormal basement membrane | For recurrent erosions | Sometimes but recurs | Reduced |

## Corneal dystrophies

Only those corneal dystrophies that affect children are described in this chapter.

## Epithelial dystrophies (Table 6.4)

Epithelial dystrophies are associated with spontaneous recurrent corneal erosions. They tend to follow an autosomal dominant pattern of inheritance and rarely reduce visual acuity. Histopathology often shows abnormalities of the epithelial basement membrane. Meesmann's dystrophy, Reis–Bücklers' dystrophy and Cogan's dystrophy all primarily involve the epithelium.

### Meesmann's epithelial dystrophy

Meesmann's dystrophy is inherited as an autosomal dominant trait with incomplete penetrance. Corneal changes develop before the age of 10 with bilateral symmetrical epithelial vesicles. Transient discomfort occurs when cysts break through the epithelial surface, but this is rare before the age of 40. Subepithelial opacities may involve the whole cornea. However, vision is rarely affected and treatment seldom required.[15] The epithelium is thickened and disordered with vesicles of degenerate cytoplasm in basal layers.

### Reis–Bücklers' dystrophy

Reis–Bücklers' dystrophy is an autosomal dominant disease with a high degree of penetrance. It causes the most severe problems of all epithelial dystrophies with painful recurrent corneal erosions occurring several times a year from childhood to middle age.[16,17] There is progressive opacification of Bowman's layer in central and mid-peripheral cornea resulting in reduced visual acuity by the age of 30–40 (Figure 6.10). Vacuoles form in basal epithelial cells with disruption of organelles. The basement membrane is absent in some areas and may also be replaced by abnormal irregular fibrils which extend into overlying cell layers.

Treatment of recurrent erosions is initially

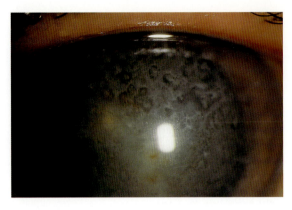

Figure 6.10   Honeycomb variant of Reis–Bücklers' corneal dystrophy (Courtesy of Mr MG Kerr Muir)

with topical lubricant ointment or bandage contact lenses. Epithelial stability can be improved by removing cells and causing mild trauma to Bowman's layer. This can be done manually although the excimer laser is a more controlled method.[18] Reduced acuity may make lamellar or penetrating keratoplasty necessary. However, the disease can recur in the donor tissue.

## Stromal dystrophies (Table 6.5)

### Granular dystrophy

Granular dystrophy is an autosomal dominant disorder. Bilateral discrete white opacities in superficial stroma become visible before the age of 10 (Figure 6.11a,b). The intervening cornea usually remains clear and vision good unless the opacities enlarge, coalesce, and extend into deep stroma. There are milder variants that present later in life, as well as more severe ones that progress rapidly and cause recurrent erosions.[17] Hyaline material consisting of protein and phospholipids accumulate in the stroma. These lesions stain with Masson trichrome, but only weakly with PAS (periodic acid–Schiff). The disease may recur in graft tissue and here crystals may form within epithelial cells. No treatment is required early in the disease, but occasionally penetrating keratoplasty is indicated to restore vision.

Table 6.5  Stromal dystrophies

| Dystrophy | Synonyms | Inheritance | Age of onset | Depth in stroma | Peripheral stroma | Intervening stroma | Vision | Pathology | Stain | Graft | Recurrence |
|---|---|---|---|---|---|---|---|---|---|---|---|
| Granular dystrophy | Groenouw 1, bread-crumb | Autosomal dominant | <10 years | Initially superficial, late deep | Clear | Initially clear | May deteriorate | Hyaline deposits | Masson | Sometimes | Sometimes |
| Lattice dystrophy type I | | Autosomal dominant | <10 years | Initially anterior, late throughout | Clear | Initially clear | Good until 40 years | Amyloid | Congo Red | Often | Frequent (affects anterior stroma only) |
| type II | | Autosomal dominant familial amyloidosis | 20–30 years | Initially anterior, late throughout | Clear | Initially clear | Good until 70 years | Amyloid | Congo Red | Sometimes | |
| type III | | Autosomal recessive | > 40 years | Initially anterior, late throughout | Clear | Initially clear | Good until 70 years | Amyloid | Congo Red | Sometimes | |
| Gelatinous drop-like dystrophy | | Sporadic or autosomal recessive | <10 years | Bowman's membrane | Clear until late | Confluent opacity | Severe impairment | Amyloid | Congo Red | Sometimes | Sometimes |
| Macular dystrophy | | Autosomal recessive | <10 years | Initially anterior, late throughout | Clear | Ground-glass appearance | May deteriorate | Mucopolysaccarides | Alcian Blue | Sometimes | Sometimes |
| Central crystalline dystrophy | Schnyder dystrophy | Autosomal dominant Some autosomal recessive | <10 years | Bowman's and anterior stroma | Clear | Variable | Usually good | Cholesterol and lipid | | Sometimes | Frequent |

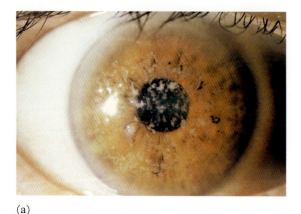

(a)

Figure 6.11 Granular dystrophy with broad beam illumination (a) and slit-lamp view (b). (Courtesy of Mr MG Kerr Muir)

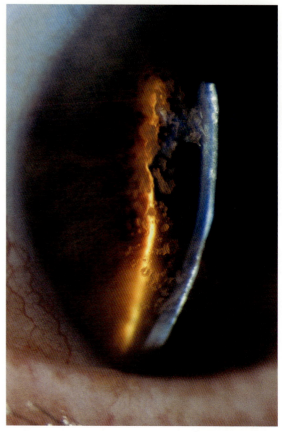

(b)

## Lattice dystrophy

Type I and II are inherited as autosomal dominant traits, but type III is recessive. Thin lines develop in the anterior stroma before 10 years of age and gradually become thicker (Figure 6.12). The intervening stroma loses clarity, eventually obscuring lattice lines. At this stage there is substantial loss of visual acuity. Recurrent erosions are common.[17] Type II is associated with familial systemic amyloidosis. Avellino corneal dystrophy is a variant which has affected several families from Avellino, Italy. They show evidence of lattice dystrophy as well as Reis–Bücklers' or granular dystrophies. The cause is thought to be a defect in keratocyte metabolism in which there is extracellular deposition of amyloid. In late disease amyloid is found throughout the stroma as well as in Desçemet's membrane.

Treatment of recurrent erosions has been described above. Many patients require penetrating keratoplasty by middle age. Recurrent disease occurs in nearly 50% and differs in that there is diffuse haze limited to the anterior stroma.

## Gelatinous drop-like dystrophy

Amyloid deposition in epithelium and Bowman's layer causes irregularities in the corneal surface with accompanying foreign-body sensation, pain, and loss of vision in both eyes. It may recur after deep lamellar, or penetrating, keratoplasty. Cases may be sporadic or inherited as an autosomal recessive trait. It is most common in Japan.

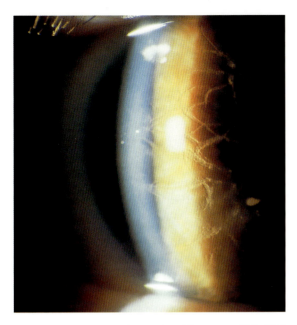

Figure 6.12   Lattice dystrophy. (Courtesy of Mr MG Kerr Muir)

## Macular dystrophy

The first signs of this autosomal recessive dystrophy are evident before the age of 10 with bilateral symmetrical diffuse opacities in the central anterior stroma (Figure 6.13). By the age of 30, there is a ground-glass appearance throughout the stroma with opacification of Descemet's membrane. Visual acuity is not usually affected until about 50 years of age when penetrating keratoplasty may be necessary.[17] The disease can recur in the donor tissue, although not as frequently as with lattice dystrophy.

A disorder in the breakdown of corneal glycosaminoglycans results in deposition of mucopolysaccharides which stain with Alcian Blue. The epithelial basement membrane is abnormal in places with degenerative changes in overlying cells.

## Central crystalline dystrophy

Both autosomal dominant and recessive forms occur, often associated with inherited hyperlipidaemia. Cholesterol and lipid deposits form throughout the central corneal stroma. The disease is usually asymptomatic.

## Other stromal dystrophies

The remaining dystrophies are uncommon and all are inherited autosomal dominant diseases. Fleck, central cloudy, and posterior amorphous corneal dystrophies may present in childhood but have good visual prognoses and do not usually require treatment.

Congenital hereditary stromal dystrophy is present at birth with bilateral dense opacity of the central superficial stroma. Early keratoplasty may be necessary to prevent severe amblyopia.

## Endothelial dystrophies

### Posterior polymorphous dystrophy

Posterior polymorphous dystrophy follows autosomal dominant inheritance. It is thought to be an abnormality of anterior segment development in which multilayered epithelial-like cells cover the posterior surface of the cornea On slit-lamp examination polymorphous opacities, some

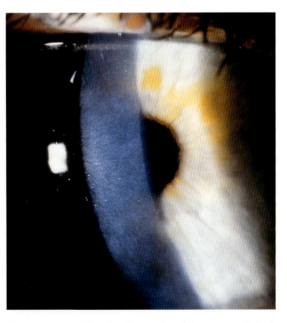

Figure 6.13   Macular dystrophy. (Courtesy of Mr A Morrell)

vesicular and surrounded by a grey halo, are seen at the level of Desçemet's membrane. There is often a "beaten metal" appearance of the entire posterior surface of the cornea. The abnormalities are evident at birth or develop early in life.[19] Patients are usually asymptomatic, and surgery rarely required. The visual prognosis is good.

Associated disorders include: broad peripheral iridocorneal lesions, raised intraocular pressure (15%), anterior chamber cleavage syndrome, band keratopathy, posterior keratoconus, and Alport syndrome.[19] Iridocorneal endothelial syndrome can be differentiated from posterior polymorphous dystrophy since it is unilateral with no family history.

### Congenital hereditary endothelial dystrophy (CHED)

CHED is an abnormality of anterior segment development *in utero*. The posterior layer of Desçemet's membrane is abnormal and endothelial cells absent or atrophic resulting in oedema of the entire cornea with substantial reduction in visual acuity. Full-thickness keratoplasty is often required within the first few months of life to prevent amblyopia. The autosomal recessive variant is present at birth, more severe, but static, while the dominant form presents within the first few years of life and is slowly progressive.[20] The important differential diagnosis is congenital glaucoma, in which there is corneal enlargement and raised intraocular pressure.

## Congenital abnormalities

A number of rare disorders resulting from abnormal development of the cornea have been described. Rarely the cornea may be completely absent, usually in association with other anterior segment abnormalities. Megalocornea is defined as a horizontal corneal diameter of greater than 12 mm in neonates or 13 mm after one year of age. It is usually seen as an X-linked recessive trait and may be associated with glaucoma, ectopia lentis and cataract later in life. Patients

tend to be myopic because of increased curvature of the cornea. Microcornea may occur as an isolated abnormality but is more usually seen in association with nanophthalmos, microphthalmos, and coloboma. In cornea plana, the cornea is relatively flat with a power of less than 43 dioptres. Values as small as 23 dioptres have been reported. Cornea plana is usually associated with microcornea or sclerocornea.

### Corneal abnormalities in anterior segment dysgenesis

A number of corneal abnormalities may be seen in association with anterior segment dysgenesis (see Chapter 5). In posterior embryotoxon, Schwalbe's line is displaced centrally so that it is visible at the periphery of the cornea. It occurs in 15–30% of otherwise normal eyes, or is associated with other developmental abnormalities of the anterior segment such as Axenfeld's anomaly and Rieger syndrome. Isolated posterior embryotoxon may be inherited as an autosomal dominant trait. Sclerocornea refers to replacement of cornea tissue with sclera. It varies from mild, with only peripheral changes, to complete opacity of the cornea. In Peters' anomaly, the central cornea of both eyes is white with adherent strands of iris (leukoma). Desçemet's membrane and endothelium are absent in this area.

### Dermoids

Dermoids are masses of tissue destined to be skin, but displaced during embryological development. They may contain keratinised epithelium, hair, sebaceous glands and other structures, even teeth. Limbal and corneal dermoids can cause profound loss of vision due to astigmatism or scarring of the visual axis. It may be associated with other developmental abnormalities, including Goldenhar syndrome.

### Other early-onset corneal abnormalities

Trauma to the cornea during birth can occur during forceps deliveries. There are ruptures in

Desçemet's membrane which heals to leave a ridge of hypertrophic membrane. Corneal oedema may clear or persist. Congenital glaucoma can lead to abnormalities of the cornea including corneal enlargement, oedema, and ruptures in Desçemet's membrane.

## Ectatic corneal disorders

### Anterior keratoconus

Keratoconus is a bilateral disease characterised by corneal thinning with localised protrusion resulting in irregular astigmatism and high myopia which cannot be corrected by spectacles. There is usually no definite pattern of inheritance, but a family history of the disease has been reported in 5–20% of cases. It is rarely inherited as an autosomal dominant or recessive trait. Some studies have reported it to be commoner in females.[21]

### Clinical features

Keratoconus usually becomes evident between 10 and 20 years of age, although it may rarely be present at birth. Early signs include progressive myopic or irregular astigmatism, and distortion of the retinoscopy reflex. Use of Placido's disc to examine the regularity of rings reflected from the corneal surface has now largely been replaced by computerised corneal topography which is more sensitive for detecting localised protrusion of the cornea. Progression of the disease is variable and asymmetrical. It tends to advance slowly for 6–10 years and then stop. Less commonly there is episodic deterioration over a longer period. In about 10% of cases the disease is unilateral.[22] Late in the disease conical distortion of the cornea is visible to the naked eye (Figure 6.14). The distortion of the lower lid on down gaze is known as Munson's sign (Figure 6.15). The apex of the cone is usually thin, eccentric, and inferionasal. There are fine superficial linear scars, deep vertical stretch lines (Vogt's striae), and increased visibility of corneal nerves. Fleischer ring, deposits

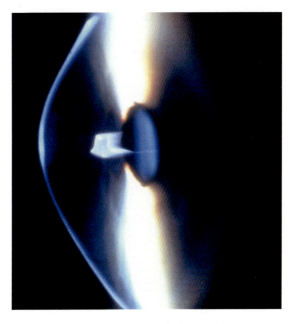

Figure 6.14    Slit-lamp view of advanced keratoconus

of ferritin in basal epithelium, may be seen at the base of the cone, especially with cobalt blue illumination.[22] Keratoconus is more common in individuals with atopy and may be associated with a number of other ocular and systemic disorders (Table 6.6.) Rarely Desçemet's membrane can rupture resulting in the sudden onset of corneal oedema (acute hydrops) as a result of breaks in the endothelial barrier to fluid influx. Visual acuity is markedly reduced.

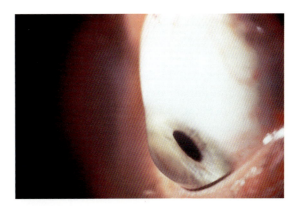

Figure 6.15    Munson's sign in same patient as Figure 6.14

77

Table 6.6   Keratoconus: associated ophthalmic and systemic disorders

| Ophthalmic disorders | Systemic disorders |
| --- | --- |
| Floppy-eyelid syndrome | Atopy |
| Pellucid marginal corneal degeneration | Down syndrome |
| Secondary corneal amyloid deposition | Marfan syndrome |
| Blue sclera | Hypothyroidism |
| Vernal keratoconjunctivitis | Osteogenesis imperfecta |
| Ectopia lentis | Apert syndrome |
| Congenital cataracts | Ehlers–Danlos syndrome |
| Aniridia | Noonan syndrome |
| Microcornea | Crouzon disease |
| Leber's congenital amaurosis | Little's disease |
| Retinitis pigmentosa | Neurofibromatosis |
| Eye rubbing | Addison disease |
| | Bardet–Biedl syndrome |
| | Van der Hoeve syndrome |

Oedema resolves spontaneously over 2–4 months, often with residual scarring.

**Pathological changes**

The pathogenesis of keratoconus is unclear. The earliest histological change is fragmentation of Bowman's and the epithelial basement membranes.[23] This may be a result of release of proteolytic enzymes from degenerate basal epithelial cells. Healing leaves fine superficial stromal scars.

Corneal thinning is a result of reduced numbers of lamellae, each being of normal thickness. An abnormality in keratocyte metabolism is presumed to be responsible for extracellular granular deposits which stain with PAS. There is overproduction of Desçemet's membrane.

**Treatment**

In early stages of the disease, it may be possible to correct the refractive error by spectacles. As the astigmatism becomes increasingly irregular, hard gas-permeable contact lenses give better results, replacing the distorted anterior surface of the cornea with a regular one. Considerable skill is required to fit lenses, particularly with eccentric oval cones. Surgery is indicated when contact lens wear becomes uncomfortable, gives insufficient correction of visual acuity or results in trauma to

the apex of the cone as it rubs on the back surface of the lens. The most common surgical procedure is penetrating keratoplasty, which has a good visual prognosis. Rejection is rare and there have been only a few reports of recurrent disease in the donor tissue. Lamellar grafts have some advantages. There is minimal risk of rejection and the integrity and strength of the globe is not compromised. Thus it may be appropriate in cases such as Down syndrome where there is risk of trauma to the eye and where detection of rejection may be difficult. Acute hydrops is usually treated with topical steroids and mydriatic agents. Once healed it may be possible to refit a contact lens, but in cases with axial scarring a corneal graft may be necessary.

**Keratoglobus**

Keratoglobus is an extremely rare bilateral condition in which the whole cornea is thinned and ectatic. It is almost always present at birth, but does not progress. Unlike keratoconus, the cornea may perforate with minor trauma and contact lenses are not used. Penetrating keratoplasty is technically difficult.

**Posterior keratoconus**

There is a steep localised concavity of the posterior surface of the cornea with a normal anterior curvature. Thus it is not a true ectatic disorder. The condition is usually sporadic, congenital, unilateral and non-progressive, and is more common in females. It is not associated with anterior keratoconus. In the area of thinning there is absence of Bowman's membrane, abnormalities of Desçemet's membrane and stromal opacification. The cause is unknown, but it is presumed to be a form of anterior segment dysgenesis.

**Metabolic diseases of the cornea**

Metabolic diseases affecting the cornea are a diverse group of disorders in which an abnormality of general metabolism results in the

Table 6.7   Metabolic diseases of the cornea

| Biochemical | Synonyms | Inheritance | Defect | Conjunctival and corneal changes | Other ocular changes | General features |
|---|---|---|---|---|---|---|
| **Protein** | | | | | | |
| Cystinosis | | Autosomal recessive | Lysosomal cystine transport, with intracellular deposition | Deposition of polychromatic cystine crystals throughout stoma | Loss of retinal pigment epithelium and deposition of cystine in RPE and choroid | Rickets, stunted growth, renal failure |
| Hypertyrosinaemia type II | Richer–Hanhart syndrome | Autosomal recessive | Absence of tyrosine aminotransferase | Conjunctival plaques chronic keratitis | Strabismus and cataracts | Skin lesions and mental retardation |
| Alkaptonuria | | Autosomal recessive | Homogentisic acid oxidase with accumulation of homogentisic acid | Pigmentation in interpalpebral area in deep epithelium and Bowman's layer | | Dark urine, arthralgia |
| **Lipid** | | | | | | |
| Mucolipidoses | | | | | | |
| I | Spranger syndrome | Autosomal recessive | Glycoprotein sialdase | Rarely fine corneal opacities | Macular cherry-red spot, cataract | Retarded growth |
| II | I-cell or inclusion cell disease | Autosomal recessive | N-acetylglucosamine phosphotransferase | Bilateral corneal haze | Cortical cataracts, glaucoma and optic atrophy | Severe growth retardation with thickened skin |
| III | Pseudo-Hurler polydystrophy | Autosomal recessive | N-acetylglucosamine phosphotransferase | Fine corneal opacities | Disc oedema, maculopathy | Musculoskeletal abnormalities and mental retardation |
| IV | Berman syndrome | Autosomal recessive (Ashkenazi Jews) | Ganglioside sialidase (neuraminidase) | Corneal opacity, pain and irregular surface present from birth | Cataract, optic atrophy, attenuated retinal vasculature | Psychomotor retardation |
| Fabry's | | X-linked recessive (female carriers mild disease) | α-galactosidase resulting in accumulation of sphingolipids | Whort like superficial corneal opacity | Retinal oedema, optic atrophy and cataracts | Skin, genitourinary, CNS and musculoskeletal involvement |
| Hyperlipoproteinaemias | (Types I–V) | Autosomal dominant or recessive | Abnormal circulating lipoproteins | Lipid keratopathy, corneal arcus | Lipaemia retinalis | Xanthelasma, coronary heart and peripheral vascular disease |
| Familial plasma cholesterol ester deficiency | | Autosomal recessive | Lecithin-cholesterol acyltransferase (LCAT) | Cloudy cornea and annular stromal opacity | | |
| Tangier's disease | | Sometimes autosomal recessive | Absent high-density lipoproteins, deposition of cholesterol | Corneal haze | | |
| **Carbohydrate** | | | | | | |
| Mucopolysaccharidoses | | | | | | |
| Hurler syndrome | Type I-H | Autosomal recessive | α-L-Iduronidase (complete) | Corneal clouding with fine grey opacities first in anterior stroma, later throughout cornea | Pigmentary retinopathy and optic atrophy | Dwarfism, grotesque face, joint contractures, mental retardation, hirsuitism |
| Scheie syndrome | Type I-S | Autosomal recessive | α-L-Iduronidase (partial) | Corneal clouding from birth | Pigmentary retinopathy and optic atrophy | Normal face, growth and mental development |
| Hunter syndrome | Type II | X-linked recessive | Iduronate sulphatase | None or mild corneal haze later in life | Pigmentary retinopathy and optic atrophy | Skeletal abnormalities, deafness, vascular disease and abnormal facies |

Table 6.7   *contd*

| Biochemical | Synonyms | Inheritance | Defect | Conjunctival and corneal changes | Other ocular changes | General features |
|---|---|---|---|---|---|---|
| **Carbohydrate** *contd* | | | | | | |
| San Filippo syndrome | Type III | Autosomal recessive | Heparan sulphate sulphamidase | None | Pigmentary retinopathy and optic atrophy | Severe mental retardation, less severe facial disfiguration than Hurler's |
| Morquio syndrome | Type IV | Autosomal recessive | N-Acetyl-α-D-glucosaminidase | Mild to severe corneal clouding | None | Dwarfism, abnormal facial appearance, deafness, hepalosplenomegaly |
| Maroteaux–Lamy syndrome | Type VI | Autosomal recessive | Arylsulphatase B | Mild-to-severe corneal clouding | No RPE changes, optic atrophy may occur | Skeletal abnormalities normal facies and mental development |
| Beta-glucuronidase deficiency | Type VII | Autosomal recessive | β-Glucuronidase | None | None | Skeletal abnormalities, hepatosplenomegaly and mental retardation |
| Glucose-6-phosphatase deficiency | Von Gierke's disease | Autosomal recessive | Glucose 6-phosphatase | Feint peripheral clouding | Perimacular lesions | Slow development, fat face, hepatomegaly and hypoglycaemic episodes |
| **Others** | | | | | | |
| Lowe syndrome | | X-linked recessive | Decreased ability of kidneys to make ammonia with acidosis and aminoaciduria | Corneal keloids | Cataract, glaucoma and miotic pupil | Mental retardation, aminoaciduria |
| Riley–Day syndrome | Familial dysautonomia | Autosomal recessive | Dopamine-β-hydroxylase | Corneal anaesthesia, epithelial erosions and tear deficiency, ulceration, perforation | Myopia, exodeviations, blepharoptosis, anisocoria, tortuosity of retinal vasculature | Dysautonomia |
| Alports syndrome | | X-linked dominant, rarely autosomal dominant or recessive | Collagen IV defects causing fragile basement membranes | Arcus, posterior polymorphous dystrophy, granular stroma | Lenticonus, cataracts, retinal flecks | Nephritis, deafness |
| Fish-eye syndrome | | Autosomal recessive | Partial lecithin-cholesterol acyltransferase (LCAT) deficiency | Corneal clouding | None | Hyperlipo-proteinaemia |
| Phenylkelonuria | | Autosomal recessive | Phenylalanine hydroxylase | Corneal opacities | Squint, cataract and albinoid fundus | Mental retardation, fits, microcephaly |
| Goldberg–Cotlier disease | Goldberg syndrome, galactosialidosis | Autosomal recessive | Both sialidase and β-galactosidase | Corneal clouding | Macular cherry-red spot | Gargoylism, skeletal abnormalities, mental retardation, fits, deafness |

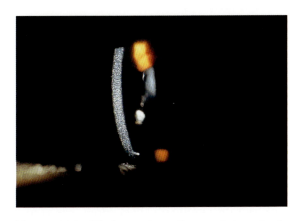

Figure 6.16   Slit-lamp view of corneal deposits in cystinosis

accumulation of abnormal substances in the cornea. In contrast to corneal dystrophies they are often inherited as autosomal recessive traits with progressive accumulation of abnormal substance in several layers of the cornea, affecting peripheral as well as central regions (Figure 6.16). They are often associated with systemic and developmental abnormalities with limited life expectancy. Details are given in Table 6.7.

## References

1  Burd EM. Bacterial keratitis and conjunctivitis. In: Smolin G and Thoft RA, eds *The Cornea: Scientific Foundations and Clinical Practice*. Chapter 5. Boston: Little, Brown, 1994: 135.

2  An BB, Adamis AP. Chlamydial ocular disease. *Int Ophthalmol Clin* 1998; **38**(1): 221–30.

3  MacCallan A. The epidemiology of trachoma. *Br J Ophthalmol* 1908; **15**: 369.

4  World Health Organization. Simplified Trachoma Grading. http: www.who.int/pbd/trachoma/gradcard/grading.htm

5  Duke-Elder S. The adenoviruses. In: Duke-Elder S, ed. *System of Ophthalmology*, Vol 8. St Louis: CV Mosby, 1965: 348.

6  Leopold I, Sery T. Epidemiology of herpes simplex keratitis. *Invest Ophthalmol Vision Sci* 1963; **2**: 498.

7  Rapoza PA, Quinn TC, Kiessling LA, Taylor HR. Epidemiology of neonatal conjunctivitis. *Ophthalmology* 1986; **93**: 456–61.

8  Fransen L, Klauss V. Neonatal ophthalmia in the developing world: epidemiology, aetiology, management and control. *Int Ophthalmol* 1988; **11**(3): 189–96.

9  Foster CS. Immunological disorders of the conjunctiva, cornea and sclera: vernal keratoconjunctivitis. In: Albert DB and Jakobiec FA, eds *Principles and Practice of Ophthalmology*, Vol 1, chapter 10, Philadelphia: WB Saunders: 1994: 193–5.

10  Verin P. Treating severe eye allergy. *Clin Exp Allergy* 1998; **28** Suppl 6: 44–8.

11  Stevens AM, Johnson FC. A new eruptive fever associated with stomatitis and ophthalmia: report of two cases in children. *Am J Dis Child* 1922; **24**: 526–33.

12  Mateos MA, Ros A, Lopez F. Erythema multiforme: a review of twenty cases. *Allergol Immunopathol* 1998; **26**(6): 283–7.

13  McDonnell PJ, Schofield OM, Spalton DJ, *et al*. The eye in dystrophic epidermolysis bullosa: clinical and immunopathological findings. *Eye* 1989; **3**(1): 79–83.

14  Allansmith MR, Ross RN. Phlyctenular keratoconjunctivitis. In: Tasman W and Jaeger EA, eds *Duane's Clinical Ophthalmology* Philadelphia: JB Lippincott chapter 8: 1990: 1–6.

15  Bron AJ, Burgess SE. Inherited recurrent corneal erosion. *Trans Ophthalmol Soc UK* 1981; **101**(2): 239–43.

16  Rice NSC, Ashton N, Jay B, Black RK. Reis–Bucklers' dystrophy: a clinicopathologic study. *Br J Ophthalmol* 1968; **52**: 577–603.

17  Miller CA, Krachmer JH. Epithelial and stromal dystrophies. In: Kaufman HE, Barron BA, McDonald MB and Waltman SR, eds *The Cornea*, chapter 15. New York: Churchill Livingstone, 1988: 383–424.

18  Liu C, Buckley R. The role of the therapeutic contact lens in the management of erosions: a review of the treatment strategies. *CLAO J.* 1996; **22**(1): 79–82.

19  Cibis GW, Krachmer JA, Phelps CD, Weingeist TA. The clinical spectrum of posterior polymorphous dystrophy. *Arch Ophthalmol* 1977; **95**: 1529–37.

20  Judisch GF, Maumenee IH. Clinical differentiation of recessive congenital hereditary endothelial dystrophy and dominant hereditary endothelial dystrophy. *Am J Ophthalmol* 1978; **85**(5): 606–12.

21  Rabinowitz YS, Keratoconus. *Surv Ophthalmol* 1998; **42**(4): 297–319.

22  Zadnik K, Barr JT, Gordon MO, Edrington TB. Biomicroscopic signs and disease severity in keratoconus. Collaborative Longitudinal Evaluation of Keratoconus (CLEK) Study Group. *Cornea* 1996; **15**(2): 139–46.

23  Chi HH, Katzin HM, Teng CC. Histopathology of keratoconus. *Am J Ophthalmol* 1956; **42**: 847.

# 7 Ocular inflammatory disease

ELIZABETH M GRAHAM, ROSALYN M STANBURY

The incidence of uveitis is estimated to be approximately 17 per 100 000 of the population per year.[1] In an epidemiological study from Switzerland,[2] 40 (9%) of 435 new patients with uveitis were under the age of 20 years. Tugal-Tutkun *et al.*[3] in a recent study of 130 patients with the onset of uveitis before the age of 17 years found that anterior uveitis (58%) and intermediate uveitis (20%) were the most common forms with posterior uveitis (14%) and panuveitis (8%) accounting for about a fifth of cases. The most important aetiological factor was juvenile idiopathic arthritis (JIA) which accounted for 41.5% of cases. Although Perkins in 1966[4] highlighted the association of anterior uveitis with Still disease it is only over the last two decades that the group of disorders now termed "juvenile idiopathic arthritis" (previously known as juvenile chronic arthritis in the United Kingdom and juvenile rheumatoid arthritis in the USA) has been recognised.

The majority of causes of uveitis in children are identical to those seen in adults. There are a few notable exceptions particularly juvenile chronic arthritis (JIA) and Kawasaki disease which are unique to children and intermediate uveitis and toxoplasmosis which are more frequent in children and young adults. Endogenous endophthalmitis in children may be caused by different organisms to that in adults. This chapter places emphasis on the disorders that predominantly affect children.

## Chronic anterior uveitis

Giles[5] in his series of articles on uveitis in childhood reports the following aetiologies for anterior uveitis from a group of 230 children seen at four teaching centres in the USA and Canada (Table 7.1). In the majority of cases, the cause of the uveitis is unknown and where a specific aetiology is identified most cases are accounted for by JIA, Fuchs' heterochromic cyclitis and sarcoidosis.

## Juvenile idiopathic arthritis (JIA)

Juvenile idiopathic arthritis is the commonest cause of juvenile arthritis, accounting for 70% of cases and is by far the most frequent systemic disease associated with uveitis in childhood. Three main subgroups, classified on the basis of mode of onset and the extent of joint involvement, are recognised (Table 7.2). Uveitis occurs in 20% of seronegative JIA patients.[6] In three-quarters it is bilateral, but if it remains unilateral for 12 months, the second eye is unlikely to become involved. The uveitis is asymptomatic, chronic

Table 7.1  Causes of anterior uveitis in the paediatric population (modified from Giles[5])

| Aetiology | Cases |
|---|---|
| Unknown | 138 (60%) |
| Juvenile rheumatoid arthritis | 46 (20%) |
| Fuchs' heterochromic cyclitis | 9 (4%) |
| Sarcoidosis | 9 (4%) |
| Syphilis | 4 (2%) |
| Tuberculosis | 4 (2%) |
| Ankylosing spondylitis | 3 (1%) |
| Trauma | 3 (1%) |
| Sympathetic ophthalmia | 2 (1%) |
| Ulcerative colitis | 1 (0.5%) |
| Reiter syndrome | 1 (0.5%) |
| Keratouveitis | |
|    Herpes simplex | 8 (3%) |
|    Herpes zoster | 2 (1%) |

Table 7.2    Subgroups of juvenile idiopathic arthritis (JIA)

| Mode of onset | Percentage of JIA population | Clinical features |
| --- | --- | --- |
| Systemic (Still disease) | 20% | Fever with one of: lymphadenopathy, hepatosplenomegaly, maculopapular rash. Arthritis may be involved |
| Polyarticular | 20% | Five or more joints are involved in the first three months; 25% are rheumatoid factor positive and their disease follows the pattern of adult rheumatoid arthritis |
| Pauciarticular | 60% | Four or fewer joints involved in the first 3 months |

and non-granulomatous (Figure 7.1). It almost never involves the posterior segment although a few cells may be seen in the anterior vitreous due to spillover from the anterior chamber. Girls with JIA are at greater risk than boys of developing uveitis. Two-thirds of JIA patients are girls but they comprise three-quarters of those with uveitis. Very occasionally the uveitis antedates the arthritis but more usually follows it and in 90% of cases it occurs within seven years of the diagnosis of JIA. The incidence of uveitis varies with the subgroup of the JIA. It occurs in 1–2% with systemic onset, 2–5% of the polyarticular onset and in 20–30% of the pauciarticular onset particularly those with extended pauciarticular disease. The risk of developing uveitis is increased if the patient is antinuclear antibody (ANA) positive. The antibody is present in 30% without eye problems and in 75% of those with uveitis.

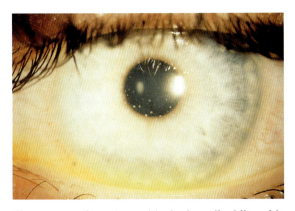

Figure 7.1    Chronic uveitis in juvenile idiopathic arthritis. The eye is not injected and there are fine keratic precipitates on the corneal endothelium. (Courtesy of Ms L Graham)

As the uveitis is usually asymptomatic, children with JIA should be screened on the slit lamp for the signs of uveitis. Initial slit-lamp examination should be performed by an ophthalmologist as soon as possible after diagnosis and repeat examinations should continue for ten years or until the age of 12 years, whichever is shorter. Table 7.3 summarises the 1994 recommendations of the joint working party of the Royal College of Ophthalmologists and the British Paediatric Association.

The mainstay of treatment of the uveitis associated with JIA is with topical steroids and mydriatics. Most cases can be controlled by topical dexamethasone 0.1% (or topical Predsol Forte). In some cases, particularly if there is difficulty instilling drops, ointment betamethasone may also be used at night. A short-acting mydriatic, such as tropicamide 1% should be used to keep the pupil mobile and prevent posterior synechiae. Very occasionally a subconjunctival steroid injection is necessary to bring the uveitis under control. Systemic steroids and cytotoxic agents have been used in severe cases but their success is limited.

Tugal-Tutkun et al.[3] found that the JIA group had significantly more complications than the other subgroups of paediatric uveitis. Glaucoma is a particular problem and may be caused by several mechanisms. Glaucoma may be steroid induced, may be secondary to peripheral anterior synechiae, may occur as a complication of posterior synechiae and iris bombe may be associated with the breakdown of the blood aqueous barrier or be due to a combination of factors.

Table 7.3   Recommendations for screening for uveitis risk in children with juvenile idiopathic arthritis (JIA)

| Risk | JIA features | Slit-lamp examination |
|---|---|---|
| High risk | Onset before 6 years. Pauciarticular and ANA-positive | 3-monthly for 1 year, then 6-monthly for 5 years, then annually |
| Medium risk | Polyarticular and ANA-positive, Pauciarticular and ANA-negative | 6-monthly for 5 years, then annually |
| Low risk | Onset after 11 years. Systemic JIA. HLA B27 | Annually |

ANA = antinuclear antibody

Peripheral anterior synechiae has been reported to occur in 14–27% of cases of anterior uveitis associated with JIA and is probably a major contributory factor.

The intraocular pressure should be monitored during treatment with steroids and if the pressure rises, a topical beta-blocker should be used. A change in topical steroid from dexamethasone to fluorometholone is of limited value as it is likely to result in worsening of the uveitis. Initial treatment for glaucoma is medical with topical beta-blockers and carbonic anhydrase inhibitors (CAIs). Topical brimonidine and latanoprost may be used when other medications fail or are contraindicated, but experience of these agents is limited in childhood. Caution should be used with systemic CAIs as these children may be taking aspirin and severe acidosis has been reported with combined CAI and aspirin use.

Surgical treatment, including filtration surgery, trabeculodialysis and cyclocryotherapy and more recently cyclodiode treatment have all been used. Kanski[6] reports the best results with trabeculodialysis, with 18 of 30 eyes (60%) having an intraocular pressure of less than 21 mmHg at 23 months follow-up. Despite optimum treatment of glaucoma, the visual prognosis is poor, with 35% of eyes with glaucoma progressing to "no perception of light".

It has been estimated that cataract occurs in 30–46% of patients with JIA. Surgery should be performed when the uveitis is quiescent but in young children who are at risk of amblyopia any delay in surgery should be minimised. The perioperative period should be covered with increased steroids. Surgery should include removal of lens, capsules and anterior vitreous; this removes any scaffold for the future development of inflammatory membranes. Intraocular lenses are not recommended at present. Visual rehabilitation postoperatively includes the use of gas-permeable contact lenses (soft contact lenses are inappropriate because of the continued need for topical treatment) or spectacles, with the treatment of any amblyopia. Kanski and Shun-Shin[7] found that 55% of eyes treated in this way achieved a vision of 6/18 or better.

Band keratopathy is a common complication, occurring in 30% of children but it rarely compromises the visual acuity. If it does require treatment this can be approached surgically with removal of the corneal epithelium and application of a chelating agent or ablation with the Excimer laser. Phthisis bulbi occurs in approximately 4% of eyes and may develop secondary to contraction of a cyclitic membrane leading to detachment of the ciliary body and reduced aqueous production.

The visual outcome in JIA is related to the severity of the inflammation at initial ocular examination and to the overall duration of the uveitis.[8] Neither the severity of the arthritis nor the level of the ANA titre is related to the visual outcome. Overall, the uveitis is mild and the outcome good in 25%, in a further 25% the uveitis is severe with the development of complications and a poor visual outcome, and in the remaining 50% the uveitis is moderate, requires prolonged treatment and results in a fair visual outcome. The main causes of a poor visual outcome are secondary glaucoma and amblyopia. Male sex and systemic immunosuppressive therapy (for arthritis) are also poor prognostic factors (personal communication, CJ Edelsten and EM Graham).

## Sarcoidosis

Sarcoidosis is a chronic, systemic, granulomatous condition of unknown aetiology. There are two clinical subsets within paediatric sarcoidosis. Before the age of 5 years, patients show a triad of uveitis, arthritis and skin rash with pulmonary disease in a third. Between the ages of 8 and 15 years, almost all have lung disease and one third have involvement of eye, skin, liver and spleen with arthritis being uncommon. Hoover *et al.*[9] has reviewed paediatric ocular sarcoid; in the 5 years and under age group 80% had anterior uveitis; of these 25% also had a posterior uveitis and 15% a focal choroiditis; no retinal phlebitis was described. The anterior uveitis may be chronic, granulomatous or acute non-granulomatous and is rarely symptomatic in the younger age group. In the 8–15-year age group, approximately one-third have an anterior uveitis.

Diagnosis depends on showing non-caseating granulomata in a biopsy specimen in association with a compatible clinical picture. In children, a skin rash is frequently present and is a convenient site to biopsy. In Hoover's study[9], 14 of 15 skin biopsies were diagnostic. The serum angiotensin-converting enzyme reflects the mass of active granulomata and is elevated in 60–90% of systemic sarcoid. The normal range for children is higher than for adults and this must be taken into consideration when interpreting results.

The treatment of the anterior uveitis is essentially the same as for JIA but intractable cases and those with posterior involvement may need systemic steroids and second-line immunosuppression.

## Tuberculosis

In recent years tuberculosis (TB) has re-emerged as a serious health problem; ophthalmic manifestations are varied and the diagnosis depends on a high index of suspicion. It is rare to see ocular TB in otherwise healthy patients or in those with isolated pulmonary TB, therefore an underlying immunodeficiency state should be considered in all patients with ocular involvement. The intraocular manifestations include a chronic granulomatous anterior uveitis, iris nodules, choroidal granulomata and retinal periphlebitis which may be associated with neovascularisation.[10] The choroidal granulomas are usually few in number but less commonly may be extensive; they range in size from one quarter of a disc to several disc diameters and are most frequently seen at the posterior pole. A definite diagnosis of TB requires identification of the organism, for example, from sputum or a lymph-node biopsy; direct biopsy of ocular material is rarely feasible. Further developments in the use of the polymerase chain reaction (PCR) may enable a diagnosis to be made from an aqueous tap or a vitreous biopsy. Treatment with at least three antituberculous drugs, depending on sensitivities, should be used. Steroids, either topically for anterior uveitis or systemically for posterior uveitis, may be required in addition.

## Congenital syphilis

The incidence of congenital syphilis has increased over the last ten years and in the USA is the highest it has been for thirty years. At birth, the fundus shows a salt-and-pepper chorioretinitis[11] which should be distinguished from mumps, rubella, herpes simplex and varicella. The disease then becomes quiescent and can reactivate later in approximately one-third of cases. Corneal neovascularisation occurs and after a few months the cornea clears leaving unperfused vessels (ghost vessels). These become reperfused when the inflammation recurs and this can be associated with an anterior uveitis. Complications include cataract (the lens may dislocate) and glaucoma – both open- and closed-angle forms can develop. Treatment of congenital syphilis includes systemic penicillin and probenecid; this has little effect on established interstitial keratitis and uveitis and local steroids are also required.

## Fuchs' heterochromic cyclitis

This condition almost always presents before the age of 45 years and in children is rarely diagnosed before the teenage years. It is usually unilateral. The signs include iris heterochromia with stromal atrophy, scattered non-pigmented keratic precipitates, mild anterior uveitis with no posterior synechiae and a few cells in the anterior vitreous. No specific treatment is required for the anterior uveitis but 20% of patients develop open-angle glaucoma requiring treatment; 70% of patients develop cataract.

## Acute anterior uveitis

### Ankylosing spondylitis

Childhood onset of ankylosing spondylitis may be complicated by attacks of acute anterior uveitis as in adult disease. Ansell[12] found uveitis to be present in 27% of her 77 juvenile patients, particularly those with peripheral arthropathy. The uveitis is usually symptomatic and in Kanski and Shun-Shin's series[7] all 46 patients with ankylosing spondylitis had acute anterior uveitis as their initial ocular problem and three then developed severe chronic anterior uveitis which was complicated by the development of cataract. As in adults, there is a strong association with human leukocyte antigen (HLA) B27 (94% in Kanski's group). The majority of patients are boys. In two large series[7,12] the mean age of onset of ankylosing spondylitis was 11.5 years and the uveitis rarely antedated the joint problems. Treatment is similar to that of the anterior uveitis associated with JIA; posterior segment involvement is extremely rare.

### Reiter's disease

The postdysenteric form of this reactive arthritis is recognised to occur in children where three-quarters have the HLA B27 histocompatibility antigen. The enteric form has a sex ratio of 1 : 1 unlike the sexually transmitted form where males predominate. Uveitis (usually acute) occurs in about 30% of cases.

### Leprosy

Conjunctivitis, keratitis, episcleritis, and scleritis are all features of leprosy and are worsened by exposure and corneal hypoaesthesia. Uveitis is common in leprosy and two clinical forms have been described. Acute, granulomatous uveitis occurs with erythema nodosum leprosum and a chronic low-grade form occurs with lepromatous leprosy.

Both types can lead to sight threatening complications and require local steroids and mydriatics in addition to systemic treatment for the leprosy as indicated.

### Kawasaki disease

Kawasaki disease is a systemic inflammatory illness of unknown aetiology. It most frequently affects children under the age of 5 years of all races but particularly the Japanese. The principal signs include a fever lasting five days or more, reddening of palms and soles which become oedematous and desquamate, a polymorphous exanthem, red lips, tongue, oral and pharyngeal mucosa and cervical lymphadenopathy. The above in the main are self-limited, but life-threatening coronary artery aneurysms can occur as a late feature in about 16% of patients. The ocular features of Kawasaki disease include:[13]

- Bilateral, bulbar conjunctival injection in 90% in the acute phase.

- Bilateral, acute non-granulomatous uveitis in 80% one week later.

- Bilateral, superficial keratitis in 20%.

- Vitreous opacification, swollen optic disc, dilated retinal vessels and subretinal haemorrhage are rare complications.

The uveitis is usually mild and self limited lasting two to three weeks. If it is severe, topical steroids may be needed. Whenever the diagnosis is considered an urgent paediatric opinion should be sought. Intravenous gamma-globulin with aspirin early in the course of the disease has been shown to reduce the risk of coronary artery abnormalities.

### Acute viral infections

Mumps, chickenpox and infectious mononucleosis can all be associated with an acute anterior uveitis.

### Tubulointerstitial nephritis and uveitis (TINU)

Acute tubulointerstitial nephritis is an uncommon renal disease that may be idiopathic or may be associated with infection, drug exposure (antibiotics and non-steroidal antiinflammatory agents) and systemic diseases such as systemic lupus erythematosus, Sjögren syndrome and sarcoidosis. The uveitis is commoner in children and females and is usually bilateral, acute and non-granulomatous. It responds well to topical treatment and the visual prognosis is good.

### Intermediate uveitis

Intermediate uveitis is predominantely a disease of young adults but may present in childhood. The usual presentation is with floaters, mild blurring of vision and slight photosensitivity, although the disorder may be asymptomatic in the early stages. There is a wide spectrum of disease severity from mild disease to a severe inflammation. The disorder is characterised by vitreous cells, exudate "snow banking" at the pars plana with variable peripheral periphlebitis and neovascularisation. The anterior chamber reaction is usually mild. Giles[14] reviewed 60 children with pars planitis and found that in over one-third the presentation was acute with red, painful, photophobic eyes, and moderate anterior chamber activity. The features of intermediate uveitis may

be seen in sarcoidosis, Lyme disease, multiple sclerosis, TB, and toxocariasis. Investigations (depending on clinical features) may include a full-blood count, erythrocyte-sedimentation rate (ESR), serum angiotensin-converting enzyme, *Toxocara* enzyme-linked immunosorbent assay (ELISA), chest *x*-ray and Mantoux. Complications can include[15] cystoid macular oedema (50%) (Figure 7.2), cataract (41%), neovascularisation (6.5%), vitreous haemorrhage and traction retinal detachment (8%), and epiretinal membrane formation (35%). Topical steroids and mydriatics are used for anterior uveitis. Periocular or systemic steroids are indicated if there is cystoid macular oedema or vitreous cellular activity causing reduction of vision to less than 6/12. Peripheral retinal cryopexy and second-line immunosuppression may be necessary if systemic steroids fail. Pars plana vitrectomy may be indicated for posterior segment complications. Overall the visual prognosis is fairly good. Malinowski *et al.*[15] found an average final visual acuity of 20/44 after 7½ years' follow-up and this was not significantly different from the presenting vision. They found no difference between the visual results for adults and children.

### Posterior uveitis

Posterior uveitis may have a variety of causes in childhood including toxoplasmosis (70%),

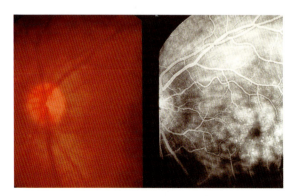

Figure 7.2 Fundus photograph and fluorescein angiogram showing cystoid macular oedema in intermediate uveitis. (Courtesy of Ms L Graham)

toxocariasis (10%), sarcoidosis, bacterial infections (for example, TB, syphilis), viral infections (for example, cytomegalovirus, rubella, herpes simplex, herpes zostor, measles), and fungal infections.[5]

## Toxoplasmosis

Toxoplasmosis is the commonest cause of posterior uveitis in the older child. The causative organism is *Toxoplasma gondii*. The cat is its definitive host and man acquires the infection by ingestion of tissue cysts in meat or oocysts from soil; 80–90% of individuals who acquire the infection are asymptomatic. Chorioretinitis due to toxoplasmosis usually results from a reactivation of a perinatally acquired infection[16] but may also complicate acquired toxoplasmosis.[17]

The typical lesion of active chorioretinitis occurs at the edge of an area of chorioretinal atrophy. It is pale and fluffy and often associated with perivasculitis (Figure 7.3). There is usually a marked vitritis with a granulomatous anterior uveitis. These episodes of activity are self-limited and resolve over weeks to a few months. The diagnosis depends largely on recognising the clinical appearances; the presence of toxoplasma antibodies confirms exposure to the organism. Treatment with pyrimethamine, folinic acid, sulphadiazine and steroids is indicated if the lesion involves the macula or optic nerve, if there is a marked vitritis impairing vision or if the patient is immunocompromised. Clindamycin can be used as an alternative antibiotic. Further reactivation may occur, usually in older children or adults, and complications can include cataract, glaucoma, macular scar or oedema, retinal detachment, optic atrophy, and subretinal neovascular membranes.

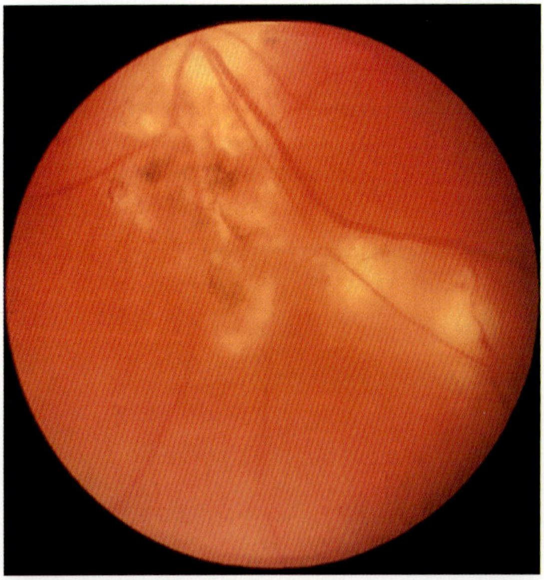

## Toxocariasis

*Toxocara canis* is a common intestinal worm found in dogs. It is acquired by man when the ova of the nematode are ingested. Larvae reach the eye by haematogenous spread. Four patterns of ocular involvement have been described: a chronic destructive endophthalmitis, a loclised posterior pole granuloma in an otherwise quiet eye, a peripheral granuloma with associated vitreous strands, and a variable degree of inflammation and a vitreoretinal abscess (Figure 7.4). Diagnosis is assisted by positive serology; an eosinophilia is rarely present with ocular disease.

Figure 7.3  Fundus photograph of *toxoplasma chorioretinitis* showing an active, pale lesion with indistinct borders adjacent to an area of old, chorioretinal atrophy. (Courtesy of Ms L Graham)

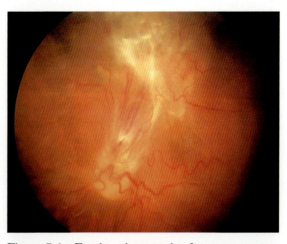

Figure 7.4  Fundus photograph of toxocara granuloma. (Courtesy of Mr MP Snead)

Treatment with local or systemic steroids reduces the inflammation. The use of specific antihelminthic drugs is controversial as there is no clear evidence that they improve the visual outcome and it is possible that death of the worm may incite more inflammation. Vitrectomy may be indicated where visual loss is due to severe vitreous involvement.

## Cytomegalovirus retinitis (CMV)

CMV causes opportunistic infections in immunocompromised hosts. It is a particular problem in the AIDS population. In the paediatric age group, the human immunodeficiency virus (HIV) is acquired congenitally or from contaminated blood or blood products. CMV retinitis is seen in 30% of adults with AIDS but in only 6% of children with AIDS[18]. Symptoms are usually those of floaters unless the CMV retinitis affects central vision. The eye is white with a very mild anterior chamber reaction and only a few cells in the vitreous. The retinitis shows as an area of white, necrotic retina with associated haemorrhage and sheathing of arterioles (Figures 7.5a,b). Diagnosis depends largely on recognition of the clinical signs, but vitreous biopsy with PCR identification of viral DNA may be used in difficult cases. The standard treatment is with intravenous ganciclovir in an induction dose of 5 mg/kg twice daily for two to three weeks then reducing to a once-daily maintenance regime. Neutropenia is the most important side effect. Foscarnet can be used in resistant cases. These drugs are virostatic and not virocidal and so treatment needs to be continued for until an efficient immune system is restored.

# Panuveitis

## Behçet's disease

The International Study Group for Behçet's disease established criteria for its diagnosis in 1990 and these include oral ulceration plus two of the following recurrent genital ulceration, eye lesions, skin lesions, or a positive pathergy test. In a recent report from Italy,[19] of 211 patients with Behçet's disease and ocular involvement a paediatric onset was seen in 7.6%. Uveitis alone or in

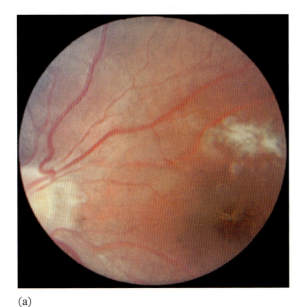

(a)

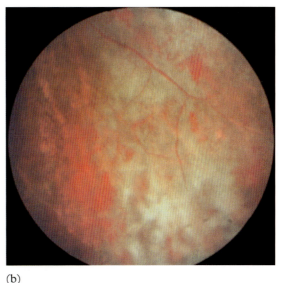

(b)

Figure 7.5  CMV retinitis involving posterior pole (a) and peripheral retina (b) in immunosuppressed child following liver transplantation

combination with other major symptoms was the presenting symptom in two-thirds of the children compared to one-third of adults, 15 of 16 children had a panuveitis and one a posterior uveitis; all had retinal vasculitis at presentation and one-third developed a hypopyon at some stage. Ocular complications (cataract, macular oedema, subretinal neovascularisation and retinal detachment) are more common in children. Treatment, as with adults, involves the use of systemic steroids and second-line immunosuppressants.

## Endogenous endophthalmitis

Endogenous endophthalmitis occurs when infection, either bacterial or fungal, spreads to the eye via the bloodstream from a primary focus elsewhere. Overwhelming bacterial infection such as meningitis (*Neisseria meningitidis* and *Haemophilus influenzae*) or pneumonia (*Streptococcus pneumoniae*) are common pathogens in childhood cases. The risk factors for endogenous candidal endophthalmitis include intravenous catheters, abdominal surgery, broad-spectrum antibiotics, immunosuppressive therapy and intravenous drug use. The clinical presentation is very variable from a mild, localised infection to one that is extensive and severe.[20]

Diagnosis depends on a high index of suspicion and investigations should include blood cultures, urine cultures, culture of other sites as indicated and either aqueous or vitreous tap depending on the site of principal infection. All patients should receive systemic antibiotics. Periocular antibiotics may be of help when the infection is predominantly anterior. Intravitreal antibiotics have revolutionised the treatment of exogenous endophthalmitis but in endogenous endophthalmitis they should be reserved for posterior disease. The prognosis depends on the pathogenicity of the organism, the site of the ocular infection and the delay before treatment is started. The non-ocular focus of infection may not be discovered but meningitis, urinary-tract infection, endocarditis, septic arthritis, and ear and chest infections must be excluded in children.

## Sympathetic ophthalmia

Sympathetic ophthalmia is a bilateral, granulomatous panuveitis that follows a penetrating injury (accidental or surgical) to one eye. The injured eye is the exciting eye and the fellow eye is the sympathising eye. The prevalence is 0.1–0.2% after penetrating trauma; 70% of cases occur within three months of injury and 90% within one year. Onset is usually insidious with slight pain, photophobia, and reduced visual acuity. Examination shows a granulomatous panuveitis with characteristic small, yellow-white lesions at the level of the retinal pigment epithelium (Dalen–Fuchs nodules) in the mid-peripheral fundus. The inflammation can be complicated by cataracts, rubeosis iridis, glaucoma, cystoid macular oedema, and serous retinal detachments. The visual outcome is often poor.

There has been much debate as to whether the injured eye should be removed, either prophylactically or as part of the treatment, once sympathetic ophthalmia has occurred. In general, an eye with the potential for useful vision should not be enucleated, but removal of a blind, severely traumatised eye may aid diagnosis and may have a beneficial effect on the inflammation in the fellow eye if performed early in the course of the disease. Initial treatment consists of high-dose local and systemic steroids. If this fails to control the disease, cyclosporin (a potent inhibitor of T-lymphocyte function) should be added with careful monitoring of blood pressure and renal function; this drug is well tolerated in children. Immunosuppressants, such as azathioprine, may be used if the other agents fail or have to be stopped because of side effects.

## Masquerade syndromes

A number of conditions including retinoblastoma, leukaemia, lymphoma, juvenile xanthogranuloma, retinal detachment, intraocular foreign body and ocular ischaemia may be associated with intraocular inflammation and may need to be excluded in children with atypical forms of uveitis or who show poor response to treatment.

## References

1 Smit RLMJ, Baarsma GS, de Vries J. Classification of 750 consecutive uveitis patients in the Rotterdam Eye Hospital. *Int Ophthalmol* 1993; **17**: 71–5.

2 Tran VT, Auer C, Guex-Crosier Y, *et al*. Epidemiological characteristics of uveitis in Switzerland *Int Ophthalmol* 1995; **18**: 293–8.

3 Tugal-Tutkun I, Havrlikova K, Power WJ, Foster CS. Changing patterns in uveitis of childhood. *Ophthalmology* 1996; **103**(3): 375–83.

4 Perkins ES. Pattern of uveitis in children. *Br J Ophthalmol* 1966; **50**: 169–85.

5 Giles CL. Uveitis in childhood. *Ann Ophthalmol* 1989; **21**: 13–28.

6 Kanski JJ. Uveitis in juvenile chronic arthritis: incidence, clinical features and prognosis. *Eye* 1988; **2**: 641–5.

7 Kanski JJ, Shun-Shin A. Systemic uveitis syndromes in childhood: an analysis of 340 cases. *Ophthalmology* 1984; **91**: 1247–52.

8 Wolf MD, Lichter PR, Ragsdale CG. Prognostic factors in the uveitis of juvenile rheumatoid arthritis. *Ophthalmology* 1987; **94**(10): 1242–8.

9 Hoover DL, Khan JA, Giangiacomo J. Pediatric ocular sarcoidosis. *Surv Ophthalmol* 1986; **30**(4): 215–28.

10 Helm CJ, Holland G. Ocular tuberculosis. *Surv Ophthalmol* 1993; **38**(3): 229–56.

11 Margo CE, Hamed LM. Ocular syphilis. *Surv Ophthalmol* 1992; **37**(3): 203–20.

12 Ansell BM. Juvenile spondylitis and related disorders. In: Moll JMH, ed. *Ankylosing Spondylitis*. Edinburgh: Churchill Livingstone, 1980; 120–36.

13 Ohno S, Miyajima T, Higuchi M, *et al*. Ocular manifestations of Kawasaki disease. *Am J Ophthalmol* 1982; **93**: 713–17.

14 Giles CL. Pediatric intermediate uveitis. *J Ped Ophthalmol Strabismus* 1989; **26**: 136–9.

15 Malinowski SM, Pulido JS, Folk JC. Long term visual outcome and complications associated with pars planitis. *Ophthalmology* 1993; **100**: 818–25.

16 Perkins ES. Ocular toxoplasmosis. *Br J Ophthalmol* 1973; **57**: 1–17.

17 Glasner PD, Silveira C, Kruszon-Moran D, *et al*. An unusually high prevalence of ocular toxoplasmosis in southern Brazil. *Am J Ophthalmol* 1992; **114**: 136–44.

18 de Smet MD, Butler KM, Rubin BI *et al*. The ocular complications of HIV in the pediatric population. Recent advances in uveitis. In: *Proceedings of the 3rd International Symposium on Uveitis*. 1992; 315–19.

19 Pivetti-Pezzi P, Accoriniti M, Abdulaziz MA, *et al*. Behçet's disease in children. *Jpn J Ophthalmol* 1995; **39**: 309–14.

20 Greenwald MJ, Wohl LG, Sell CH. Metastatic bacterial endophthalmitis: a contemporary reappraisal. *Surv Ophthalmol* 1986; **31**(2): 81–101.

# 8  The paediatric glaucomas

PENG T KHAW, ANDREW NARITA, RODOLFO ARMAS, TONY WELLS, MARIA PAPADOPOULOS

Like the adult glaucomas, the paediatric glaucomas are not a single condition but a diverse group of conditions.[1,2] Preservation of a lifetime of vision for these patients is dependent on rapid accurate diagnosis followed by the appropriate treatment. The approach to this group of disorders is different from adults partly because the disorders are different in their behaviour and response to therapy and also because the management of eye disorders in children also differs.[3] There has been a dramatic improvement in the prognosis for these patients, particularly those with very refractory forms, due to changes in the techniques available for treatment.

## Incidence

The paediatric glaucomas are uncommon. A consultant ophthalmologist in the United Kingdom would expect to see only one case every few years. The most common form, primary congenital glaucoma, has an incidence of about 1 in 10 000 live births. The incidence is higher in areas where consanguineous marriages are more common. Despite their relative rarity, the paediatric glaucomas account for 2–15% of individuals in blind institutions for children around the world in both developed and developing countries. The 1994 WHO/World Bank survey estimated that there were 300 000 cases of the paediatric glaucomas worldwide, of whom 200 000 were blind.

## Clinical presentation

The paediatric glaucomas have one thing in common – raised intraocular pressure – and

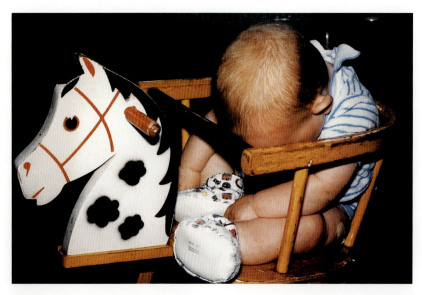

Figure 8.1 Photophobic child with primary congenital glaucoma. (Courtesy of Prof PT Khaw)

affected children usually present with symptoms and signs of raised intraocular pressure. If the pressure is high or has risen rapidly, the symptoms and signs are more dramatic (Figure 8.1). The patients may also present because of associated ocular abnormalities or for screening if they have a family history of childhood glaucoma. The main reason for a delay in diagnosis after first seeking medical advice is failure to think about the possibility of paediatric glaucoma due to its rarity. The differential diagnoses of patients presenting with the possible signs and symptoms of the paediatric glaucomas are detailed in Table 8.1.

## Types of glaucoma

The different types of childhood glaucoma are summarised in Table 8.2. There are many different classifications of childhood glaucoma, mainly because there is still an incomplete understanding of the pathophysiology of many of the variants.[1,2-6] The childhood glaucomas can be primary in which there is a developmental abnormality of the anterior chamber angle, or secondary. In the case of secondary glaucomas, this can be in association with developmental

Table 8.1 Common signs of the paediatric glaucomas: differential diagnosis

Corneal splits
  Birth trauma
  Hydrops
Corneal oedema or opacity
  Birth trauma
  Congenital hereditary endothelial dystrophy
  Metabolic, e.g. mucopolysaccharidoses
  Sclerocornea
  Rubella
  Infections including herpes simplex keratitis
Enlarged cornea
  Axial myopia
  Megalocornea/megalophthalmos
  Osteogenesis imperfecta
  Connective tissue disorder (e.g. fibrillin mutation)
Watering and "red eye"
  Conjunctivitis
  Nasolacrimal duct obstruction
  Corneal epithelial defect, abrasion, very occasionally dystrophy
  Ocular inflammation

Table 8.2 The paediatric glaucomas

Primary glaucoma
  Primary congenital glaucoma/trabeculodysgenesis
  Juvenile-onset open-angle glaucoma
Secondary glaucoma
  Associated with anterior segment dysgenesis
    Trabeculodysgenesis (Axenfeld–Rieger)
    Irido-corneo-trabeculo-dysgenesis (Peters')
    Aniridia
    Iris hypoplasia
    Microphthalmos
    Ectropion uveae
  Associated with ocular disease/treatment
    Following congenital cataract surgery (especially after full lensectomy)
    Persistent hyperplastic vitreous
    Retinopathy of prematurity
    Trauma
      Hyphaema
      Angle recession
  Associated with phakomatoses
    Neurofibromatosis
    Sturge–Weber syndrome
      Port wine stains
      Cutis marmorata telangiectasia congenita
      Klippel–Trenaunay–Weber syndrome
      Oculodermal melanocytosis
      Von Hippel–Lindau
  Associated with metabolic disease
    Lowe syndrome
    Homocystinuria
    Mucopolysaccharidoses, e.g. Hurler syndrome
  Associated with inflammatory/infective disease
    Seronegative arthritis
    Congenital rubella, cytomegalovirus and other infective causes
  Associated with ocular tumours
    Benign, e.g. iris cysts, juvenile xanthogranuloma
    Malignant, e.g. retinoblastoma, leukaemia
  Associated with chromosomal/systemic disorders
    Down syndrome (trisomy 21)
    Patau syndrome (Trisomy D13–15)
    Turner syndrome (XO)
    Rubinstein–Taybi syndrome
    Pierre Robin syndrome
  Associated with connective-tissue abnormality
    Marfan syndrome
    Weill–Marchesani syndrome
    Homocystinuria
    Ehlers–Danlos syndrome
    Sulphite oxidase deficiency

abnormalities of the eye or secondary to obstruction of aqueous outflow due to a variety of causes.

### Primary congenital glaucoma

The commonest form of paediatric glaucoma is primary congenital glaucoma (also called trabeculodysgenesis). In this form of glaucoma, the problem lies in the drainage angle which does not develop normally. There are no other ocular or systemic abnormalities apart from the changes induced by raised intraocular pressure such as buphthalmos. The classic symptoms are due to raised intraocular pressure (Table 8.3) When corneal oedema resolves, most of the symptoms resolve but the patient may be mildly photophobic for life particularly if many corneal splits remain. In milder cases, parents may get constant comments about how beautiful and large their children's eyes are, or asymmetry may be noted (Figure 8.2).

The condition is more usually bilateral, although the intraocular pressure may only be raised in one eye in up to 25% of patients. In the majority of cases of primary congenital glaucoma, there is no family history of glaucoma. The figures from our own unit reveal that the risk for parents who have had one child with primary congenital glaucoma of having another affected child in the absence of a family history is less than 2%. Other authors have suggested that about 10% of cases are hereditary and, in most cases, the condition is autosomal recessive. Mutations on the *CYP1B1* gene on chromosome 2 have been found in a number of affected fami-

Table 8.3   Presentation of the paediatric glaucomas

---

Usually associated with the paediatric glaucomas presenting in the first few years of life:
  Epiphora
  Photophobia
  Blepharospasm
  Enlarged eye (buphthalmos)
  One eye larger than the other
  Corneal clouding/opacification (secondary to pressure or
    associated abnormality)
  Other incidental ocular abnormality
  (Screening due to family history of early-onset familial
    glaucoma or other ocular disease with associated
    glaucoma, e.g. Sturge–Weber)
If these symptoms and signs are minimal, diagnosis may be delayed. This may lead to later diagnosis with presentation due to:
  Reduced vision
  Nystagmus
  Strabismus, particularly divergence
  Rapidly increasing myopia
  Screening at optometrist visit

---

lies with primary congenital glaucoma.[7,8] Most of the children with primary congenital glaucoma respond extremely well to goniotomy.

### Juvenile-onset open-angle glaucoma

"Juvenile glaucoma" is the term that has traditionally been used to describe a group of patients presenting after the age of 3 and before the age of 35 years. Some of these patients may

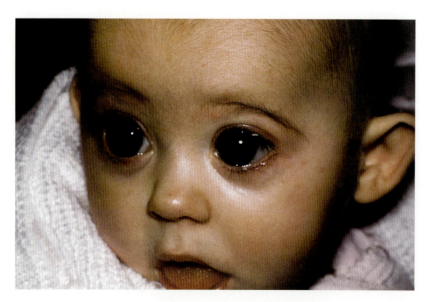

Figure 8.2 Child with bilateral primary congenital glaucoma who presented with eye enlargement, epiphora, and photophobia. (Courtesy of Prof PT Khaw)

be misclassified and have late-onset primary congenital glaucoma or mild variants of the other secondary paediatric glaucomas. There is a subgroup of patients who have juvenile-onset glaucoma associated with a distinctive hypoplastic iris stroma (Figure 8.3): it may be that this group overlaps with the Rieger anomaly patients as linkage has been found in one family to 4q25, a region previously shown to harbour one of the genes associated with Rieger's anomaly.[7,8]

There is also a distinct group of patients who have no anterior segment abnormalities and present in their later childhood years with glaucoma. There is often a family history of glaucoma. Several of these families show mutations at the *GLC1A* locus on chromosome 1q.[8,7] There is a suggestion that these patients do not respond well to medical or laser treatment but do well with drainage surgery. In our experience, these patients do well with trabeculectomy and adjunctive beta-radiation.

## Axenfeld–Rieger anomaly/syndrome

There is some confusion regarding the terminology of these conditions. Axenfeld's anomaly refers to anterior segment abnormalities including iris and angle defects, Rieger anomaly to anterior segment defects with iris and angle abnormalities and Rieger syndrome to ocular changes with systemic abnormalites such as abnormal teeth and facial abnormalities particularly hypertelorism. Due to the wide overlap in features, the term "Axenfeld–Rieger syndrome" (also known as irido-trabeculo-dysgenesis) is now used to encompass the whole spectrum of abnormalities. The spectrum varies from mild involvement with a posterior embryotoxon to the more severe forms with iris involvement including a flat, featureless, hypoplastic appearance, atrophy, polycoria, and ectropion uveae. They are all associated with the formation of a posterior embryotoxon (Figure 8.4) or an abnormal thickening in Schwalbe's line, which may also occur as an isolated abnormality in up to 10% of normal individuals. Axenfeld–Rieger patients usually develop glaucoma later than patients with primary congenital glaucoma but still have to be followed regularly. If there is any doubt, the children have to be examined under anaesthesia to exclude glaucoma as this will develop in up to 50% of cases. The inheritance pattern of this group is usually autosomal dominant. Two loci have been identified, *RIEG 1* at 4q25 and *RIEG2* at 13q14[8].

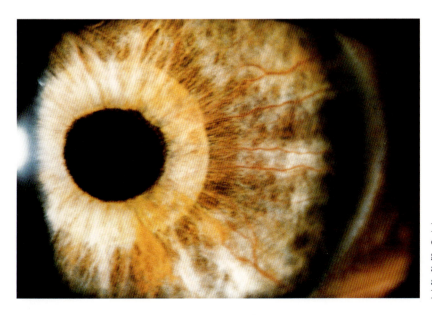

Figure 8.3   Iris hypoplasia in child with juvenile onset glaucoma. Note moth-eaten appearance, prominent vessels and collarette. (Courtesy of Prof PT Khaw)

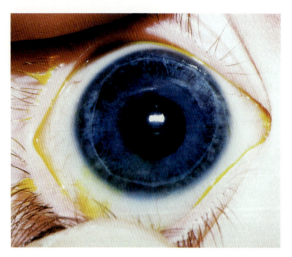

Figure 8.4 Prominent posterior embryotoxon in Axenfeld–Rieger syndrome. (Courtesy of Prof PT Khaw)

## Peters' anomaly

The term "Peters' anomaly" (also known as irido-corneo-trabeculo-dysgenesis) is used when there is a central defect in Desçemet's membrane and corneal endothelium with thinning and opacification of the adjacent corneal stroma. Other iris and anterior segment abnormalities may also be present. The condition is usually bilateral and sporadic. Up to 50% of these patients will develop glaucoma. Corneal grafting is very rarely indicated. Treatment of the glaucoma may often improve the central opacity particularly if intraocular pressure can be reduced to the low teens with antimetabolite-assisted trabeculectomy, and a broad iridectomy may be useful to achieve a clear optical axis.

Goniotomy does not work well in Axenfeld–Rieger syndrome and is usually not possible in Peters' anomaly and in these conditions primary trabeculotomy or trabeculectomy may be more appropriate (Figure 8.5). A significantly abnormal anterior segment is associated with a high risk of surgical failure with any form of surgery.

## Aniridia

Congenital aniridia is an autosomal dominant disorder in which there is abnormal development of the iris; the degree of iris involvement varies from complete aniridia to an intact iris with abnormalities of stromal architecture. Other findings include corneal pannus and neovascularisation, cataract, foveal hypoplasia, nystagmus, and strabismus. Development of glaucoma may be associated with progressive angle anomalies. The incidence of glaucoma is variable and is quoted as occurring in between 50 and 75% of cases. Aniridia is associated with mutations of the PAX6 gene on chromosome 11p13. Although some affected individuals have a family history, many do not and the latter represent new autosomal dominant mutations. Individuals with sporadic aniridia have an increased risk of developing Wilms' tumour due to the fact that they have large deletions of 11p13 which encompass both the PAX6 gene and the adjacent Wilms' tumour locus. In the past, such children would have regular screening for Wilms' tumour but it is now possible to exclude deletion of the Wilms' tumour locus using fluorescent *in situ* hybridisation techniques (FISH).

Glaucoma in patients with aniridia is often very refractory to treatment. Prophylactic goniotomy has been advocated to prevent gradual angle closure and glaucoma as has drainage surgery. However, drainage surgery is difficult and prophylactic measures such as tight

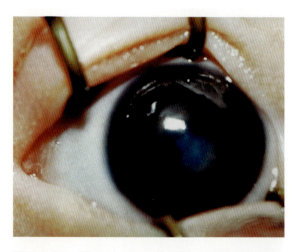

Figure 8.5 Peters' anomaly after trabeculectomy. Opacities may improve spontaneously and with pressure lowering. (Courtesy of Prof PT Khaw)

releasable sutures and the use of viscoelastics should be taken to avoid a postoperative flat anterior chamber which will damage both lens and cornea due to the absence of an iris.

## Aphakic glaucoma

Raised intraocular pressure may complicate surgery for congenital cataract.[9] This may occur in more than a quarter of the patients if the cataracts are operated on within the first few months of life. Occasional cases may be due to pupil block but in the majority of cases the angle is open and the mechanism of glaucoma is presumed to be microscopic blockage of the trabecular meshwork. The incidence of glaucoma where the posterior capsule is spared appears to be much lower than when the capsule is removed. Aphakic glaucoma is difficult to manage. All patients who have had congenital cataracts removed should have their intraocular pressures measured at least yearly in clinic. Generally speaking, if glaucoma develops within the first few years after cataract removal, some form of laser or surgical treatment is likely to be necessary. Diode cycloablation is effective but needs to be repeated and medical treatment almost always needs to be continued. Trabeculectomy with weaker intraoperative antimetabolities such as 5-fluorouracil (5-FU) or beta-radiation has a poor success rate. Adjunctive mitomycin-C increases the success rate but makes contact lens wear risky because of the cystic avascular bleb that results. Therefore the surgical procedure of choice in this unit is drainage tube surgery (which we combine with mitomycin-C) which results in a posteriorly placed thicker bleb which permits subsequent contact lens wear if necessary.[10] Extensive measures should be taken to prevent hypotony in these eyes which have a significantly increased risk of choroidal haemorrhage.

## The phakomatoses (see Chapter 17)

The most common phakomatosis associated with glaucoma is the Sturge–Weber syndrome.

Glaucoma occurs in up to 50% of patients, particularly if both the ophthalmic and maxillary divisions of the trigeminal nerve are affected. All neonates with Sturge–Weber syndrome should have glaucoma excluded. Glaucoma may arise as a result of changes in uveoscleral pressure but there may also be changes in the angle at the macro- and microscopic level. There are two peaks of incidence in this disease. The first peak occurs at about 1–2 years of age with the second peak occurring at around 5–6 years of age. It is the former group that may respond to goniotomy as a primary treatment, as there is often a goniodysgenesis which gives rise to the glaucoma. However, the response rate to goniotomy is inferior to that seen in primary congenital glaucoma. The second peak group tends not to respond to goniotomy and requires primary trabeculectomy. Due to high episcleral venous pressures, choroidal effusions often develop after any form of pressure-lowering surgery. Too sudden a decompression of the globe may give rise to expulsive choroidal haemorrhages. Filtration surgery in these patients must be coupled with extensive measures to minimise any period of hypotony, such as an intraoperative infusion and tight releasable sutures.

The other phakomatoses may be associated with glaucoma although with a lower incidence than Sturge–Weber syndrome. Management depends on the individual patient characteristics, although angle procedures such as goniotomy or trabeculotomy are not usually effective.

## Inflammatory disease (see Chapter 7)

Inflammation as a cause of paediatric glaucoma is rare and may complicate intraocular inflammation from any cause. Juvenile chronic arthritis is the commonest cause of childhood uveitis and patients with this disorder need to be monitored for the development of ocular hypertension and glaucoma. Intraocular inflammation may give rise to glaucoma by a variety of mechanisms including chronic trabecular obstruction,

97

pupil block, and following topical steroid usage. If chronic steroid usage is an essential part of the disease management, then it is best to manage the intraocular pressure as if the steroids were an integral part of the disease, rather than constant changing of the steroid regimen in an attempt to reduce intraocular pressure. Unassisted trabeculectomy does not work well in the inflammatory glaucomas, and Mitomycin-C (MMC) trabeculectomy or tube surgery may be indicated.

### Lens subluxation (see Chapter 9)

A variety of diseases such as Marfan syndrome, Weill–Marchesani syndrome, homocystinuria and high myopia may give rise to paediatric glaucoma which may be due to abnormalities in the trabecular meshwork or a subluxed lens, although as a rule glaucoma in childhood is unusual. Early-onset glaucoma in these conditions is usually associated with lens displacement. A prophylactic iridectomy may sometimes be required.

### Miscellaneous

A wide variety of other conditions are associated with paediatric glaucoma. Many syndromes and congenital malformations are associated with glaucoma. Many of these are rare and there is very little precedent in the literature defining the right treatment for these glaucomas. The best treatment plan is arrived at by a thorough history and examination and devising a plan based on a rational assessment of all the factors. It is important to mention that childhood tumours such as juvenile xanthogranuloma of the iris, leukaemia or retinoblastoma which may give rise to glaucoma by way of obstruction of the outflow tracts from tumour cells or secondary haemorrhage. These rare conditions are important in that the primary disorder must be diagnosed because inadvertent surgery may worsen the prognosis, e.g. in retinoblastoma. The treatment is generally conservative and involves treating the primary disorder.

## Assessing a child with suspected or known glaucoma

There is no substitute for time spent eliciting an accurate history and examination in the clinic (Table 8.1). This usually provides the correct diagnosis in the majority of cases. It is also vital for building the relationship between the ophthalmologist and the patient and his/her parents. It is important at this stage to inquire about age of onset, a family history of childhood onset glaucoma, any associated congenital defects or general problems, and any history of maternal problems during pregnancy including the birth history. A complete general examination may also be important to detect any systemic abnormalities which may be associated with the glaucoma. It is important to work closely with a paediatrician and geneticist who are highly experienced in the assessment, care and counselling of patients with various systemic disorders associated with childhood glaucoma. It is important to develop a teamwork approach to the management of the paediatric glaucomas (Table 8.4).

Observing the child in clinic, it may be possible to assess the relative and actual sizes of both eyes, the presence or absence of corneal oedema and the presence of lacrimation, photophobia, and blepharospasm. If a neonate has recently been fed it may be possible to carry out

Table 8.4  The Moorfields Eye Hospital paediatric glaucoma service team

---

Ophthalmologist (paediatric glaucoma)
Paediatric anaesthetist
Paediatrician (with a special interest in syndromes
   associated with glaucoma)
Geneticist (with a special interest in ocular genetic disease)
Paediatric nurse coordinator (coordinates child and family
   care)
Orthoptist (sees patients pre- and postexamination/refraction and supervises
occlusion therapy)
Optometrist (special skills in assessing vision and refraction
   in children with glaucoma)
Care coordinator for children with visual problems (social
   support, education)
Play supervisor

---

quite a thorough examination including applanation tonometry, particularly if a tonopen is used. In an older child, examination and applanation tonometry on the slit lamp microscope may be possible from the age of 3 years in exceptional cases but in the majority examination under anaesthesia is necessary until about the age of 5 years. Although it is important to get the child used to the concept of the slit lamp, the surgeon must gain the confidence of the child and parents so that the child does not develop a phobia about future examinations. If there is any doubt and there is possible glaucoma, then the child should be examined under general anaesthesia.

It is important to examine the child's parents wherever possible as the presence of subtle signs of anterior segment dysgenesis in the parents, such as an abnormal iris and posterior embryotoxon, may change the genetic advice that the parents receive and may alter the management of subsequent siblings. Families should be referred for genetic counselling if there is any chance of a genetic component, or if there are specific worries in this area.

Following the consultation, it is important to explain at the beginning to parents the nature of the condition, and that their child will probably require life-long follow-up. When explaining the need for an examination under anaesthetic, it should be explained to the parents that surgical intervention such as goniotomy may be required at the same time. At each follow-up anaesthetic a further procedure may be required, as a subsequent rise in intraocular pressure may not be readily detected clinically without an examination under anaesthetic. It is also useful to ask the parents if they are worried about specific issues, as often occur and result in severe anxiety and misconceptions can be addressed. An illustrated booklet explaining in lay terms the nature of the condition and the various treatments is helpful.[11] Other investigations such as ultrasound can be carried out before examination under anaesthesia if indicated to exclude posterior segment pathology, document axial length, and occasionally detect optic disc cupping if it is marked.

## Examination under anaesthesia

Most anaesthetic agents alter the intraocular pressure, and in particular halothane can lower the intraocular pressure substantially (up to 20–30 mmHg). It is important to use a consistent anaesthetic regimen so that the normal range for the chosen anaesthetic regimen can be established. We use ketamine hydrochloride (Ketalar) given intramuscularly at 5–10 mg/kg (usually 7 mg/kg) or intravenously if the child is older and the intramuscular volume is too large. Ketamine can cause a transient rise in intraocular pressure, and readings are then obtained after the child is anaesthetised, which is about 10 min after the injection is given. We convert to full anaesthesia with assisted ventilation if surgery is required. Under anaesthesia, we carry out any general examination that is not possible while the patient is awake, venesection for laboratory investigation, and any other investigations such as keratometry, pachymetry and ultrasound which are indicated.

## Measuring intraocular pressure

Local anaesthetic drops are used before applanation as patients may still be sensitive to corneal applanation. The gold standard for tonometry is the Perkins hand-held tonometer with a blue filter after fluorescein has been instilled in the eye. The tonopen is more expensive but has the advantage of being relatively convenient and requiring only a small area of contact and therefore may be useful if the cornea has a central opacity, e.g. Peters' anomaly or is extensively scarred. The majority of normal eyes have pressures less than 22 mmHg with this regimen, but the readings are taken in context with all the other clinical findings. Corneal thickness needs to be taken into account when measuring intraocular pressure particularly if they are very thick (overread) or thin (underread).

## Cornea/lens

The cornea is examined under magnification for the presence of oedema, opacities and splits

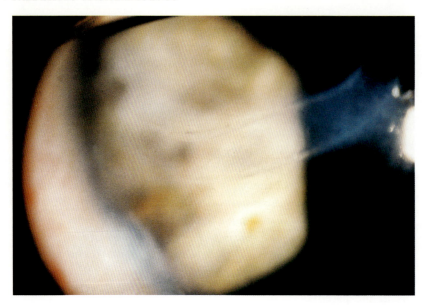

Figure 8.6 Split in Desçemet's membrane (Haab's striae). Together with an enlarged cornea, these are virtually pathognomonic of a raised intraocular pressure in an infant. (Courtesy of Prof PT Khaw)

in Desçemet's membrane which are virtually pathognomonic of glaucoma (Figure 8.6) A portable slit lamp with oblique illumination is useful, otherwise a diagnosis may be missed in more subtle cases. Other causes such as the corneal dystrophies may give rise to symptoms such as lacrimation, photophobia, and blepharospasm. The corneal diameter is then measured along the horizontal meridian with calipers from edge to edge where cornea transparency begins. The normal horizontal paediatric corneal diameter is 10.5 mm increasing by about 1 mm in the first year of life. A diameter greater than 12.5 mm is very suggestive of raised intraocular pressure. This measurement is important not only for diagnosis. If the corneal diameter is increasing, this is an indication of persistently raised intraocular pressure requiring treatment.

Corneal oedema is also a sign that the glaucoma may not be controlled. However, occasionally, corneal oedema may persist for a few weeks after lowering of the intraocular pressure. If the endothelium has been compromised by excessive eye enlargement and pressure damage or multiple operations, pressures in the low teens may be required before the oedema clears and this has implications for the type of surgery indicated.

There may also be associated abnormalities such as the limbal pannus associated with aniridia.

Lens opacities which are associated with irido-corneo-trabecular dysgenesis and other secondary infantile glaucomas may occasionally be present. If they are visually significant, they may require treatment. If cataract extraction in patients with congenital glaucoma is required, it is vital to preserve the posterior capsule if possible as this makes the pressure easier to control. It is very important to check for lens subluxation, particularly if there is the possibility of vitreous prolapse into the anterior chamber. This is seen in severe cases of childhood glaucoma in association with ocular enlargement, also in aniridia, microspherophakia, and Marfan syndrome. A laser or surgical peripheral iridectomy may be required if there is a danger of pupil block. The presence of significant lens subluxation considerably worsens the surgical prognosis and may require extensive surgical intervention such as vitreolensectomy and tube surgery.

## Iris and drainage angle

Examination of the iris, angle and lens may provide clues which are vital in the management

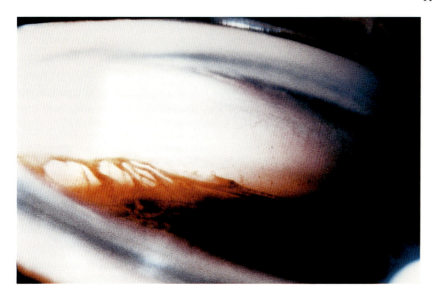

Figure 8.7 Iridocorneal abnormality in angle on gonioscopy. Therefore this child does not have primary congenital glaucoma and will probably not respond well to goniotomy. (Courtesy of Prof PT Khaw)

of the child's glaucoma. Abnormalities of the iris such as an abnormal stroma and pupil such as corectropia, may suggest iridotrabecular dysgenesis rather than simple primary congenital glaucoma. Gonioscopy will confirm the presence or absence of irido-angle abnormalities (Figure 8.7). This is important for management (iridotrabecular dysgenesis responds better to trabeculotomy than goniotomy) and genetic counselling as conditions with iridotrabecular dysgenesis are usually autosomal dominant in contrast with primary congenital glaucoma which is usually sporadic or recessive. The presence of abnormal masses may suggest secondary glaucoma due to malignant or inflammatory conditions. Gonioscopy is not so useful in follow up as there is no obvious correlation of postoperative appearance with pressure control.

**Optic disc and fundus**

The optic disc is one of the most important parameters available to aid the diagnosis and to monitor the progression of visual damage caused by the raised intraocular pressure. Direct ophthalmoscopy can be carried out with a non-dilated pupil, and an indirect ophthalmoscope, particularly one with a small pupil facility, can be very helpful in obtaining a binocular view of the disc. Dilatation of the pupils preoperatively is not recommended as this may alter and mask the angle appearance, may spuriously increase the intraocular pressure, and increase the risk of lens damage if surgery is required. The appearance of the optic disc is carefully recorded with drawings or with photographs if possible, and the horizontal and vertical cup/disc ratios noted. An increase in the size of the cup nearly always indicates that the glaucoma is not controlled and that further treatment is necessary. Conversely, a stable cup/disc ratio with borderline intraocular pressures and stable corneal diameters suggests that a more conservative approach may be appropriate.

The cup/disc ratio is a useful indicator of disease in children even in an outpatient setting. A cup/disc ratio of >0.3 is found in only 2.6% of newborn infant eyes, while a cup/disc ratio greater than 0.3 is found in 68% of eyes with congenital glaucoma. The rest of the fundus should also be examined for any associated abnormalities such as foveal hypoplasia in aniridia.

**Refraction**

After a full examination, the pupils are dilated with cyclopentolate 0.5% and retinoscopy performed. A lens rack with multiple lenses is particularly useful in this context. Buphthalmic eyes are usually myopic, but usually less than the axial length would suggest, due to simultaneous changes reducing the curvature of the cornea. The state of refraction is useful as a prognostic sign with respect to the risk of amblyopia and will indicate the need for occlusion therapy.[12] Rapidly progressing myopia may also suggest that the intraocular pressure is not optimally controlled.

## Treatment

In uncontrolled paediatric glaucoma, we know from historical data that the prognosis is very poor without appropriate treatment. The decision to treat is based on the overall clinical situation, and specifically on the three most important findings, those of corneal enlargement, optic nerve head changes and the intraocular pressure.[5,13] The finding of an enlarged corneal diameter, raised intraocular pressure and a cupped optic disc usually leaves no doubt that immediate treatment is necessary. If the corneal diameter and cup/disc ratio is increasing, it is probably indicated even if the intraocular pressure is borderline or normal. On the other hand, if the intraocular pressure is slightly raised or borderline but there is no change in disc or corneal diameter further, measures need not be introduced immediately. As with all clinical situations, the risks of treatment have to be balanced against the risk of disease damage.

### Medical therapy

The primary treatment of the childhood glaucomas is surgical. However, medical therapy may be useful as a temporising measure if surgical treatment is not possible, before surgical treatment can be undertaken or as an adjunct to maximise intraocular pressure lowering after surgery. Children may run a higher risk of cardiovascular side effects as high blood drug levels may be achieved following topical administration of drops, approaching therapeutic levels after oral administration in adults. Children have smaller blood volumes and immature metabolic systems which may result in a drug half life two to six times longer than in the adult. We advise the parents to use punctal occlusion for 3–5 min after instilling any drops to reduce the chance of systemic toxicity.

### Pilocarpine

One drop of pilocarpine 1% every 6–8 h can be used for temporary treatment before surgical intervention in infants. At this dose, systemic toxicity has not been a problem, although it remains a possibility. The drops are usually stopped the night before surgery to allow the intraocular pressure to return to actual levels for assessment. For longer-term use, it is important to bear in mind that topical pilocarpine may increase the long-term risk of surgical failure.

### Beta-blockers

Topical beta-blockers have also been used with some success in patients with childhood glaucoma, but inevitably this is in patients who have already undergone previous surgery. Topical beta-blockers in the neonates and infants should be avoided because of the risk of systemic side effects. If these drugs are used, we advise punctal occlusion and using a cardioselective agent such as betaxolol may reduce side effects. In older children it is important to inquire about respiratory symptoms of asthma which at this age may present as nocturnal coughing. Parents should be told to report symptoms of respiratory problems and to stop the drops if these become a problem, and return for reassessment.

### Newer topical agents

The recent advent of a topical carbonic anhydrase inhibitor may be useful because of the reduced systemic side effects, and it may replace pilocarpine as our first-line temporising agent, although caution must be used, particularly in a compromised cornea where the endothelial pump may not be working optimally. The role of topical alpha-agonists and the newer prostaglandin analogues is not yet clear but they may be useful adjuncts in the future. Adrenergic agents such as adrenaline or dipivefrine hydrochloride (Propine) are not useful because of the minimal effects on intraocular pressure in addition to beta blockers and the very deleterious effects on the conjunctiva.

### Acetazolamide

Oral acetazolamide has been used by other centres but should be used with caution in neonates and infants. Children on oral carbonic anhydrase inhibitors may have unusual side effects such as bed wetting, disturbed hyperactive behaviour and failure to thrive.

### Surgical therapy

All surgical procedures have advantages and disadvantages and varying indications. The treatment of choice for the different types of glaucoma depends on the age of the patient, the type of glaucoma, associated ocular disease, and the experience of the surgeon. Paediatric surgery differs in several ways, but particularly in that direct trabecular meshwork surgery (goniotomy or trabeculotomy) can be carried out.

#### Angle surgery

**Goniotomy** Goniotomy is the operation of choice where there is primary trabecular meshwork dysgenesis (primary congenital glaucoma) without other anterior segment dysgenesis.[3,13-15] It is an extremely effective operation with over 90% of patients having controlled intraocular pressure at five years postsurgery. Unlike trabeculotomy or trabeculectomy, goniotomy does not damage the conjunctiva; previous conjunctival incisional surgery appears to increase the chance of subsequent failure of trabeculectomy due to scarring. However, goniotomy is a difficult procedure to perform because it requires surgical techniques not commonly used. Although safe in experienced hands, potential complications include lens and corneal damage, inadvertent cyclodialysis and scleral perforation. It cannot be performed safely without an operating microscope and special instruments.

When performing goniotomy, the cornea can usually be cleared by removing the epithelium with alcohol or with a dehydrating agent such as glycerol. A contact lens such as the Barkan is used which allows direct visualisation of the angle. Using a sharp knife such as the Barkan, which is tapered to prevent loss of aqueous from the anterior chamber as the knife is passed into the eye, the angle is incised over about 90–120° and the iris is often seen to gently fall back (Figure 8.8). The knife is then gently withdrawn. The procedure can then be repeated during subsequent examinations with the eye intorted or extorted to treat a new part of the angle. The Q-switched Nd-YAG laser is not useful as a tool for goniotomy.

**Trabeculotomy** Trabeculotomy can, in theory, be used for any condition where a

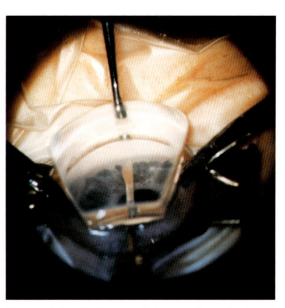

Figure 8.8 Goniotomy being performed viewed through an irrigating Barkan lens. The response to goniotomy in primary congenital glaucoma is extremely good (>90% over five years) and it preserves conjunctiva for future surgery. (Courtesy of Prof PT Khaw).

goniotomy is required. It is particularly useful where a goniotomy cannot be performed due to corneal opacification.[15] It may be more effective in very early onset primary congenital glaucoma and in patients with iridotrabecular and irido-corneo-trabecular dysgenesis (e.g. Axenfeld–Rieger syndrome and Peters' anomaly). Like goniotomy, primary angle-opening procedures are not likely to work if the patients are older (over 4 years). Many surgeons use trabeculotomy as the primary procedure in all patients with primary congenital glaucoma, but we do not do so because of the increased trauma associated with the procedure compared with goniotomy, and the long-term prejudicial effect on future trabeculectomy.

Some authors have suggested that trabeculotomy combined with trabeculectomy may be superior. However, this is a more complex operation and there are theoretical reasons why a working trabeculectomy may result in closure of a trabeculotomy cleft including inadequate flow of aqueous through the trabecular meshwork. Furthermore, combined surgery technically requires the placement of a scleral flap closer to the iris root with an increased risk of iris/ciliary process prolapse and incarceration.

Trabeculotomy has the advantage of being technically possible even if the cornea is opaque. It also involves some surgical techniques and approaches (conjunctival flap, scleral flap) which are more familiar to ophthalmic surgeons than goniotomy. However, despite having some techniques in common with trabeculectomy, the trabeculotomy technique is difficult particularly for the surgeon who only sees the occasional case of congenital glaucoma. The conjunctiva is damaged which prejudices future glaucoma filtration surgery near the area, and it is essentially more traumatic than a goniotomy.

When performing a trabeculotomy an operating microscope is essential as are special trabeculotomes. A trabeculectomy flap is cut and Schlemm's canal is located by gently cutting down in the limbal area. The canal is then cannulated with a trabeculotome and swept into the anterior chamber (Figure 8.9). This is then repeated on the other side of the canal. The canal cannot be found in up to 15% of cases. Hyphaema is usually seen although it usually clears. Complications include tears of Desçemet's membrane, persistent hyphaema and cyclodialysis. We prefer to use the inferotemporal quadrant to spare the superior conjunctiva for any possible future surgery.

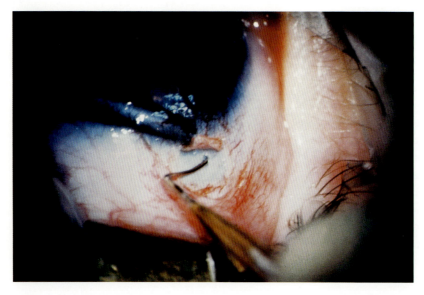

Figure 8.9 Trabeculotomy being performed. Inferotemporal area is used to preserve superior conjunctiva

### Drainage surgery

**Trabeculectomy** Drainage surgery is generally performed if patients have failed goniotomy or trabeculotomy. Trabeculectomy can be a primary procedure in situations where the patient is unlikely to respond sufficiently to goniotomy or trabeculotomy. These include patients older than 4 years of age, and patients who need a very low intraocular pressure (very cupped discs/corneal opacification) which can only be achieved by drainage surgery and strong antiscarring agents. Filtration surgery has the advantage that most general ophthalmologists have experience performing this procedure in adults with glaucoma, and are performing this surgery much more regularly.

If the operating surgeon has no or minimal experience of goniotomy or trabeculotomy and it is not possible to refer the patient to a specialised centre, it would be safer to carry out a trabeculectomy. The disadvantage is that filtration surgery is the most invasive procedure compared to goniotomy and trabeculotomy and probably has the highest complication rate of the three procedures in the hands of surgeons experienced in carrying out all three procedures. It is a more difficult procedure in patients with childhood glaucoma compared with adult glaucoma due to the distorted anatomy. The failure rate of primary surgery appears higher than primary trabeculotomy and goniotomy.[17] There are exceptions in the literature, but patients who do well with primary trabeculectomy would do very well with goniotomy or trabeculotomy.

The surgical technique for trabeculectomy in a child is a modified version of that used in adults. A corneal traction suture (7/0 black silk) is used rather than a superior rectus traction suture (this has to be placed with great care as the coats of the eye are much thinner than normal). A fornix-based flap affords good exposure and reduces surgical trauma to the conjunctiva and episclera. Superiorly positioned flaps are preferred as inferior or interpalpebral blebs carry too high a risk of endophthalmitis. A scleral flap (about $3-4 \times 2-3$ mm) is raised. It is important to know in advance where the true limbus is located as many eyes have conjunctivalisation of the cornea. Transillumination may be helpful. The flap is located so that the sclerostomy is in the corneal area. This reduces the chance of bleeding and iris, ciliary body and vitreous prolapse. Sutures are pre-placed to minimise the period of hypotony which is dangerous in these large eyes. A paracentesis is then made, which has to have a long intracorneal path or leakage will occur in large eyes with thin corneas.

A sclerostomy is then swiftly cut using a scleral punch (Duckworth and Kent, UK), a peripheral iridectomy cut and the flap closed rapidly with between two and five 10/0 nylon sutures depending on what antiscarring agent is used and the conjunctiva is closed. At least one releasable suture is also used which expedites easy removal in the future under anaesthetic not requiring a laser. All patients with childhood glaucoma undergoing glaucoma filtration surgery then receive at least 750 cGy (rads) of beta-radiation postoperatively. If patients are high risk they receive intraoperative mitomycin-C 0.2 or 0.4 mg/ml. Postoperative treatments include antibiotic and steroid eyedrops. We continue steroid eyedrops for at least two months after surgery.

**Antifibrosis treatment** The long-term success rate of patients with childhood glaucoma undergoing glaucoma filtration surgery is reduced compared to adults due to scarring at the site of surgery.[17] The use of postoperative injections of 5-FU has considerably increased the success rate for adult patients who have a high risk of failing glaucoma filtration surgery. However, the regular and frequent injections of 5-FU in the early postoperative period are not a practical proposition in the children with glaucoma. A variety of single application intraoperative regimens can be used for the prevention of postoperative fibrosis, depending on the risk factors (Table 8.5).

**Intraoperative beta-radiation** All children with glaucoma whom we treat with filtration

Table 8.5 Risk factors for trabeculectomy failure in the paediatric glaucomas (even with adjunctive beta-radiation or 5-FU)

- Corneal diameter >14 mm
- Very disordered anterior segment (e.g. Axenfeld–Rieger syndrome with marked iris/angle abnormalities)
- Previous conjunctival surgery (including squint/retinal detachment surgery and trabeculotomy)
- Indian subcontinent origin
- Red eye/persistent ocular inflammation
- Aphakia
- Neovascularisation
- Previous failed trabeculectomy with beta-radiation or 5-FU
- Very early onset disease (at birth or "before")
- Recent previous surgery including laser

surgery for the first time receive adjunctive intra-operative beta-radiation. The use of beta-radiation has considerably increased the success rate of glaucoma filtration surgery in this group since its introduction with virtually no associated complications even in the very long term.[18] A single application of 750 cGy of beta-radiation can inhibit the proliferation of Tenon's capsule fibroblasts for several weeks without resulting in massive cell death.[19] A semicircular strontium-90 probe (Amersham International) is gently placed over the filtration area at the end of surgery and left there for the time required to deliver a surface dose of 750 cGy (rads) of radiation (Figure 8.10).

**Intraoperative topical antimetabolites**

Laboratory studies have shown that mitomycin-C (MMC) has long-term relatively irreversible effects on local Tenon's capsule fibroblasts including widespread cell death with a permanent reduction in cellular number.[20] In adults, we use a titratable regimen of 5-min intraoperative exposures to either 5-FU 50 mg/ml or MMC 0.2 or 0.4 mg/ml is used in an attempt to achieve maximal benefit with a minimum of side effects. Cell culture and adult clinical studies suggest that intraoperative 5-FU is equivalent to the effect of beta-radiation, but intraoperative beta-radiation is preferred in children because of the long record of safety and the more diffuse less cystic blebs compared to 5-FU (Figure 8.11).

MMC 0.4 mg/ml is considered for patients who have failed filtration surgery with previous adjunctive beta-radiation or 5-FU or have a combination of high-risk characteristics (Table 8.5). The 0.4 mg/ml dose is used unless the subconjunctival tissues are thin, or there is a particular worry about hypotony or endophthalmitis, in which case MMC 0.2 mg/ml is used. The resultant blebs were previously thin and avascular with potential for hypotony and endophthalmitis, although the recent conversion to large surface areas of anti-metabolite, large

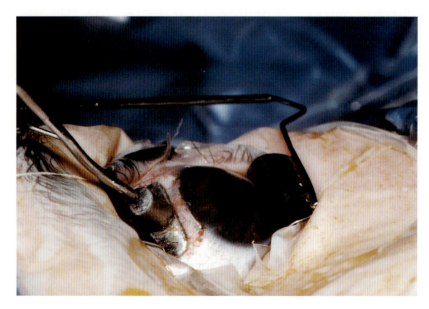

Figure 8.10 Beta-radiation being applied using a strontium-90 probe at the end of the filtration surgery operation. (Courtesy of Prof PT Khaw)

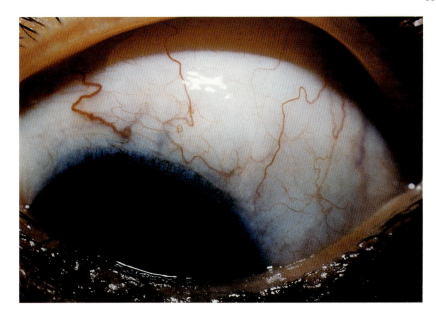

Figure 8.11 Beta-radiation bleb – more diffuse and non-cystic than blebs associated with 5-FU or MMC which are thinner and more cystic. This makes these blebs less prone to complications such as endophthalmitis. (Courtesy of Prof PT Khaw)

scleral flaps and fornix-based conjunctival flaps has changed this considerably.

MMC should not be used unless clearly indicated in paediatric glaucoma as the risks are high both in the short and particularly the long term. The aim of varying concentrations is to minimise side effects while gaining from the convenient single-dose antiscarring effect. Controlling the area of treatment may also have similar effects. It is important that these antimetabolites are delivered appropriately and we use a special clamp (John Weiss, UK) to protect the conjunctival edge (Figure 8.12).

**Postoperative antimetabolites** Subconjunctival injections of 5-FU can be given while the patient is under anaesthesia for examination. If intraoperative antiscarring treatment is used,

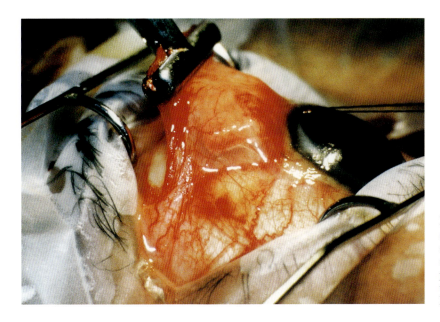

Figure 8.12 MMC being applied on sponge between conjunctiva and sclera. Note special conjunctival clamp to protect cut edge of conjunctiva. (Courtesy of Prof PT Khaw)

this may prolong the period in which postoperative subconjunctival injections of 5-FU may be useful up to several months. Usually 0.1–0.2 ml of 5-FU 50 mg/ml is given adjacent to the bleb, but not into the bleb, because of the danger of intraocular entry; 5-FU has a pH of 9.0 (Figure 8.13). Sometimes this is combined with healon–GV™ to prevent tear film leakage and prolong the drug delivery.

### Tube drainage devices

Drainage tubes have been used with some success in paediatric glaucoma.[10] However, specific precautions need to be taken as there are complications associated with these procedures including hypotony, choroidal effusions, and haemorrhages, particularly in patients with large eyes and reduced scleral rigidity. Trabeculectomy with MMC has now replaced tubes in many situations. However, tubes are useful in aphakic eyes that have developed glaucoma following congenital cataract surgery, and in eyes that have failed MMC trabeculectomy. The success rate of trabeculectomy with 5-FU or even MMC is much lower than phakic eyes. Furthermore, a working MMC-enhanced trabeculectomy in an aphakic eye is usually avascular and cystic, increasing the chance of endophthalmitis which will proceed straight through to the vitreous cavity unchecked.

This type of bleb rules out contact lens wear. The bleb in an eye with a tube in position is far less avascular even when MMC is used (Figure 8.14).

If a tube is to be used without antiscarring agents, a large surface area plate is required (i.e. a two-plate rather than single-plate Molteno implant). Measures should be taken to avoid prolonged hypotony such as a tubal occlusive suture (6/0 Vicryl) which can be combined with an intraluminal 3/0 Supramid suture particularly if adjunctive MMC is used. If MMC is used, the sclera is protected because of the larger sponge used and the risk of intraocular toxicity. Tube surgery in aphakic eyes should be combined with vitrectomy to prevent tube blockage and 20% $C_3F_8$ (after clearing anaesthetic nitrous oxide from the circulation) left in to prevent choroidal detachment and haemorrhage in these high-risk eyes. As large buphthalmic eyes and aphakic eyes have an increased chance of hypotony associated complications, a continuous intraoperative infusion through an anterior chamber paracentesis is used.

**Cyclodestruction** Cyclocryotherapy has previously been used in the management of paediatric glaucoma. However, cyclocryotherapy is associated with complications, particularly

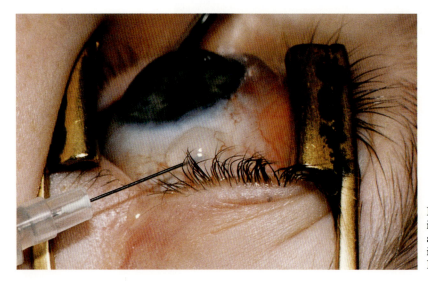

Figure 8.13 Subconjunctival injection of 5-FU being applied adjacent to but not into the bleb. (Courtesy of Prof PT Khaw)

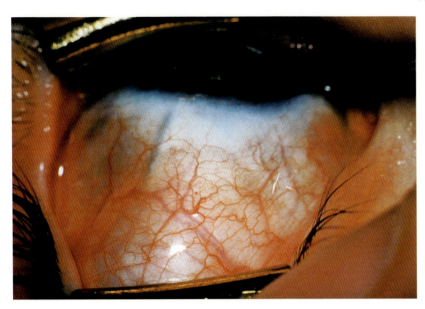

Figure 8.14 Bleb following Molteno drainage tube and plate insertion with adjunctive MMC 0.5 mg/ml. Note relatively vascular conjunctiva compared with limbal MMC bleb. (Courtesy of Prof PT Khaw)

significant postoperative discomfort, inflammation, and phthisis. Cyclodestructive procedures are reserved for eyes with poor visual prognoses, where any form of drainage surgery may carry a high risk, e.g. large aphakic eyes or where drainage surgery is technically not possible (e.g. severely scarred conjunctiva). Cyclocryotherapy and Nd-YAG cyclodestruction have been replaced with the use of the contact diode laser cyclophotocoagulation. In using the diode laser, it is important to transilluminate the eye to ensure accurate placement of the laser burns on the ciliary body, as the normal anatomical landmarks are often distorted. The probe is then placed over the eye in the appropriate position. Using the iris medical laser with a G-probe, a dose of approximately 1500 to 2500 mW for 1500 to 2500 mS delivering forty burns over 360° sparing the 3 and 9 o'clock areas is given. This regimen is based on uptake in enucleated eyes and appears to achieve a similar pressure lowering to cyclocryotherapy but continued medical therapy and further top-up treatment are usually required.

## Long-term follow-up

After a surgical procedure the patient is examined again under anaesthesia about one to three weeks later, and then at increasing intervals after that if progress is satisfactory. This follow-up is increasingly important because of the procedures that can now be carried out. If the pressure is rising after trabeculectomy, releasable sutures can be pulled or cut, needlings of the bleb area can be performed, and subconjunctival 5-FU can be given. Parents are told to return if they notice worsening symptoms such as photophobia or blepharospasm, or signs such as an increase in corneal oedema or diameter.

As children get older, they should be introduced to the concept of slit-lamp examination and tonometry without unduly stressing or frightening them for further visits. Usually, the majority of children can be examined at the slit lamp by the time they are 5 years old, although some may require examination under anaesthesia for a longer period. Conversely, some children may allow a complete examination from as early as 3 years of age.

Patients need life-long follow-up as they continue to relapse for several decades after the primary treatment, and this must be stressed to the parents. If patients are likely to have significantly impaired acuity in the longer term, it is important that arrangements are made for the early assessment of any special schooling requirements. In the UK, registration as blind or partially sighted with statementing alerts the appropriate authorities and mechanisms.

## Amblyopia, refractive correction and occlusion therapy

Amblyopia is a significant complication of paediatric glaucoma and is important as a cause of poor vision in these patients.[12] Vision can be significantly improved in patients with childhood glaucoma if a regimen of occlusion of the better eye is commenced. The patients are assessed by an orthoptist. Findings which suggest the need for occlusion therapy include visual acuity not equal in both eyes, strabismus (vision is almost always worse in the squinting eye) and anisometropia on refraction of more than 1 dioptre. The amblyopic eye is usually the most ametropic. Correction of any refractive error is carried out as soon as is practically possible. The orthoptist plays a critical role as part of the team in managing these patients. It is essential to have accurate estimates of visual acuity in these children and to tailor the occlusion regime to the individual patient taking into account the depth of amblyopia and the age of the child (Figure 8.15).

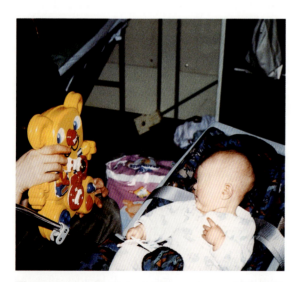

Fiureg 8.15 Occlusion therapy in a child with unilateral primary congenital glaucoma. (Courtesy of Prof PT Khaw)

## References

1 Shaffer RN, Weiss DI. *The Congenital and Pediatric Glaucomas*. St Louis: CV Mosby, 1970.
2 Kwitko ML. *Glaucoma in Infants and Children*. New York: Appleton-Century-Crofts, 1973.
3 Rice NSCR. Management of infantile glaucoma. *Br J Ophthalmol* 1972; **56**: 294–8.
4 Hoskins H, Hetherington J, Shaffer R, Welling A. Developmental glaucomas: diagnosis and classification. In: *Symposium on Glaucoma. Transactions of New Orleans Academy of Ophthalmology*. CV Mosby: St Louis, 1975: 194–7.
5 DeLuise VP, Anderson DR. Primary infantile glaucoma (congenital glaucoma). *Surv Ophthalmol* 1983; **28**: 1–19.
6 Khaw PT, Rice NCS, Baez KA. The congenital glaucomas. In: El Sayyad F, ed. *The Refractory Glaucomas*. Dallas: Igaku-Shoin Medical Publishers, 1995: 1–21.
7 Sarfarazi M. Recent advances in molecular genetics of glaucomas. *Hum Mol Genet* 1997; **6**: 1667–77.
8 Friedman JS, Walter MA. Glaucoma genetics; present and future. *Clin Genet* 1999; **55**: 71–9.
9 Asrami SG, Wilensky JT. Glaucoma after congenital cataract surgery. *Ophthalmology* 1995; **102**: 863–7.
10 Netland PA, Walton DS. Glaucoma drainage implants in paediatric patients. *Ophthal Surg* 1993; **24**: 723–9.
11 The childhood glaucomas: a guide for parents. 2000. Available from childrens ward, Moorfields Eye Hospital or on http//www.moorfields.org.uk.
12 Clothier CM, Rice, NS, Dobinson P, Wakefield R. Amblyopia in congenital glaucoma. *Trans Ophthalmol Soc UK* 1979; **99**: 427–31.
13 Morin JD. Congenital glaucoma. *Trans Am Ophthalmol Soc* 1980; **78**: 123.
14 Khaw PT. What is the best primary surgical treatment for the infantile glaucomas? *Br J Ophthalmol* 1996; **80**: 495–6.
15 Richardson KT, Ferguson WJJ, Shaffer RN. Long term functional results in infantile glaucoma. *Trans Am Acad Ophthalmol* 1967; **71**: 833–6.
16 Fulcher T, Chan J, Lanigan B, *et al*. Long term follow-up of primary trabeculectomy for infantile glaucoma. *Br J Ophthalmol* 1996; **50**: 499–502.
17 Beauchamp GR, Parks MM. Filtering surgery in children; barriers to success. *Ophthalmology* 1979; **86**: 170–80.
18 Miller MH, Rice NSC. Trabeculectomy combined with beta irradiation for congenital glaucoma. *Br J Ophthalmol* 1991; **75**: 584–90.
19 Constable PH, Crowston JG, Occleston NL, *et al*. Long term growth arrest of human Tenon's fibroblasts following single application of beta radiation. *Br J Ophthalmol* 1998; **82**: 448–52.
20 Cordeiro MF, Occleston NK, Khaw PT. New concepts: manipulation of the wound-healing response. *Dev Ophthalmol* 1997; **28**: 242–60.

# 9 Disorders of the lens

ISABELLE M RUSSELL-EGGITT

Congenital cataracts occur in about 3 in 10 000 live births; there are about 250 new cases per year in the UK and about two-thirds are bilateral. Congenital cataract is the most common treatable cause of childhood visual impairment and despite advances in surgical techniques, the visual results are often unsatisfactory due to the presence of stimulus deprivation amblyopia. The single most important factor determining the visual prognosis is the age at which cataracts are first detected and treatment started. In most cases, the lens opacities are present at birth and it is important that all neonates are examined with an ophthalmoscope at the discharge examination so that any abnormalities of the red reflex that may indicate opacities of the lens are detected. The prompt identification of congenital cataract and referral to a paediatric ophthalmologist will have major impact on the long-term visual prognosis.

## Aetiology

Congenital cataract may occur as an isolated ocular abnormality, may be associated with another developmental abnormality of the eye (most commonly microphthalmos), or may occur as part of a systemic disorder or syndrome. Most unilateral cataracts occur as an isolated abnormality in an otherwise normal child but some are seen in association with persistent hyperplastic primary vitreous (PHPV) (see Chapter 10) or posterior lenticonus. Bilateral congenital cataract may result from genetic mutations (most commonly autosomal dominant) or may be associated with a variety of disorders including chromosomal abnormalities, intrauterine infection, metabolic syndromes and genetically determined systemic disorders (Table 9.1). In about 40% of cases the underlying cause is not identified.

## Inherited congenital cataract

Most genetic forms of cataract are inherited as an autosomal dominant trait but rare autosomal

Table 9.1 Aetiology of bilateral congenital cataract

| |
| --- |
| Idiopathic |
| Congenital infection |
|   Rubella |
|   Varicella |
|   Toxoplasmosis |
| Inherited |
|   Autosomal dominant |
|   X-linked recessive |
|   Autosomal recessive |
| Chromosomal disorders |
|   Trisomy 21 |
|   Trisomy 13 |
| Metabolic disease |
|   Hypocalcaemia |
|   Galactosaemia |
|   Hypoglycaemia |
|   Hereditary hyperferritinaemia |
|   Peroxisomal disorders |
|   Mitochondrial disorders |
| Systemic syndromes |
|   Lowe syndrome |
|   Nance–Horan syndrome |
|   Hallerman–Streiff syndrome |
|   COFS syndrome |
|   Cockayne syndrome |
| Other ocular disorders |
|   Aniridia |
|   Microphthalmos |

recessive and X-linked recessive dominant forms are seen. In autosomal dominant congenital cataract (ADCC), a wide variety of phenotypes are seen (Figures 9.1a,b–9.3a,b). Most are partial rather than complete at birth but may progress in later childhood. The phenotypes can be broadly divided into those affecting the anterior (Figure 9.1) or posterior pole of the lens, those affecting the nucleus and those affecting one lamella of the lens including the cortex (Figure 9.3). In general, the phenotype is consistent within families but can vary in severity. In one large study[1] of ADCC, eight different phenotypes could be distinguished (Table 9.2) and many of the underlying genetic mutations have now been identified[2].

## Syndromes associated with congenital cataract

There are a large number of syndromes associated with childhood cataract.[3–5] This chapter

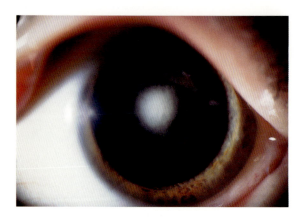

Figure 9.2    Nuclear cataract

will consider some of those associated with infantile onset. Syndromes associated with congenital cataract are usually, but not always, inherited. Cataract may also complicate chromosomal disorders.

- The commonest syndrome associated with childhood onset of cataract is *trisomy 21 (Down syndrome)*. The cataracts are usually symmetrical and are frequently dense and pearly white at birth, but may develop later in childhood. It has been suggested that the lens opacity in Down syndrome is due to increased free-radical production in the lens as the gene for Cu/Zn superoxide dismutase (which produces hydroxyl ions) which is expressed in lens is encoded on chromosome 21. Other chromosomal disorders, for example trisomy 13 (Patau syndrome) may also have associated cataract but the diagnosis is usually apparent from other dysmorphic features.

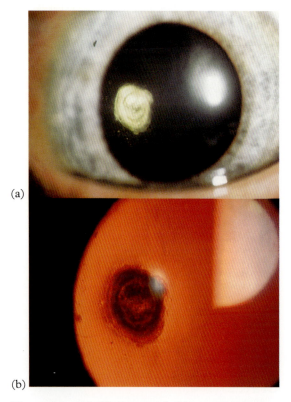

(a)

(b)

Figure 9.1    (a) Slit-lamp and (b) retroillumination view of anterior polar cataract

Table 9.2    Phenotype classification of autosomal dominant congenital cataract[4]

| |
| --- |
| Anterior polar |
| Posterior polar |
| Cortical |
| Nuclear |
| Lamellar |
| Cerulean ("blue dot") |
| Coralliform |
| Pulverulent |

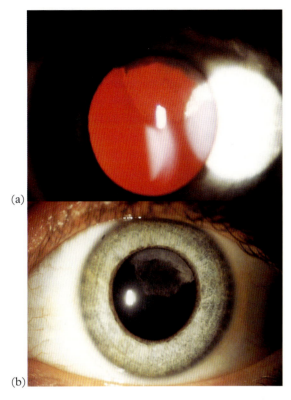

Figure 9.3 (a) Slit-lamp and (b) retroillumination view of cortical cataract affecting superior cortex

- One of the commonest causes of X-linked cataract is the *Nance–Horan syndrome*. In this disorder, affected males have cataract, abnormal dentition and a characteristic facies with prominent ears. The congenital cataract is dense and often associated with mild microphthalmos. The iris is also abnormal and tends to become adherent to operative incision sites. Female carriers may show mild tadpole-shaped sutural lens opacities and abnormal teeth.

- In *Lowe syndrome*, another X-linked disorder, cataracts are associated with hypotonia, variable developmental delay, aminoaciduria and a characteristic facial appearance that is evident in later childhood. Congenital dense nuclear cataract is an almost invariable feature in affected males and other ocular features may include microphakia, posterior lenticonus, congenital glaucoma, and blue sclerae.

Even optimally managed cases may develop nystagmus and only achieve moderate acuity levels. The diagnosis may be missed in early infancy as aminoaciduria may be intermittent. Carrier females may have multiple dot lens opacities (Figure 9.4a,b).

- *Hallerman–Streiff syndrome* appears to occur sporadically in a child with normal intellect in 85% of cases. There is a typical facial appearance with frontal prominence, small chin and a thin pointed nose which develops thin-veined skin and a progeric appearance. Cataracts

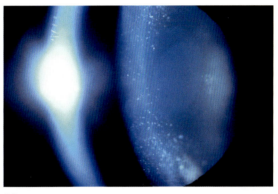

(a)

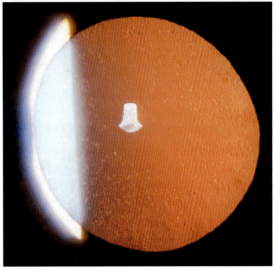

(b)

Figure 9.4 Slit-lamp (a) and retroillumination view (b) of carrier of Lowe syndrome showing multiple punctate lens opacities

113

occur in infancy in about 85% with the majority of eyes being mildly microphthalmic.

- *Conradi–Hunermann syndrome* (chondrodysplasia punctata) is a genetically heterogeneous disorder in which there is asymmetric bone shortening with characteristic punctate calcification of the epiphyses on *x* ray. There are patchy skin changes, alopecia, and congenital cataracts often with microspherophakia. Optic atrophy may develop later.

- If an infant with cataract fails to thrive, particularly if there is jaundice, a diagnosis of *galactosaemia* should be considered. Galactosaemia is caused by a mutation within the gene encoding galactose-1-phosphate uridyl transferase which results in impaired galactose utilisation and manifests as severe failure to thrive in infancy with hypotonia, hepatosplenomegaly, and jaundice. Inheritance is autosomal recessive. Increased formation of the polar alcohol galactitol from galactose has a hyperosmotic effect, leading to lens fibre swelling. The earliest lens change is the "oil droplet" appearance of the red reflex due to refractive changes in the lens nucleus. This is reversible with dietary control, but otherwise progresses to cataract. Swollen lens fibres rupture, appearing as lens vacuoles, before opacities develop. In affected infants lens clarity should be monitored together with metabolic control.

## Investigation in infantile cataract

All infants with bilateral congenital cataracts should be referred to a paediatrician or clinical dysmorphologist. Systemic examination including measurement of head circumference (severe microcephaly in Cockayne syndrome) and appropriate investigations such as estimation of 7-dehydrocholesterol in cases with 2/3 syndactyly (Smith–Lemli–Opitz syndrome) and assessment of muscle tone (poor in Down syndrome) should enable most syndromic forms of cataract to be identified. When this fails to suggest a diagnosis, a TORCH (TOxoplasm, Rubella, Cytomegalovirus, Herpes viruses) screen (to rule out intrauterine infection), urinary amino acids or, more specifically, estimation of renal tubular protein excretion (to exclude Lowe syndrome) and urinary reducing sugars (to exclude galactosaemia) should be performed. It is also important to examine the parents and siblings on the slit-lamp to exclude inherited forms of cataract. Dominantly inherited cataract may show a wide range of clinical expression and some affected individuals may have minor lens opacities that are asymptomatic.[1] Similarly, female carriers of Lowe syndrome and the Nance–Horan syndrome may have classical lens opacities which do not give rise to symptoms. In eyes which are anatomically abnormal, ultrasound examination is helpful in assessing the state of the posterior segment and electrodiagnostic studies are helpful in conditions such as the peroxisomal disorders and Cockayne syndrome where there may be an associated retinal dystrophy.

## Childhood-onset cataract

Some infantile cataracts are partial and do not give rise to visual problems until later childhood. For example, many of the dominantly inherited forms of cataract are mild in infancy but progress in later childhood as do some cataracts in children with Down syndrome. Surgery then becomes necessary in later childhood. Some forms of inherited cataract, for example the cerulean or "blue dot" cataract (Figure 9.5) do not appear until the teens or early adult life. Galactotinase deficiency, posterior lenticonus and the rare cardiomyopathy-cataract and hyperferritinaemia-cataract syndromes should be considered in developmental cataracts. Other forms of childhood cataract, for example those associated with trauma or inflammatory eye disease (see Chapter 7) and those caused by prolonged treatment with systemic steroids or secondary to radiotherapy, occur for the first time in later childhood. Similarly, posterior

114

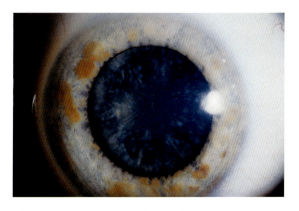

Figure 9.5  Cerulean ("blue dot") cataract

subcapsular lens opacities complicate many of the forms of early-onset retinal dystrophies. Childhood-onset cataract usually causes fewer problems with diagnosis and management and the visual prognosis is better.

## Management

### Bilateral cataracts

A priority is to ascertain the cause of the cataracts. For example, if an infant has Down syndrome or rubella embryopathy, there may be an underlying heart defect which should be investigated before a general anaesthetic is given. Once a diagnosis is made, the ophthalmologist must decide whether early surgery is appropriate or whether initial conservative management is more appropriate. Such a decision is rarely problematic in older children who can cooperate with standard visual acuity testing but may be very difficult in infants with congenital cataract.

Complete bilateral congenital cataract in an infant requires early surgery. In infants born with partial cataracts, surgery is not always indicated and the decision whether or not to operate has to be mainly based on an assessment of the morphology of the lens opacity. Lamellar, mild anterior or posterior and multiple dot lens opacities have a good visual prognosis if surgery is postponed until the child is older. If there is a family history, comparison with other relatives

may be helpful but is of limited value if there is a wide range of phenotypic expression in the family. Dense partial cataracts will need early surgery but in lesser degrees of opacity, it is better to defer surgery and monitor the lens opacities and visual function, intervening in later childhood if vision deteriorates. If nystagmus is already present, then the optimal time for surgery may have already have been missed. In some children with partial cataract there may be associated high refractive error which requires correction with spectacles. If the degree of opacity varies between the two eyes, occlusion therapy may be necessary to prevent amblyopia.

If surgery is undertaken, the majority of ophthalmologists would advise lensectomy without lens implantation in the child under the age of one year. However, in carefully selected eyes early lens implantation is now being investigated in major centres. Aphakia is usually corrected with contact lenses. At surgery, it is important to examine the eye and record the corneal diameters, any anterior segment anomalies, the type of lens opacity, and the intraocular pressure. It is important to exclude any conjunctivitis or lacrimal sac infection; if present, surgery is postponed until they have been adequately treated. Most surgeons use a peripheral corneal approach and perform a lensectomy and anterior vitrectomy in infant eyes. If preserved, the posterior capsule invariably opacifies quickly in infants and may hinder accurate refraction and cause amblyopia.

One method of lens extraction is to place a small self-retaining infusion before a can-opener capsulotomy or capsulorhexis is performed via a separate incision which is then enlarged to 20 gauge to allow aspiration of the lens and followed by a primary posterior capsulotomy and anterior vitrectomy. In cases of persistent hyperplastic primary vitreous (PHPV) the vessels may bleed so that intraocular cautery may be helpful. It is also used if an iridectomy is required as the infant iris is often very vascular. The incisions are then closed with a single fine suture such as 10/0 Vicryl.

In children over the age of one year, intraocular lens implantation, particularly in asymmetrical or uniocular cases, is becoming more common.[6] The anterior capsule is more elastic the younger the child, and with no formed nucleus, an anterior capsulorhexis is difficult to perform. To perform a manual capsulorhexis it is essential to put the capsule under tension with instillation of a viscoelastic substance in the anterior chamber. Mechanical capsulotomy with a diathermy, radiowave or even a standard vitrector can form a round opening, but with slightly less strength than a perfect manual capsulorhexis. It is important to place the implant within the capsular bag to avoid pupil capture, lens decentration, or tilt. Heparin coating reduces postoperative inflammation. Heparin can also be added to the balanced salt solution infusion and adrenaline helps to maintain pupil dilation. The infant pupil, in particular in small eyes with anterior segment malformation or in cases of the Cockayne, Lowe and Marfan syndromes, may have hypoplasia of the iris dilator muscle and may be difficult to dilate. In such cases, as in the bound-down pupils of uveitis and trauma, self-retaining iris hooks are helpful. Anterior chamber injection of TPA (recombinant tissue plasminogen activator) a few days after primary surgery may play a role in treating fibrinous uveitis post surgery, but carries the risk of intraocular haemorrhage.

Posterior capsule opacification is still problematic in children following lens implantation. The incidence may be reduced by primary posterior capsulotomy or preferably posterior capsulorhexis accompanied by anterior vitrectomy in infants (as the vitreous face acts as a scaffold for lens fibres). Placing the implant optic through the posterior capsulotomy may retard opacification of the vitreous face.

Children undergoing intraocular lens implantation should undergo preoperative or intraoperative biometry to allow an informed choice of implant power. Since there is a myopic shift in refraction following lens implantation in children, most surgeons plan to leave eyes initially moderately hypermetropic and correct the immediate residual refractive error with bifocal glasses or contact lenses.

In dense bilateral congenital cataracts, it is important that dense cataract is not only removed by six weeks of age, but that refractive correction is provided quickly. Spectacles can be effective, but may be difficult to make and fit especially if of high prescription and may not be worn well in young infants. Aphakic glasses have the advantage of acting as a low visual aid with the magnification factor due to the hypermetropic correction being in front of the focal point of the eye. The aniseikonia produced by this effect makes spectacles of limited use in unilateral aphakia. Contact lens wear may rarely be complicated by serious infection and is expensive, but in the developed world is usually the preferred option for aphakic infants.[7,8] Risks are low with daily wear and careful supervision and training of the family. Intraocular lenses are not generally used under one year of age and then generally only at the primary operation and are placed in the capsular bag. An enhanced inflammatory response is dampened by heparin coating of the lens and topical steroids postoperatively. There is an unpredictable myopic shift in refraction with increasing age.

Amblyopia is of prime importance. Acuity, compliance with occlusion therapy, fixation preference, strabismus, clarity of the visual axis, and refraction should be regularly assessed. Examination should include corneal clarity and size, intraocular pressure, retinal and optic disc appearance at least every four months and the angle appearance noted if a general anaesthetic is required. Aphakic glaucoma may occur as a result of associated angle anomaly, early pupil block due to retained lens matter or inadequate anterior vitrectomy or it may be a delayed "open-angle" form. The latter is particularly difficult to manage (see Chapter 8).

**Unilateral cataract**

If dense unilateral congenital cataract is detected after 16 weeks of age, then amblyopia cannot be reversed and surgical treatment is inadvisable. If the cataract is detected before eight weeks then good acuity can be achieved in many cases with prompt surgical treatment, optical rehabilitation and intensive occlusion.[9-11] The parents need to be informed that the amblyopia treatment will involve occlusion of the phakic eye for at least half the waking hours for the next five years.[12] This is not without risk to the phakic eye as mild loss of acuity, particularly contrast sensitivity, may occur. Strabismus is common even with early treatment. Glaucoma may be a late complication in up to 50% of these eyes. Results are poor if there are associated ocular anomalies such as moderate microphthalmos (a corneal diameter > 1 mm less than the fellow eye).

## Lens subluxation

Lens subluxation (displacement of the lens within the pupillary space), except when traumatic, is almost always bilateral, but often asymmetrical in children. This displacement may progress to dislocation of the lens into the anterior or posterior segment. Lens subluxation is generally due to a weakness or defect in the zonule which may result from a number of different causes including:

- congenital absence of a portion of the zonule (for example, in colobomatous defects);

- an abnormality of the structure of the fibres of the zonule (for example, in Marfan syndrome); or

- zonule stretching in an abnormally large anterior segment or with an abnormally small lens or in association with trauma to a previously normal eye.

### Aetiology

In most children with lens subluxation, there is an underlying weakness of the zonule which is genetically determined but in some cases there may be local ocular factors that are responsible (Table 9.3).

Table 9.3   Lens subluxation in children

Genetic disorders
  Simple ectopia lentis*
  Ectopia lentis et pupillae**
  Marfan syndrome*
  Homocystinuria**
  Sulphite oxidase deficiency**
  Hyperlysinaemia**
  Weill–Marchesani syndrome**
  Ehlers-Danlos syndrome (heterogeneous)

Trauma
  Ocular abnormalities
  Bupthalmos
  Megalocornea
  Aniridia
  High myopia

*Autosomal dominant
**Autosomal recessive

### Marfan syndrome

Marfan syndrome is one of the commonest causes of ectopia lentis in childhood. It is a dominantly inherited disorder caused by mutations of the type 1 fibrillin gene encoded on chromosome 15. The incidence is about 1 per 10 000 live births. Lens subluxation occurs in about two-thirds of eyes. Lenses may rarely be congenitally dislocated into the vitreous, but more usually progressively sublux during childhood and adult life; the subluxation usually occurs in a superonasal direction (Figure 9.6). Presentation is often with high and fluctuating

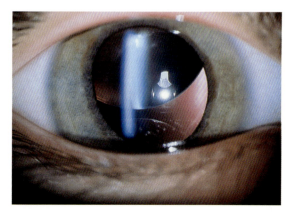

Figure 9.6   Superiorly subluxed lens in child with Marfan syndrome

myopic astigmatism. The pupil often dilates poorly as the iris dilator muscle is hypoplastic. The eyelids may be floppy due to an abnormality of the tarsal plate. Almost all patients have abnormal aortic echo studies and the mitral valve may be floppy. It is important to make the diagnosis as the vascular associations are life-threatening. Other features of Marfan syndrome include tall stature, scoliosis, chest-wall deformity, arachnodactyly (Figure 9.7a,b), joint laxity, and inguinal herniae.

### Homocystinuria

This metabolic disorder, inherited as an autosomal recessive trait, is characterised by deficiency of cystathione synthetase. Affected individuals have high blood and urine levels of homocysteine and methionine. The disorder

results in a weak zonular structure and lens progressive subluxation occurs in up to 90% of eyes. Lens subluxation is rare under three years of age. Lens subluxation may be complicated by pupil-block glaucoma and occasionally the lens may dislocate into the anterior chamber. In contrast to Marfan syndrome the lens often dislocates inferiorly (Figure 9.8). Other features of homocystinuria include mental retardation in late-treated cases, malar flush, and fair hair. General anaesthesia in homocystinuria carries an increased risk of vascular thrombosis which can be reduced with dietary control, pyridoxine, folic acid, and aspirin. Dehydration should be avoided by infusion of intravenous fluids during preoperative starvation.

### Other metabolic causes

Subluxated lenses may also be seen in a number of rare recessive disorders including sulphite oxidase deficiency, molybdenum co-factor deficiency and hyperlysinaemia. In these rare disorders, the ectopia lentis is associated with severe neurological abnormalities.

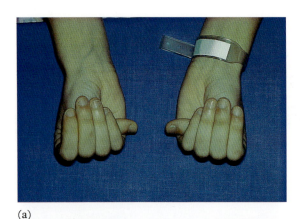

(a)

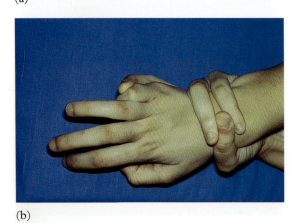

(b)

Figure 9.7(a)(b)   Arachnodactyly in a 14-year-old girl with Marfan syndrome

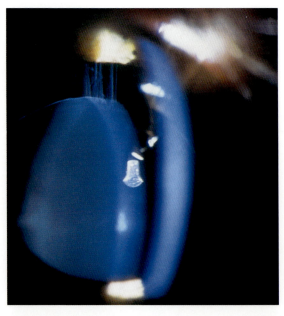

Figure 9.8   Inferiorly subluxed lens in a 4-year-old boy with homocystinuria

## Ectopia lentis et pupillae

This disorder is not associated with any systemic abnormalities. Inheritance is usually autosomal recessive, but may be autosomal dominant with variable expression. The pupils are oval or slit-like and dilate poorly. There may be a persistent pupillary membrane and the iris may be translucent. The lens often subluxes in the opposite direction to the pupil deviation.

### Simple ectopia lentis

This is a diagnosis of exclusion; the findings are of ectopia lentis in a child without evidence of any systemic abnormalities. The eye examination is otherwise normal. It is usually inherited as an autosomal dominant trait but autosomal recessive inheritance has also been reported.

### Weill–Marchesani syndrome

The Weill–Marchesani syndrome is an autosomal recessive disorder characterised by short stature, short fingers and toes (brachydactyly), myopia, glaucoma, and microspherophakia with lens subluxation. Lens dislocation into the anterior chamber may occur.

### Ocular abnormalities

Lens subluxation has been reported in aniridia, buphthalmos, ocular coloboma and following blunt trauma to the eye. In these disorders, the subluxation is often unilateral. Bilateral subluxation may also complicate megalocornea or anterior megalophthalmos.

## Clinical symptoms and signs

When symptomatic, lens subluxation usually presents with reduced visual acuity. The zonular weakness leads to the lens becoming more spherical and unstable within the eye, giving rise to fluctuating myopia and astigmatism. Amblyopia and secondary strabismus is common. An early sign is iridodonesis (tremulous iris) and occasionally parents may notice the eye appearing to "wobble" with movement and this complaint may prompt referral. In some children, for example with Marfan syndrome, the lens subluxation may be first identified at screening examinations. Rarely, the presentation may be with the symptoms and signs of an acute secondary glaucoma when the displaced lens causes pupil block. The child presents with a painful, red, tearing eye with corneal oedema and reduced vision.

Lens subluxation is easily diagnosed on slit-lamp examination but if the pupils are not well dilated, early changes may be missed. A thorough systemic examination should be performed in all cases of ectopia lentis and all children should be referred to a paediatrician so that systemic disorders causing it can be excluded.

## Management

Initially, it is important to establish the correct diagnosis and it is particularly important to exclude homocystinuria before any operative procedures are considered because of the risk of general anaesthesia in that disorder. Most children with lens subluxation can be managed conservatively with accurate refraction and treatment of any amblyopia. The intraocular pressure should also be monitored regularly. Contact lenses may be helpful for high ametropia or anisometropia particularly when one or both lenses have dislocated into the vitreous causing aphakia. They are, however, of limited value in correcting lenticular astigmatism.

In a minority of children the lens subluxation may be such that it is impossible to achieve an accurate refraction and maintain good visual acuity with spectacle correction. Surgery then becomes inevitable. Surgery is also indicated for lenses which dislocate regularly into the anterior chamber. The results of surgery using modern vitrectomy instrumentation are excellent.[13-15] Most children who undergo lensectomy are managed with spectacles or contact lenses postoperatively.[16] In the future it may be possible to stabilise the capsular bag by placing a fixation device such as a Morscher ring, allowing stable intraocular lens implantation.

The complications of dislocated lenses are mainly those of complete dislocation into the anterior or posterior segment or pupil-block glaucoma. Posterior segment dislocation rarely gives rise to problems and surgery is usually not necessary. Anterior dislocation is managed by dilating the pupils, posturing and treatment for raised intraocular pressure. Lensectomy is generally carried out once the inflammation has settled. Pupil-block glaucoma is similarly managed by the use of mydriatics and medical therapy to control the intraocular pressure.

Overall, the visual prognosis in children with subluxated lenses is very good. With modern microsurgical instruments and vitrectomy equipment, the results are excellent. Amblyopia related to high refractive errors remains the major cause of visual impairment.

## References

1 Ionides A, Francis P, Berry V, *et al.* Relationship between phenotype and genotype in autosomal dominant cataract in man. *Br J Ophthalmol* 1999; **83**: 802–8.

2 Francis P, Berry V, Moore AT, Bhattacharya S. Lens biology development and human cataractogenesis. *Trends Genet* 1999; **15**: 191–6.

3 Lambert S. The Lens. In Taylor DSI, ed. *Paediatric Ophthalmology*. Oxford: Blackwell Scientific Publications, 1997: 445–76.

4 Lambert SR, Drack AV. Infantile cataract. *Surv Ophthalmol* 1996; **40**: 427–58.

5 Cassidy L, Taylor D. Congenital cataract and multisystem disorders. *Eye* 1999; **13**: 464–73.

6 Crouch ER Jr, Pressman SH, Crouch ER. Posterior chamber intraocular lenses: long term results in paediatric cataract patients. *J Ped Ophthalmol Strabismus* 1995; **32**: 210–18.

7 Amaya LG, Speedwell L, Taylor D. Contact lenses for infant aphakia. *Br J Ophthalmol* 1990; **74**: 150–4.

8 Baker JD, Hiles DA, Morgan KS. Viewpoint: visual rehabilitation of aphakic children. *Surv Ophthalmol* 1990; **34**: 366–84.

9 Beller R, Hoyt CS, Marg E, *et al.* Good visual function after neonatal surgery for congenital monocular cataracts. *Am J Ophthalmol* 1981; **91**: 559–65.

10 Birch EE, Stager DR. The critical period for surgical treatment of dense congenital unilateral cataract. *Invest Ophthalmol Vis Sci* 1996; **37**: 1532–8.

11 Lambert S. Management of monocular congenital cataracts. *Eye* 1999; **13**: 474–9.

12 Lloyd IC, Kriss A, Speedwell L, *et al.* Modulation of amblyopia therapy following early surgery for unilateral congenital cataracts. *Br J Ophthalmol* 1995; **79**: 802–6.

13 Bekhi R, Noel LP, Clarke WN. Limbal lensectomy in the management of ectopia lentis in children. *Arch Ophthalmol* 1990; **108**: 809–11.

14 Hakin M, Jacobs M, Rosen P, *et al.* Management of the subluxed crystalline lens. *Ophthalmology* 1992; **99**: 542–5.

15 Ruttum MS. Managing situations involving children with ectopia lentis. *J Pediatr Ophthalmol Strabismus* 1995; **32**: 74–5.

16 Speedwell L, Russell-Eggitt I. Improvement in visual acuity in children with ectopia lentis. *J Pediatr Ophthalmol Strabismus* 1995; **32**: 94–7.

# 10 Disorders of the vitreous and retina

ANTHONY T MOORE

A wide variety of different disorders may result in abnormal retinal structure and function in childhood. Broadly speaking, they may be present at birth when they are usually due to disordered development of the retina or they may be acquired during early infancy or childhood. Some of the disorders which become symptomatic after birth are acquired as a result of trauma, infection or other direct insults which affect the structural integrity of the retina, but many later-onset disorders are the result of genetic mutations which, although present from birth, do not cause retinal dysfunction until later childhood. Disorders of the vitreous are less common and are generally seen as developmental abnormalities; vitreous opacities may, however, develop in later childhood as a result of haemorrhage, infection, inflammation or rarely, involvement with tumour.

## Congenital abnormalities:

### Congenital abnormalities of the vitreous

Persistence of the primary vitreous or hyaloid system may give rise to a number of congenital abnormalities of the eye. Survival of remnants of the hyaloid vascular system is a common finding especially in premature infants. It is rare for the complete hyaloid artery to remain but posterior remnants may be seen projecting from the disc into the anterior vitreous and anterior remnants are seen as the so-called Mittendorf dot, a small white opacity on the posterior aspect of the lens.

Vitreous cysts are another uncommon remnant of the hyaloid system; they are usually unilateral and seen in otherwise normal eyes.[1]

A more profound disorder of vitreous development is seen in persistent hyperplastic primary vitreous (PHPV). In this disorder, which is unilateral, the affected eye is microphthalmic, there is a retrolental opacity and there is often an associated posterior polar lens cataract.[1] The usual presentation is with leucocoria or microphthalmos in early infancy. A careful examination under anaesthetic and ultrasound examination will help distinguish this disorder from other causes of leucocoria. The management of PHPV depends on the age at presentation. In infants presenting after three months of age the management is conservative and lensectomy is only indicated if there is shallowing of the anterior chamber and the eye is at risk of pupil-block glaucoma. In younger infants the parents should be offered the option of early lensectomy and anterior vitrectomy and subsequent contact lens fitting and occlusion therapy. Some good visual results have been reported in PHPV following early surgery and aggressive management of the amblyopia but it demands a great deal of parental commitment and this approach should be used only after a full discussion with the parents.[2]

### Congenital abnormalities of the retina and retinal pigment epithelium

Congenital hypertrophy of the retinal pigment epithelium (CHRPE) is usually seen as an isolated, well-circumscribed, pigmented lesion about 1–2 disc diameters in size.[3] It is usually solitary, slightly raised and often has a depigmented halo around the edge of the lesion. It rarely gives rise to symptoms and is usually detected on routine clinical examination. Histopathologically, the hamartoma is composed of thickened retinal pigment epithelium (RPE) cells with increased numbers of pigment granules; there is often overlying photoreceptor atrophy. Multiple CHRPEs, often atypical in appearance (Figure 10.1), may be seen in association with familial adenomatous polyposis coli (FAPC) a dominantly inherited disorder in which there are multiple polyps of the colon and a greatly increased risk of colon cancer. Ophthalmoscopic examination of at risk individuals from families with FAPC may help assign their genetic status.

Grouped pigmentation of the retinal pigment epithelium (bear-track retinopathy) is seen as multiple areas of pigmentation confined to one sector of the fundus which shows some resemblance to animal footprints. They are usually confined to one eye and are not associated with any systemic abnormalities. The histopathological appearance is similar to that seen in CHRPE.

Congenital hyperplasia of the RPE is seen as an isolated, small, circular, highly pigmented lesion in the peripheral retina. The lesion is non-progressive and seen in otherwise normal individuals where it is usually detected on routine examination.

Combined hamartoma of the retina and retinal pigment epithelium usually presents in infancy or early childhood with strabismus of the affected eye. Less commonly the abnormality is found on routine examination. The hamartoma may involve the disc and macula or peripheral retina. Most commonly the hamartoma is seen as a raised, peripapillary, pigmented lesion with vascular tortuosity and associated epiretinal membrane formation (Figure 10.2a,b). The vision in the affected eye is usually poor unless the macula is spared. The condition is usually non-progressive.

## Retinal coloboma (see Chapter 5)

Ocular colobomas occur as a result of a developmental failure of closure of the foetal fissure. The coloboma can involve the iris, optic nerve and retina or may be confined to only one of these tissues. Affected eyes are often microphthalmic. Optic nerve colobomas may be complicated by retinal detachment. Retinal colobomas are seen as pale defects in the retina, retinal pigment epithelium and choriocapillaris inferior to the optic disc usually at the 6 o'clock position (Figure 10.3). The size of the defect is very variable and the visual prognosis is mainly related to the degree of co-existent optic nerve involvement. Ocular colobomas may be unilateral or bilateral and are most commonly seen in otherwise normal children. A family history is uncommon. Colobomas are a common finding in chromosomal disorders and may be seen in a number of systemic disorders such as the CHARGE syndrome, focal dermal hypoplasia, and the branchio-oculo-facial syndrome.[4]

## Myelinated nerve fibres (see Chapter 5)

Normally, myelination of the optic nerve stops at the cribriform plate but in a minority of individuals the ganglion cells within the eye retain a

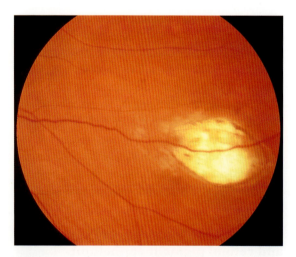

Figure 10.1 Atypical congenital hypertrophy of the RPE lesions in patient with familial adenomatous polyposis coli.

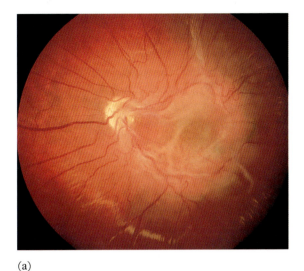

(a)

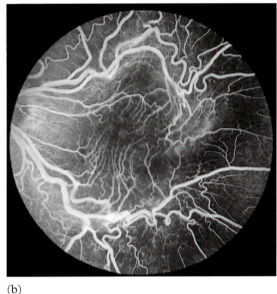

(b)

Figure 10.2   (a) Combined hamartoma of retina and retinal pigment epithelium. Note the tortuous, distorted retinal vessels on angiography (b)

myelin sheath. Such myelinated nerve fibres are seen as a white feathery opacity in the superficial retina which can be seen to follow the line of optic nerve fibres running towards the disc (Figure 10.4). Extensive myelinated nerve fibres may be seen in association with unilateral high myopia and amblyopia. Most cases are found on routine examination in otherwise normal individuals.

## Retinal dysplasia

In retinal dysplasia, there is a failure of retinal and vitreous development resulting in bilateral retinal detachment which is present at birth. Most cases are seen in male infants with Norrie's disease but retinal dysplasia may also be seen in incontinentia pigmenti, Walker–Warburg syndrome, osteoporosis–pseuodoglioma–mental retardation syndrome and

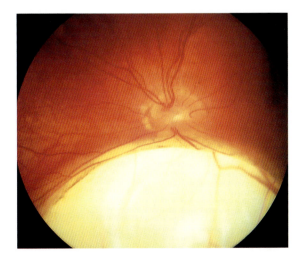

Figure 10.3   Typical retinal coloboma

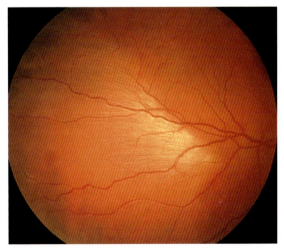

Figure 10.4   Myelinated nerve fibres in peripheral fundus

chromosomal disorders, notably trisomy 13.[1] The clinical presentation is with bilateral leucocoria which is present from birth. Clinical examination shows bilateral retrolental masses and ultrasound examination shows evidence of bilateral retinal detachment without evidence of intraocular calcification. Affected infants are blind and have roving eye movements. Surgery is only indicated if there is shallowing of the anterior chamber causing pupil-block glaucoma when a lensectomy is the operation of choice. Norrie's disease is an X-linked recessive disorder in which there is bilateral retinal dysplasia; about 25% of affected males are mentally retarded and about a third subsequently develop hearing loss. The diagnosis is straightforward when there is a family history of another affected male relative. In many cases, there is no family history but the gene for Norrie's disease has been identified and molecular genetic diagnosis of affected males and carrier females is possible.[5]

## Congenital infections

A number of maternal infections including toxoplasmosis, rubella, syphilis, cytomegalovirus, varicella and HIV may affect the foetus. The infection may be acquired through transplacental spread via the blood supply or as a result of infection from the genital tract directly. These congenital infections commonly result in damage to the developing retina. Maternal infection with rubella in the first trimester may lead to infection of the foetus resulting in a number of serious abnormalities which comprise the congenital rubella syndrome. The clinical findings include growth retardation, congenital heart defects, deafness, mental retardation, hepatosplenomegaly, thrombocytopenia and ocular abnormalities. The ophthalmological abnormalities include cataract, keratitis, glaucoma, and retinal changes. The most common ocular abnormality is a diffuse pigmentary retinopathy which is bilateral and most marked at the posterior pole. The electroretinogram (ERG) and electro-oculogram (EOG) are usually normal. Vision is usually surprisingly good given the

clinical appearance but older children with rubella retinopathy may develop choroidal neovascularisation which may lead to loss of macular function. Congenital rubella is now uncommon in Europe due to vaccination programmes but it is still an important cause of childhood blindness in some parts of the world.

Congenital toxoplasmosis is the commonest congenital infection to be encountered by the ophthalmologist. Chorioretinitis is the commonest feature of the congenital toxoplasmosis syndrome but other abnormalities include microcephaly, intracranial calcification, hydrocephalus, failure to thrive, anaemia and hepatosplenomegaly. The congenital infection occurs when a non-immune mother develops toxoplasmosis in pregnancy; the severe manifestations of the syndrome are seen in infants who were infected in the first trimester; infections later in pregnancy may have minimal effects. The ocular complications of congenital toxoplasmosis include chorioretinitis and less commonly microphthalmos, optic atrophy and cataract. Chorioretinitis may be the only manifestation in some cases. The chorioretinal scarring is seen as focal areas of retinal, RPE and choriocapillaris atrophy, usually with a pigmented border (Figure 10.5). The vision is severely affected if there is involvement of the macula.

Congenital cytomegalovirus (CMV) infection only rarely gives rise to ophthalmological abnormalities but when they occur the findings are of microphthalmos, chorioretinitis, and optic atrophy. Congenital varicella infection may also give rise to chorioretinitis which may resemble the lesions seen in toxoplasmosis and CMV infection. Other abnormalities include cataract, herpes zoster ophthalmicus and Horner syndrome. Infants who develop congenital herpes infection usually acquire herpes virus type 2 infection during the delivery through the birth canal. The common findings are of a cutaneous vesicular eruption but about half the infants will develop systemic infection including CNS involvement. Chorioretinitis and optic atrophy may be seen in infants with CNS

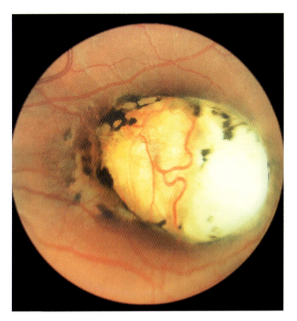

Figure 10.5    Chorioretinal scarring due to congenital toxoplasmosis

involvement. Congenital syphilis is rarely seen in the UK but when it does occur, a variety of ocular manifestations including chorioretinitis, interstitial keratitis, uveitis, and optic atrophy are seen. A high proportion of infants born to mothers infected with HIV are infected themselves. However the ocular manifestations of HIV infection are much less common in children. When retinal abnormalities occur it is generally as a result of CMV or less commonly toxoplasmosis infection when the clinical signs are similar to those seen in adults with HIV.

## Vascular abnormalities

Capillary haemangiomas of the optic disc and retina are usually seen as part of Von Hippel–Lindau disease (see Chapter 17) but may rarely occur as an isolated abnormality[6] (see Chapter 11). Multiple angiomas are indicative of Von Hippel–Lindau disease. Angiomas usually present with blurred vision but may be identified during routine fundoscopic screening of patients with the disease. The retinal angiomas vary in size and are seen as raised vascular lesions often

with a dilated feeder vessel and draining vein. Optic disc haemangiomas are seen as raised vascular tumours on the surface of the disc. Visual loss may occur as a result of retinal exudation, vitreous haemorrhage, and epiretinal membrane formation. Retinal haemangiomas respond well to treatment with cryotherapy or argon laser photocoagulation. The treatment of optic disc lesions is problematic; asymptomatic angiomas are best observed and treatment with laser is reserved for those causing visual loss.

Other congenital vascular malformations of the retina including cavernous haemangioma, retinal arteriovenous malformations and familial retinal arteriolar tortuosity may occur but are very uncommon (see Chapter 11).

## Coats' disease

Coats' disease is an uncommon unilateral disorder, usually seen in young boys, which is characterised by retinal teliangectasis and vascular exudation. The usual presentation is with leucocoria and strabismus. Fundus examination shows typical teliangectasis vessels and associated retinal exudates and often exudative retinal detachment (Figure 10.6a-c). There are often glistening cholesterol crystals in the subretinal space. Fluorescein angiography typically shows dilated irregular beading of the retinal vessels often with associated capillary non-perfusion and vascular leakage (Figure 10.6a-c). Treatment of the vascular abnormalities with argon laser or cryotherapy can prevent progression to extensive retinal detachment and rubeosis iridis. The major differential diagnosis is from familial exudative vitreoretinopathy, a dominantly inherited disorder in which the vascular changes are bilateral but often asymmetric.

## Familial exudative vitreoretinopathy (FEVR)

FEVR is a dominantly inherited disorder which results in abnormal retinal vascular

125

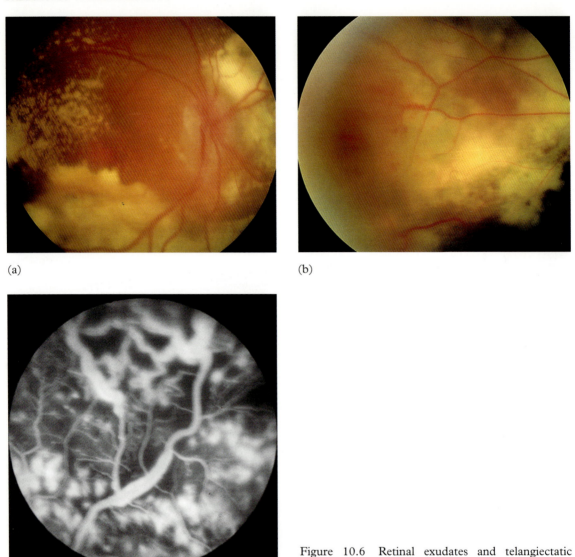

(a)

(b)

(c)

Figure 10.6 Retinal exudates and telangiectatic vessels seen in Coats' disease at posterior pole (a) and peripheral retina (b). The fluorescein angiogram (c) highlights the retinovascular abnormalities

development. There is a wide range of clinical expression from mild asymptomatic disease to extensive retinal folds (Figure 10.7a–d), vascular leakage and retinal detachment.[1] Fluorescein angiography is the most sensitive method of detecting gene carriers; angiographic changes are more marked in the temporal retina and include vascular tortuosity, capillary closure, and peripheral retinal neovascularisation (Figure 10.7a–d). Vascular changes similar to those seen in FEVR may complicate incontinentia pigmenti and fascio-scapulo-humeral dystrophy.

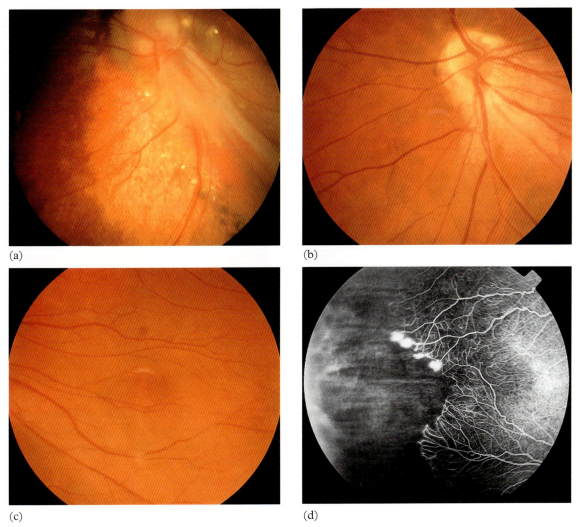

(a)

(b)

(c)

(d)

Figure 10.7 Extensive retinal fold in a child with autosomal dominant familial exudative vitreoretinopathy (a). His father has mild retinovascular changes with "dragging" of the retinal vessels towards the temporal periphery (b,c). Fluorescein angiogram in an asymptomatic patient shows typical peripheral vascular abnormalities (d)

# Acquired disorders of the vitreous and retina:

## Retinopathy of prematurity

Retinopathy of prematurity (ROP) is a vaso-proliferative retinopathy which may develop in very premature infants. In most infants, the disease is mild and undergoes spontaneous regression but in a small minority the disorder progresses to total retinal detachment and blindness.

## Risk factors for the development of ROP

Retinal vascularisation starts from the optic disc at 16 weeks' gestation and the vessels grow towards the retinal periphery reaching the nasal side by about 32 weeks and the temporal side at term. The developing retinal vessels are vulnerable to a number of different influences which may lead to disordered growth and ROP. A number of risk factors for the development of ROP have been identified (Table 10.1). The

127

Table 10.1   Possible risk factors for retinopathy of prematurity

Low birthweight
Low gestational age
Inspired oxygen
Recurrent apnoea
Exchange transfusions
Surfactant use
Vitamin E deficiency
Genetic predisposition

most important of these are birthweight and gestational age (which reflects the degree of immaturity of the retinal vessels) and the use of inspired oxygen. Other factors which have been suggested to be important in the development of ROP include exchange transfusions, surfactant usage, vitamin E deficiency, light exposure, and blood viscosity but none has been confirmed.[7]

Most ROP is seen in very low-birthweight infants. The incidence and severity of ROP is inversely related to birthweight and gestational age. About 70% of infants of <1000 g birthweight develop acute ROP, whereas in those >1500 g the incidence falls to <10%. Severe cicatricial disease is seen almost exclusively in those infants <1000 g birthweight.

Oxygen administration is the other important risk factor. The early studies in the 1950s showed that the incidence of severe ROP in premature infants exposed to high levels of inspired oxygen was much greater than in those exposed to restricted oxygen. Since then, further studies have attempted to define the optimum levels of arterial oxygen, i.e. one which will prevent morbidity from hypoxia but at the same time minimise the risk of developing severe ROP. It has not been possible to define a safe level of oxygen although it is important for neonatologists to avoid high and fluctuating levels of arterial oxygen.

## Pathogenesis of ROP

The two most important factors in the development of ROP are the degree of retinal vascular immaturity and the level of arterial oxygen.

Investigations in animal models of ROP have established that the effect of oxygen on immature retinal blood vessels is to cause vasoconstriction and this occurs as a result of downregulation of vascular endothelial growth factor (VEGF) which is a critical vascular survival factor in the immature retina.[8] Local retinal hypoxia occurring as a result of oxygen-induced vasoconstriction leads to increased VEGF production by retinal astroglial cells and retinal capillary proliferation. VEGF production appears to be a critical factor in the development of ROP and it may be possible in the future to modify the course of acute ROP by suppressing VEGF production or blocking the activation of VEGF receptors on capillary endothelial cells.[8]

It has also been suggested that oxygen may have a direct toxic effect on developing retinal blood vessels by the production of transient free radicals and that this effect may be ameliorated by the use of natural antioxidants such as vitamin E and bilirubin. There have now been a large number of trials investigating the effect of supplemental vitamin E on the development of ROP and there is, as yet, no evidence that supplemental vitamin E reduces the incidence of ROP but it may have an effect on severity of disease.[9] At present, the risks of using high-dose vitamin E outweigh the possible benefits.

## Classification of ROP

There is an internationally agreed classification of acute ROP which allows the severity, location and extent of the disease to be recorded (Table 10.2). The disease is classified into five stages on the basis of findings on indirect

Table 10.2   Classification of ROP

| Stage 1 | Demarcation line |
|---|---|
| Stage 2 | Ridge |
| Stage 3 | Ridge with neovascularisation |
| Stage 4 | Subtotal retinal detachment |
| | 4a: without foveal involvement |
| | 4b: with foveal involvement |
| Stage 5 | Total retinal detachment |

ophthalmoscopy. In the normal premature infant the peripheral retina is incompletely vascularised and has a grey–white appearance. Stage 1 ROP is reached when there is a clear demarcation line between vascularised and non-vascularised retina (Figure 10.8). In stage 2, the line is replaced by a ridge which projects anteriorly into the vitreous (Figure 10.9), and in stage 3 fragile new vessels are seen projecting from the ridge forwards into the vitreous (Figure 10.10a,b). In stages 4 and 5, the retina is partially or completely detached. An eye with "plus" disease has marked dilatation and tortuosity of the posterior retinal vessels (Figure 10.10a,b), vascular engorgement of the iris blood vessels, vitreous haze and pupillary rigidity.

The retina is divided into three zones centred on the optic disc, with zone 1 posteriorly, zone 3 peripherally, and zone 2 in between, so that the location of the disease can be defined. The extent of disease is recorded as clock hours of

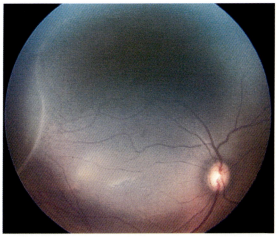

Figure 10.8    Stage I ROP showing demarcation line in peripheral retina. (Courtesy of Professor A Fielder)

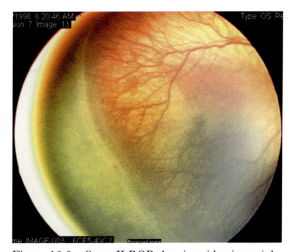

Figure 10.9    Stage II ROP showing ridge in peripheral retina. (Courtesy of Professor A Fielder)

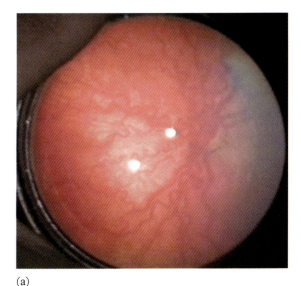

(a)

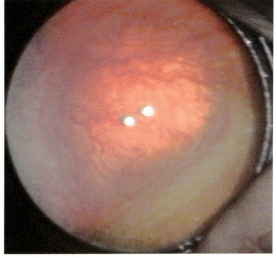

(b)

Figure 10.10    Posterior pole (a) and peripheral fundus (b) in infant with stage III ROP with "plus" disease

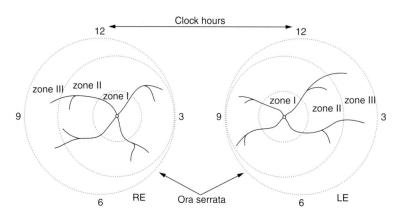

Figure 10.11    Location of disease in ROP

retinal circumference affected; as the examiner looks at the eyes, the 3 o'clock position is on the right, i.e. the nasal side of the right eye and temporal side of the left (Figure 10.11).

## Screening for ROP

It is essential that all infants at risk of developing severe ROP are identified and screened at the appropriate time by an experienced ophthalmologist. Screening can be confined to infants <1500 g birthweight or 32 weeks' gestational age. Retinal examinations should start at about 6 weeks' postnatally and continue until 36 weeks' postnatally if there is no evidence of ROP or until regression has occurred or treatment is necessary in those infants who develop retinopathy. The pupils should be dilated with cyclopentolate 0.5% and phenylephrine 2.5% 30 min before the examination and the use of a lid speculum, binocular indirect ophthalmoscopy and, in selected cases, a scleral depressor will facilitate examination of the peripheral retina. In most infants with stage 1 and stage 2 disease the ROP will regress without cicatrisation but stage 3 disease may require treatment.

## Management

Cryotherapy of peripheral avascular retina has been shown to be effective in stage 3 in reducing

the progression to blinding disease.[10] The rationale for treatment follows that for other retinovascular disorders: ablation of the peripheral retina using either cryotherapy or laser photocoagulation is thought to reduce the level of angiogenic factors produced by hypoxic retina and allows regression of new vessels. Treatment is indicated if there is stage 3 threshold disease (defined as stage 3 ROP in zone 1 or zone 2 involving five contiguous or eight cumulative clock hours with evidence of "plus disease"). Laser therapy using either the diode or argon laser appears to be as effective as cryotherapy and is easier to use in treating zone 1 disease.[11] The treatment of retinal detachment in advanced disease is controversial; although it is possible, in some cases, to re-attach the retina with surgery, the visual results are generally poor.

## Prognosis

The prognosis for most infants who develop acute ROP is excellent; most stage 1 and stage 2 disease regresses spontaneously without cicatrisation. Infants with stage 3 ROP that is confined to zone 3 also have a good prognosis. Infants who develop stage 3 threshold disease have, without treatment, a 50% risk of progressing to total retinal detachment or severe retinal scarring. Prompt treatment once threshold disease has been reached halves the risk of developing such an outcome. About 20% of eyes with threshold disease will however progress to retinal detachment or severe cicatricial changes even with optimum treatment. The prognosis is worse if disease is in zone 1. Longer-term follow-up of patients enrolled in the Cryo-ROP study has shown that the anatomical results of treatment have remained constant but the differences in functional outcome (as assessed by measurement of visual acuity) between treated and control eyes have narrowed.[12] This is probably related to co-existent ischemic damage to the visual pathways which may complicate extreme prematurity.

# Inherited retinal dystrophies

There are a large number of different inherited retinal dystrophies that become symptomatic in childhood. Some are non-progressive, for example the various forms of achromatopsia and congenital stationary night blindness (Table 10.3), but the majority show gradual deterioration over time. Both groups of disorders show abnormalities of photoreceptor or inner retinal function on electrodiagnostic testing (see Chapter 3). The majority of children with retinal dystrophies are otherwise normal but there are a number of inherited syndromes in which the abnormal retinal function is part of a more widespread systemic disorder. Some of these are summarised in Table 10.4. Recently, there have been tremendous advances in our understanding of the underlying pathogenesis of the retinal dystrophies particularly in the area of molecular genetics. It is not possible to cover these in this short account but several good reviews have been published to which the reader is referred.[13–15]

Table 10.3  Stationary retinal dystrophies

Disorders presenting with night blindness
  Congenital stationary night blindness
    Autosomal dominant
    Autosomal recessive
    X-linked recessive
  Ogouchi's disease (autosomal recessive)
  Fundus albipunctatus (antosomal recessive)
Stationary cone dystrophies
  Rod monochromatism (autosomal recessive)
  Blue cone monochromatism (X-linked recessive)
Central receptor dystrophies
  North Carolina macular dystrophy (autosomal dominant)

Table 10.4  Syndromes with associated retinal dystrophy

| Syndrome | Inheritance | Non-retinal features |
| --- | --- | --- |
| Usher syndrome | Autosomal recessive inheritance | Congenital deafness |
| Bardet–Biedl syndrome | Autosomal recessive inheritance | Obesity, polydactyly, variable mental retardation, hypogonadism |
| Refsum disease | Autosomal recessive inheritance | Ataxia, polyneuropathy, deafness, anosmia, ichthyosis, raised plasma phytanic acid |
| Abetalipoproteinaemia | Autosomal recessive inheritance | Failure to thrive, acanthocytosis, fat malabsorption, ataxia, absence of plasma low-density lipoproteins |
| Kearns–Sayre syndrome | Mitochondrial inheritance | Ptosis, ophthalmoplegia, heart block |
| Cockayne syndrome | Autosomal recessive inheritance | Deafness, growth retardation, mental retardation, presenile appearance, cutaneous photosensitivity |
| Peroxisomal disorders Infantile Refsum syndrome Neonatal adrenoleucodystrophy Zellweger syndrome | Autosomal recessive inheritance | Facial dysmorphism, severe neurological abnormalities, developmental delay, renal cysts, metabolic disturbance, increased levels of very long-chain fatty acids |
| Joubert syndrome | Autosomal recessive inheritance | Tachypnoea, cerebellar vermis hypoplasia, developmental delay, renal cysts, ocular coloboma |
| Juvenile Batten disease | Autosomal recessive inheritance | Seizures, intellectual regression, progressive neurological deterioration |
| Alström syndrome | Autosomal recessive inheritance | Diabetes mellitus, deafness, obesity, cardiomyopathy |

# Stationary retinal dystrophies

## Congenital stationary night blindness

Congenital stationary night blindness (CSNB) may be inherited as an autosomal dominant, autosomal recessive or X-linked recessive disorder. The autosomal dominant form is the least common; affected individuals have normal visual acuity, have no nystagmus but have poor night vision. Fundus examination is normal but the flash ERG shows reduced scotopic responses with well preserved cone function. The X-linked and recessive forms of CSNB usually present with nystagmus in infancy. Affected children are usually myopic, have moderately reduced acuity, and mild colour vision disturbance. Fundus examination is usually normal although tilted optic discs may be seen. A flash ERG shows poor scotopic responses but in contrast to the dominant form, there is usually a reduced b-wave in response to a bright white flash, a so-called negative-wave ERG (see Chapter 3). In most forms of CSNB, the fundus examination is normal but in two rare autosomal recessive forms of CSNB, there are characteristic fundus abnormalities. In fundus albipunctatus there is a fleck retinal appearance with multiple yellow-white flecks at the level of the RPE and in Ogouchi disease there is a green-yellow discoloration of the fundus that reverts to normal on prolonged dark adaptation.

## Achromatopsia

Two main forms of achromatopsia are seen.

- In autosomal recessive achromatopsia (rod monochromatism) there are no functioning cone photoreceptors in the retina. Affected individuals present in infancy with reduced vision, severe photophobia and rapid, fine nystagmus. There is often a high hyperopic refractive error and fundus examination is usually normal. The diagnosis is confirmed by the finding of absent cone responses on ERG; the scotopic responses are normal (see Chapter 3). When the children are old enough to be formally tested, the vision is about the level of 6/60 and there is no true colour vision. The condition is non-progressive.

- The X-linked recessive form of achromatopsia (blue cone monochromatism) is less common and milder. The clinical presentation and the ERG changes are similar to rod monochromatism but in the X-linked form the affected children are usually myopic, have better visual acuity, and evidence of residual blue cone function.

# Progressive retinal dystrophies

There are a large number of different retinal dystrophies which are progressive in nature. Although for some forms the underlying genetic mutation is known,[15] for most little is known about the disease mechanisms. They are conveniently classified according to whether there is predominantly central retinal involvement (central receptor dystrophies) or more generalised disease. The latter are subdivided on the basis of which classes of photoreceptor are predominantly affected early in the disease (rod–cone and cone–rod dystrophies) and by the age of onset.

## Infantile rod–cone dystrophy (Leber's amaurosis)

Leber's amaurosis is an autosomal recessive infantile rod–cone dystrophy which presents in the first few months of life with poor vision and nystagmus or roving eye movements. The infants are often highly hyperopic, have poor pupil responses to light, and a normal fundus examination. The diagnosis is confirmed by the finding of a very subnormal or more usually non-recordable ERG. Leber's amaurosis is not a single disorder but mutations in several different genes may give rise to a similar clinical picture.[15] Most infants with Leber's amaurosis are otherwise normal but some may show developmental

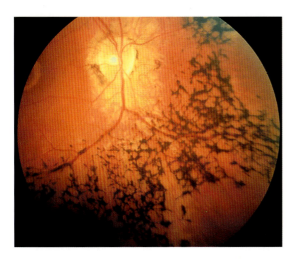

Figure 10.12 Typical fundus appearance of retinitis pigmentosa with retinal pigment epithelial atrophy and retinal pigmentation

delay or other neurological abnormalities. Such children should be referred for a paediatric opinion so that rare syndromes such as Joubert syndrome or a peroxisomal disorder can be excluded (Table 10.4).

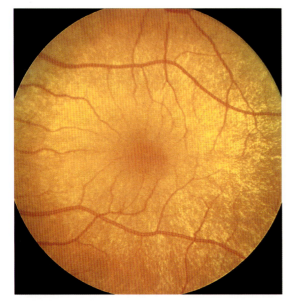

Figure 10.13 Tapetal reflex in a female carrier of X-linked retinitis pigmentosa

## Retinitis pigmentosa

Retinitis pigmentosa is the name given to a heterogeneous group of disorders in which there is a progressive rod–cone dystrophy. The age of onset and visual prognosis is very variable. The mode of inheritance may be autosomal dominant, autosomal recessive or X-linked recessive but there is considerable genetic heterogeneity even amongst these subtypes. X-linked recessive disease tends to be of early onset and severe whereas most forms of autosomal dominant retinitis pigmentosa are of later onset and have a better visual prognosis. Recessive retinitis pigmentosa shows a very variable phenotype. Many of the causative genetic mutations have now been identified.[15] Affected individuals usually present with difficulties with night vision and subsequently there is evidence of mid-peripheral field loss and retinal atrophy and pigmentation (Figure 10.12). The scotopic ERG is abnormal early in the disease with later evidence of cone involvement. In children, the retinal signs may be very subtle in the early stages, so ERG is extremely helpful in confirming the diagnosis. Female carriers of the X-linked from of the disease often show mild peripheral retinal atrophy and pigmentation. The flash ERG may show mild abnormalities. Less commonly, there may be an abnormal "tapetal" reflex from the posterior retina (Figure 10.13).

The natural history of retinitis pigmentosa is for gradual deterioration. The initial symptoms are of night blindness and in the early stages there is mild mid-peripheral field loss which is not symptomatic. Later there is progressive field loss leading to marked constriction of the visual field. Ultimately, central vision may be lost if the dystrophic process involves the macula.

Visual loss in retinitis pigmentosa may occur as a result of cataract, macular oedema or involvement of the central receptors in the dystrophic process. Although there is as yet no specific treatment for the underlying retinal dystrophy, the secondary cataract responds well to surgery and

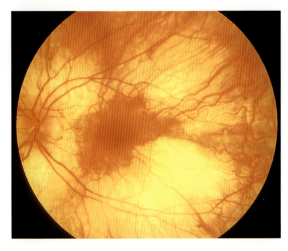

Figure 10.14   Typical fundus appearance of choroideremia with atrophy of the RPE and choriocapillaris

macular oedema may be helped by treatment with systemic acetazolamide or systemic steroids.

## Systemic associations of retinitis pigmentosa

A progressive rod–cone dystrophy may be seen in a large variety of genetic disorders, some of which are summarised in Table 10.4. In the majority of these syndromes, there is no treatment which will affect the rate of progression of the retinal dystrophy. However in Refsum's disease, dietary treatment to lower plasma levels of phytanic acid and in abetalipoproteinemia treatment with vitamin A and E may slow deterioration in retinal function.

## Choroideremia

Choroideremia is a rare progressive X-linked retinal dystrophy which presents in childhood with nyctalopia; later there is development of peripheral field loss and ultimately loss of central vision. Although in the early stages the fundus appearance may be confused with retinitis pigmentosa, later in the disease there is a characteristic fundus appearance with extensive atrophy of the choriocapillaris and retinal pigment epithelium (Figure 10.14). The rod and cone ERG shows reduced amplitude early in the disease and is extinguished at a late stage. Female carriers have a characteristic fundus appearance, with patchy peripheral pigmentary change (Figure 10.15). The visual prognosis in choroideremia is better than in X-linked retinitis pigmentosa and most affected males keep good central vision until their fifth decade.

## Gyrate atrophy of the choroid and retina

In this rare recessively inherited disorder there is a deficiency of the mitochondrial enzyme ornithine aminotransferase (OAT) (due to mutations in the *OAT* gene); this results in raised levels of plasma ornithine and progressive choroidal retinal pigment epithelial and photoreceptor atrophy leading to a characteristic fundus appearance. It is still unclear whether the retinal abnormalities are related to the high levels of ornithine in the retina or are due to some other metabolic consequence of the OAT deficiency. The usual presentation is with night blindness or progressive myopia. Affected children are

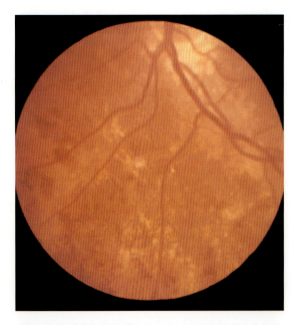

Figure 10.15  Typical fundus change in female carrier of choroideremia

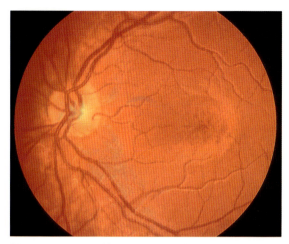

Figure 10.16 Characteristic foveal schisis in X-linked juvenile retinoschisis

usually myopic, have peripheral field loss which is progressive and have areas of retinal atrophy which are first seen in the mid-periphery. The EOG is abnormal early in the disease process and the ERG becomes abnormal as the disease progresses. It is very important to consider this diagnosis in children with a recessive retinal dystrophy as treatment may slow the rate of

progression. Measurement of plasma ornithine levels will allow the diagnosis to be confirmed and an appropriate referral made to a metabolic physician. Some patients respond to supplemental pyridoxine and show reduced ornithine levels and slowing of progression of their retinal dystrophy. The majority do not and need to follow an arginine-restricted diet.[16]

## Central receptor dystrophies

There is a large number of retinal dystrophies which predominantly affect the macular region. They show considerable clinical and genetic heterogeneity and only the more common dystrophies will be considered here. The usual presentation is with reduced acuity, usually in childhood or early adult life, and fundoscopy usually reveals an abnormal appearance of the macular region. The visual prognosis varies widely amongst the different disorders.

## X-linked juvenile retinoschisis

X-linked juvenile retinoschisis is probably the most common inherited macular dystrophy affecting males.[17] It usually presents in childhood with reduced acuity often discovered on routine vision testing at school. Less commonly, it can present with large bullous schisis in infancy or with vitreous haemorrhage. The typical foveal schisis (Figure 10.16) is seen in almost all affected individuals and about 50–70% will show peripheral retinoschisis or other peripheral retinal abnormalities such as an inner retinal sheen (Figure 10.17), vascular closure and pigmentation. The foveal schisis is subtle and easily missed unless the posterior retina is examined carefully; it is more obvious when the fundus is examined with a red-free light. The ERG usually shows a "negative waveform" in response to a bright white flash and this is helpful in confirming the diagnosis (see Chapter 3). The long-term prognosis is generally very good although severe visual loss may occur if there is extensive peripheral schisis, or

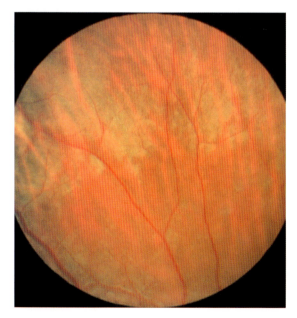

Figure 10.17 Inner retinal silvery sheen in X-linked juvenile retinoschisis

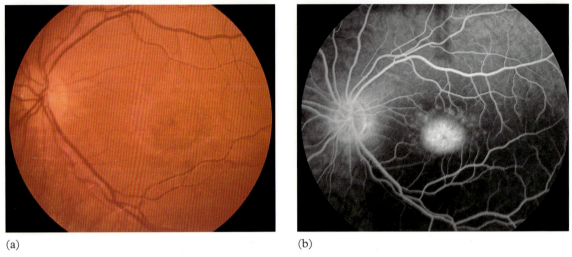

(a)                                                    (b)

Figure 10.18    Macular atrophy (a) with window defect on fluorescein angiography (b) in Stargardt disease

if there are complications such as vitreous haemorrhage or retinal detachment. Female heterozygotes are generally asymptomatic and have a normal fundus examination and normal ERG. However, the gene causing X-linked juvenile retinoschisis has recently been identified and molecular genetic diagnosis may be helpful in genetic counselling of females in families with X-linked juvenile retinoschisis who are of uncertain status.

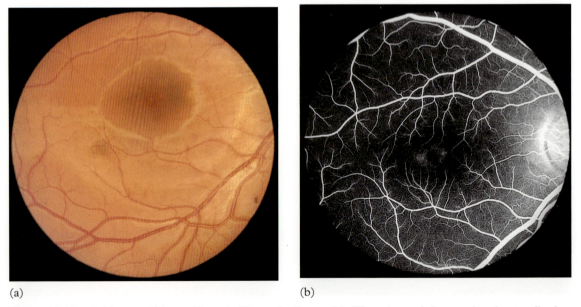

(a)                                                    (b)

Figure 10.19    A 12-year-old boy with early Stargardt disease (a). There is a subtle macular abnormality but fluorescein angiography clearly demonstrates a dark choroid (b) which helps confirm the diagnosis

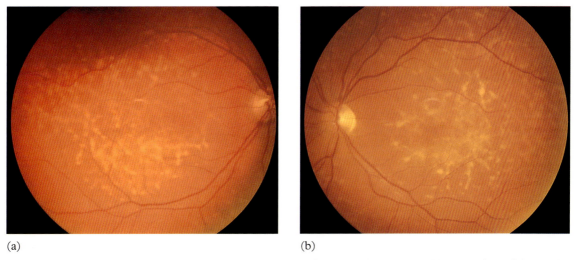

(a)                                                                          (b)

Figure 10.20    Multiple white flecks in a young girl with Stargardt disease (a). There is also mild macular atrophy (b)

## Stargardt disease

Stargardt disease is an autosomal recessive macular dystrophy in which there is loss of central vision and macular atrophy. Although some patients may present in early adult life the usual presentation is with loss of central vision in school-age children. Fundus examination usually shows a typical bull's eye maculopathy (Figure 10.18a,b) often with associated white flecks at the level of the retinal pigment epithelium.[18] Fluorescein angiography highlights the central atrophy (Figure

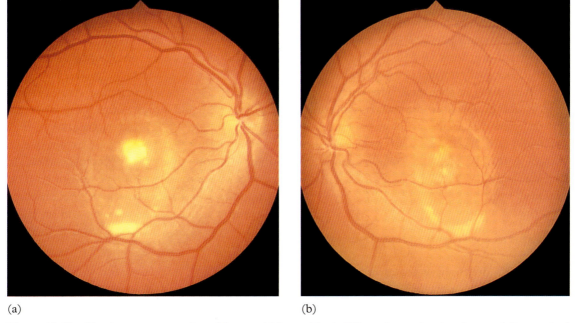

(a)                                                                          (b)

Figure 10.21    Fundus appearance in a 15-year-old boy with vitelliform dystrophy showing partially resorbed subretinal yellow deposits at the macula

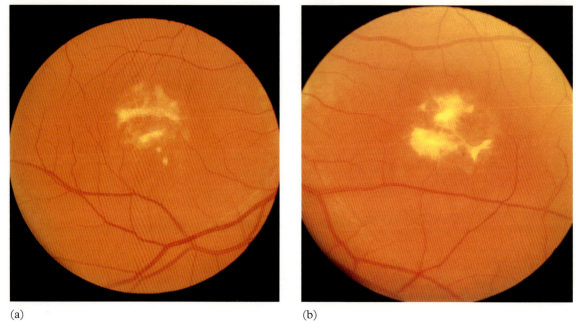

(a)                                                      (b)

Figure 10.22    Right and left fundus showing subretinal fibrosis in Best disease

10.18a,b) and also often shows the so-called "dark choroid" appearance when an abnormal absorbing layer at the level of the RPE blocks the underlying choroidal fluorescence (Figure 10.19a,b). Some affected individuals have a flecked retinal appearance without maculopathy (fundus flavimaculatus) and this variant has a better visual prognosis (Figure 10.20a,b). The flash ERG is usually normal in the early stages but the pattern ERG is abnormal. The visual prognosis in most cases is poor; the vision usually deteriorates relatively rapidly and most patients have vision of 6/60 or less by their early twenties. Later in the disease, there may be nyctalopia, peripheral field loss, and reduced scotopic and photopic ERG responses.

## Vitelliform dystrophy (Best disease)

Vitelliform dystrophy is an uncommon autosomal dominant macular dystrophy which usually presents in childhood or early adult life with mild visual loss.[19] There is a wide range of clinical expression in those carrying the causative mutation; the macular appearances range from a normal macula to the typical subretinal yellow ("egg yolk") deposits in the macular region. The ERG is usually normal but all gene carriers show a reduced light rise on EOG. The typical yellow deposits are usually circular in shape and block the underlying choroidal fluorescence on fluorescein angiography. The yellow deposits gradually resorb (Figure 10.21), leaving a circular area of retinal pigment epithelial atrophy often with subretinal fibrosis (Figure 10.22) and pigmentation. The visual prognosis is generally good except in eyes which develop subretinal neovascularisation. In view of the variable phenotype and often mild symptoms, it is important in genetic counselling to perform a fundus examination and an EOG in all at-risk family members, even if they are asymptomatic.

## North Carolina macular dystrophy

North Carolina macular dystrophy (NCMD) is an early-onset macular dystrophy which is

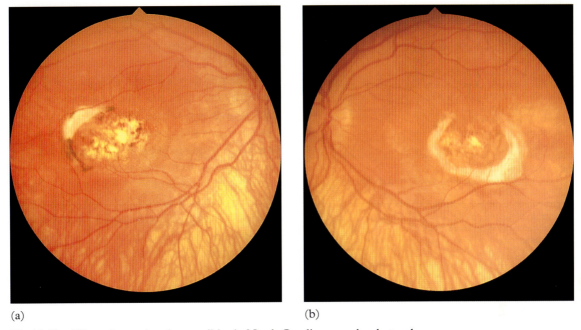

(a)                                               (b)

Fig 10.23    Bilateral macular abnormalities in North Carolina macular dystrophy

non-progressive. The causative gene is thought to be fully penetrant but there is a wide variability of clinical expression. At the severe end of the spectrum, there is a large area of focal atrophy of the macular region (grade 3) with a similar appearance to so-called macular colobomas (Figure 10.23a,b). The visual acuity is often better than the macular appearance would suggest. In more mildly affected individuals there are drusen-like deposits at the posterior pole (grade 1) which may be confluent (grade 2). EOG, ERG and colour vision testing are all normal. The long-term prognosis is good.

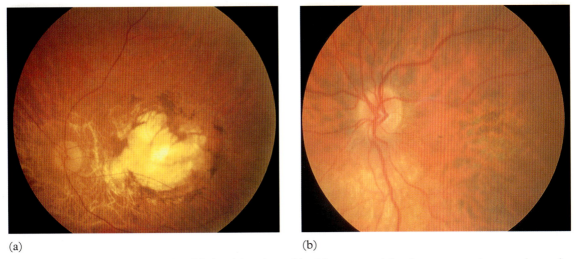

(a)                                               (b)

Figure 10.24  Fundus photographs of father (a) and son (b) with autosomal dominant progressive cone dystrophy

Table 10.5  Flecked retina syndromes

Inherited dystrophies
   Stargardt disease (fundus flavimaculatus)
   Fundus albipunctatus
   Kandori's flecked retinal syndrome
   Retinitis puctata albescens (retinitis pigmentosa)
   Dominant drusen (Doyne's honeycombe dystrophy;
     mallatia levantinesi)
   Bietti's crystalline dystrophy
   Abetalipoproteinaemia
   Alport syndrome

Acquired disease
   Type II mesangiocapillary glomerulonephritis
   Vitamin A deficiency
   Drug deposition in the retina
     tamoxifen
     methoxyfluorane anaesthesia
     canxanthine
     talc

## Cone and cone–rod dystrophies

The progressive cone dystrophies present with photophobia, reduced vision and often with nystagmus in early-onset forms.[20] Fundus examination usually shows macular atrophy similar to that seen in Stargardt disease. Cone dystrophy may be distinguished from Stargardt disease by the early loss of colour vision and the finding of reduced or absent photopic responses on ERG. Although the early symptoms and signs are suggestive of pure cone involvement, most patients later develop night blindness and show evidence of reduced scotopic responses on ERG. The fundus appearance in the late stages of the disease shows more marked macular atrophy or may be indistinguishable from retinitis pigmentosa. The cone dystrophies may show autosomal recessive, autosomal dominant (Figure 10.24a,b) and X-linked recessive inheritance and there is considerable genetic heterogeneity amongst the different subtypes.[20] Overall, the long-term visual prognosis is poor.

## Fleck retina syndromes

A variety of retinal dystrophies may give rise to multiple yellow or yellow-white flecks scattered throughout the retina.[21] These include Stargardt macular dystrophy (fundus flavimaculatus) (Figure 10.20a,b), fundus albipunctatus, Kandori's fleck retina syndrome and the retinopathy seen in Alport syndrome (Table 10.5).

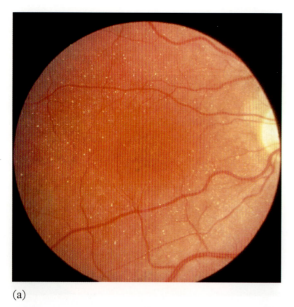

(a)

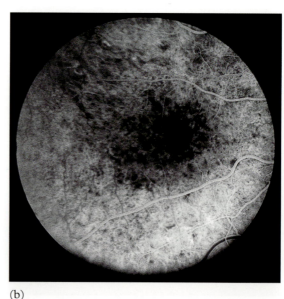

(b)

Figure 10.25    (a) Crystalline retinal deposits in Bietti's crystalline dystrophy. (b) Fluorescein angiogram shows atrophy of the underlying RPE

Multiple white deposits at the level of the RPE are sometimes seen in early retinitis pigmentosa (when the appearance is termed "retinitis punctata albescens") and less commonly in Leber's amaurosis. Multiple crystalline deposits in the retina, seen for example in oxallosis and Bietti's crystalline dystrophy (Figure 10.25a,b), may give a similar appearance. Acquired disease, for example vitamin A deficiency, may also result in a flecked retina syndrome and some drugs, for example canxanthine, may deposit in the retina giving rise to crystalline deposits. The different causes of the fleck retina syndrome can be distinguished on the basis of mode of inheritance, electrophysiological abnormalities and associated systemic abnormalities.

## Retinal detachment in childhood

Retinal detachment is very uncommon in childhood and usually occurs in anatomically abnormal eyes or secondary to trauma.[22] The detachment may be rhegmatogenous, tractional or exudative.

- Rhegmatogenous detachment may occur in developmentally abnormal eyes, for example in aphakia, PHPV, and optic disc and retinal coloboma, and may occur as a late

Table 10.6 Disorders associated with angioid streaks

Pseudoxanthoma elasticum
Paget's disease
Ehlers–Danlos syndrome
Lead poisoning
Hyperparathyroidism
Hyperphosphataemia
Haematological disorders
   Sickle-cell disease
   Beta-thalassaemia
   Spherocytosis

complication of retinopathy of prematurity. There is also an increased risk of retinal detachment in a number of inherited disorders including Stickler syndrome, FEVR, incontinentia pigmenti, juvenile X-linked retinoschisis and Marfan syndrome.

- Traumatic retinal detachment may complicate both blunt and penetrating trauma.

- Exudative retinal detachment is rare and may be associated with a number of different causes including Coats' disease, FEVR, choroidal haemangioma, posterior scleritis, and toxocariasis.

Retinal detachment in childhood often occurs in anatomically abnormal eyes and may be associated with complex intraocular pathology. The best results are achieved if such children are referred to specialist centres.

## Angioid streaks

Angioid streaks are thought to represent breaks in Bruch's membrane and are seen clinically as irregular pigmented or depigmented streaks which radiate out from the optic disc into the posterior fundus (Figure 10.26).[23] They are seen in a variety of disorders including pseudoxanthoma elasticum and haematological disorders such as sickle-cell disease and beta-thalassaemia (Table 10.6). In pseudoxanthoma elasticum, other abnormalities such as a "peau d'orange" RPE pigmentation and optic disc drusen may be

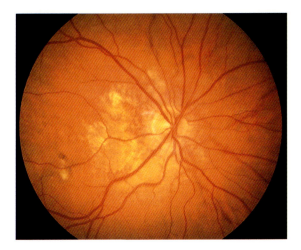

Figure 10.26 Angioid streaks in patient with pseudoxanthoma elasticum

seen. Angioid streaks are rare in childhood and usually become apparent in early adult life. They may be associated with choroidal neovascularisation and submacular haemorrhage.

## Retinal haemorrhages

Ophthalmologists are often asked to review infants who are suspected to have non-accidental injury for evidence of retinal or subhyaloid haemorrhages which may support the diagnosis. Retinal, subhyaloid and vitreous haemorrhages are a common finding in shaking injuries and are often associated with intracranial haemorrhage. Such haemorrhages are very rare in accidental injury, are not seen in children who have had seizures and occur uncommonly in children who have required resuscitation after accidental head trauma or illness. They may, however, be seen in leukaemia (see Chapter 11) or other haematological disorders. Extensive retinal haemorrhages are therefore not diagnostic of non-accidental injury. The finding of retinal haemorrhages must be interpreted in the light of the clinical history, other clinical findings and the results of haematological tests including a clotting screen.

## References

1  Moore AT. In: Taylor DSI, ed. *Vitreous in Pediatric Ophthalmology*, 2nd edn. Oxford: Blackwell Scientific Publications, 1997; 498–519.

2  Karr DJ, Scott WE. Visual results following treatment of persistent hyperplastic primary vitreous. *Arch Ophthalmol* 1986; **104**: 662–7.

3  Moore AT. Congenital and vascular abnormalities of the retina. In: Taylor DSI, ed. *Pediatric Ophthalmology*, 2nd edn. Oxford: Blackwell Scientific Publications, 1997; 614–26.

4  Warburg M. An update on microphthalmos and coloboma: a brief survey of genetic disorders with microphthalmos and coloboma. *Ophthalmic Paediatr Genet* 1991; **12**: 57–63.

5  Black G, Redmond RM. The molecular biology of Norrie's disease. *Eye* 1994; **8**: 491–6.

6  Webster AR, Maher ER, Moore AT. Retinal angiomatosis in von Hippel–Lindau disease. *Arch Ophthalmol* 1999; **117**: 371–8.

7  Ben-Sira I, Niseenkorn I, Kremer I. Retinopathy of prematurity. *Surv Ophthalmol* 1988; **33**: 1–16.

8  Aiello LP. Vascular endothelial growth factor; 20th century mechanism, 21st century therapies. *Invest Ophthalmol Vis Sci* 1997; **38**: 1647–52.

9  Raju TN, Langenberg P, Bhutani V, Quinn G. Vitamin E prophylaxis to reduce retinopathy of prematurity: a reappraisal of published trials. *J Pediatr* 1997; **131**: 844–50.

10  Cryotherapy for Retinopathy of Prematurity Co-operative Group. Multicentre trial of cryotherapy for retinopathy of prematurity: preliminary results. *Arch Ophthalmol* 1988; **106**: 471–9.

11  Connolly BP, McNamara JA, Sharma S, *et al.* Comparison of laser photocoagulation with trans-scleral cryotherapy in the treatment of threshold retinopathy of prematurity. *Ophthalmology* 1998; **105**: 1628–31.

12  Cryotherapy for Retinopathy of Prematurity Co-operative Group. Multicentre trial of cryotherapy for retinopathy of prematurity: Snellen visual acuity and structural outcome at 5½ years after randomisation. *Arch Ophthalmol* 1996; **114**: 417–24.

13  Moore AT. Inherited retinal dystrophies. In: Taylor DSI, ed. *Pediatric Ophthalmology*, 2nd edn. Oxford: Blackwell Scientific Publications, 1997; 557–98.

14  Heckenlively JR. *Retinitis Pigmentosa*. Philadelphia: JB Lippincott, 1988.

15  Inglehearn C. Molecular genetics of human retinal dystrophies. *Eye* 1998; **1**: 571–9.

16  Kaiser-Kupfer MI, de Monasterio FM, Valle D, *et al.* Gyrate atrophy of the choroid and retina: improved visual function following reduction of plasma ornithine by diet. *Science* 1980; **210**: 1128–31.

17  George NG, Yates JRW, Moore AT. Clinical features of affected males in juvenile X-linked retinoschisis. *Arch Ophthalmol* 1996; **114**: 274–80.

18  Fishman GA, Stone EM, Grover S, *et al.* Variation of clinical expression in patients with Stargardt dystrophy and sequence variations in the *ABCR* gene. *Arch Ophthalmol* 1999; **117**: 504–10.

19  Blodi CF, Stone E. Best's vitelliform dystrophy. *Ophthalmic Paediatr Genet* 1990; **11**: 49–59.

20  Simunovic MP, Moore AT. The cone dystrophies. *Eye* 1998; **12**: 553–65.

21  Moore AT. Flecked retina syndromes. In: Taylor DSI, ed. *Pediatric Ophthalmology*, 2nd edn. Oxford: Blackwell Scientific Publications, 1997: 640–8.

22  Moore AT, Snead M. Retinal detachment in childhood. In: Taylor DSI, ed. *Pediatric Ophthalmology*, 2nd edn. Oxford: Blackwell Scientific Publications, 1997: 627–39.

23  Clarkson JG, Altman RD. Angioid streaks. *Surv Ophthalmol* 1982; **26**: 235–46.

# 11 Intraocular tumours

ANTHONY T MOORE

Intraocular tumours are rare in childhood. Malignant tumours include retinoblastoma and the various intraocular manifestations of leukaemia. Benign tumours are more common and include the hamartomatous lesions of the iris and retina seen in the phakomatoses (see Chapter 17) and histiocytic disorders such as juvenile xanthogranuloma and Langerhan's cell histiocytosis.

## Retinoblastoma

Retinoblastoma is the commonest intraocular malignancy of childhood but it is nevertheless rare, occurring in about 1 in 20 000 live births.[1] About half the cases are due to mutations of the retinoblastoma (RB1) gene and the other cases are due to non-heritable somatic changes within developing retinal cells. The latter group present later with unilateral disease. Most children with the heritable form of retinoblastoma represent new mutations but about 25% will have a positive family history. Retinoblastoma is almost universally fatal when untreated but has a good prognosis with modern methods of treatment with radiotherapy and chemotherapy. It is very important therefore that children with retinoblastoma are diagnosed early and referred to specialist centres for optimum treatment.

## Pathogenesis

Children are recognised clinically as having the heritable form of retinoblastoma when they have one or more of the following:

- bilateral or multifocal disease;

- a positive family history;

- an associated second non-ocular malignancy; or

- a cytogenetically visible deletion of chromosome 13q14 which involves the RB1 locus.

Although most children with unilateral retinoblastoma have the non-heritable form, about 10–15% have an underlying RB1 germ line mutation. The mutations that induce retinoblastoma are very variable and include both large, cytogenetically visible deletions and single nucleotide changes.[2] Most mutations result in a truncated non-functional protein product.

Knudson in 1971, on the basis of clinical observations that bilateral retinoblastoma occurred at an earlier age than unilateral retinoblastoma, proposed that two mutational events were required for tumourogenesis in retinoblastoma.[3] Subsequent molecular genetic research has confirmed Knudson's two-hit hypothesis. The molecular basis of tumourogenesis is the loss of function of both RB1 loci. In the heritable form of retinoblastoma, all cells in the body have a mutation at the RB1 locus and it requires only a second spontaneous genetic rearrangement at the normal allele in a developing retinal cell for tumour formation to occur. Such events may occur in more than one retinocyte giving rise to multiple tumours. The second "hit" is usually a large deletion of DNA around the *RB1* locus. In the non-heritable form of retinoblastoma, two distinct somatic mutational events need to occur in the same retinocyte in order to give rise to tumour formation. This is very unlikely to occur in more than one retinal cell so that non-heritable retinoblastoma usually gives rise to a single tumour.

The RB1 protein product has an important role in regulating the cell cycle; it acts to inhibit cell proliferation and *RB1* was the first of a family of similar tumour suppresser genes to be discovered. *RB1* can also have important functions in tissues outside the eye and patients with the genetic form of retinoblastoma have an increased risk of second non-ocular tumours, especially sarcomas. About 2% of children with *RB1* mutations develop malignant tumours of the pineal gland; such tumours usually present with the symptoms and signs of raised intracranial pressure and have a poor prognosis. The lifetime risk of developing associated non-ocular malignancies is about 25–30% and these tumours are a more important cause of death in patients with *RB1* mutations than disseminated retinoblastoma. Mutations of the *RB1* gene may also give rise to retinomas, a benign disordered proliferation of the retina and retinal pigment epithelium. They may resemble treated retinoblastoma and their major significance is that their presence in a close relative of a child with retinoblastoma indicates that the individual is carrying the *RB1* mutation.

## Histopathology

On histological examination, retinoblastoma is usually seen as poorly differentiated malignant neuroblastic tumour composed of cells with large hyperchromatic nuclei. Necrosis and calcification within the tumour are common. Some tumours are better differentiated and may show the typical Flexner–Wintersteiner rosettes. Tumour growth within the eye may be exophytic, with tumour material lying predominantly within the subretinal space. Endophytic tumours grow forwards into the vitreous cavity,

giving rise to vitreous seeding or to a large tumour mass occupying the vitreous cavity (Figure 11.1a–c). Rarely there may be diffuse intraocular infiltration with retinoblastoma which may lead to difficulty with diagnosis. Extraocular spread of retinoblastoma occurs either via the optic nerve to the intracranial cavity or via the choroidal vessels to the orbit or systemic circulation. The bone marrow is the commonest site for retinoblastoma metastasis.

## Clinical presentation

Most children with retinoblastoma present either with strabismus or with an abnormal pupillary reflex which is evident to the parents.[4] Less commonly, the presentation is with a painful red eye, proptosis or uveitis (Table 11.1). Tumours in children with a family history of retinoblastoma are usually discovered at an early stage during screening examinations. All children with suspected retinoblastoma should have a careful examination under anaesthetic (EUA) with indirect ophthalmoscopy and scleral indentation so that the whole retina is examined. A number of other disorders may simulate retinoblastoma (Table 11.2). In children in whom there is a clear view of the fundus there is rarely difficulty in arriving at the correct diagnosis at EUA. If there is doubt about whether a solitary lesion is retinoblastoma or not, a period of observation and repeat EUA will usually allow the correct diagnosis to be made; retinoblastoma usually shows rapid growth whereas other disorders such as astrocytic hamartoma do not. When there is an opaque vitreous at presentation

Table 11.1 Presenting symptoms and signs of retinoblastoma

Leucoria
Strabismus
Glaucoma
Orbital cellulitis
Unilateral mydriasis
Heterochromia
Hyphaema
Uveitis

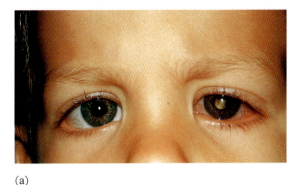

(a)

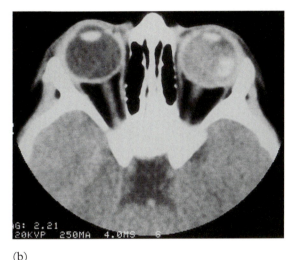

(b)

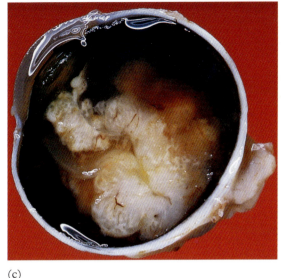

(c)

Figure 11.1    (a) Two-year-old boy who presented with a left convergent squint. The eye is inflamed and there is a white reflex in the pupil. (b) A CT scan of the orbit showed an intraocular mass with calcification confirming the diagnosis of retinoblastoma. The eye was enucleated and was shown to contain a large tumour (c)

(Figure 11.1(a)), diagnosis may depend upon the results of specialised investigations, although it is very important to examine the fellow eye carefully as the finding of small tumours will help to clinch the diagnosis of retinoblastoma.

## Investigation

It is helpful, when there is an intraocular mass or retinal detachment or an opaque vitreous preventing a clear view of the fundus, to perform a computed tomography (CT) or ultrasound scan of the eye and orbit to look for intraocular calcification (Figure 11.b). Calcification is common in retinoblastoma but rare in other disorders with a similar fundus appearance; it is important, however, to remember that the absence of calcification does not exclude retinoblastoma. In suspected inflammatory eye disease, toxoplasma and toxocara serology may be helpful. In children with large tumours that require enucleation, a bone-marrow examination and lumbar puncture should be performed at the time of surgery to exclude evidence of extraocular spread of tumour.

## Treatment

In most cases of unilateral retinoblastoma, the tumour is advanced at presentation and enucleation is the treatment of choice (Figure 11.1.c). In bilateral retinoblastoma the presenting eye usually has a large tumour which requires enucleation. The second eye will usually have smaller tumours which will respond to other treatment modalities. It is rare to have to

Table 11.2 Differential diagnosis of retinoblastoma

Tumours
    Astrocytic hamartoma
    Combined hamartoma of the retina and retinal pigment
        epithelium
    Choroidal haemangioma
    Dictyoma

Inherited disorders
    Retinal dysplasia
    Familial exudative vitreoretinopathy

Developmental disorders
    Persistent hyperplastic primary vitritis
    Coloboma
    Cataract
    Myelinated nerve fibres

Inflammatory disorders
    Toxocariasis
    Toxoplasmosis
    Endophthalmitis
    Orbital cellulitis

Others
    Retinopathy of prematurity
    Coats' disease
    Retinal detachment
    Vitreous haemorrhage

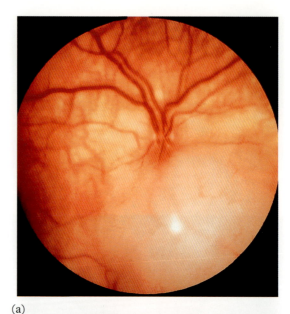

(a)

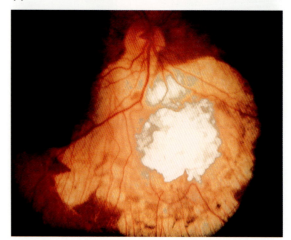

(b)

Figure 11.2 Retinoblastoma adjacent to disc (a) treatment with external beam shows good response to treatment with type 1 regression pattern (b) (Courtesy of Dr J Dudgeon)

perform bilateral enucleations at initial presentation but enucleation of an only eye may become necessary when there is recurrent tumour in an eye that has been treated with radiotherapy and/or chemotherapy. When enucleation is necessary it is important that the procedure is performed as atraumatically as possible and that at least 8–10 mm of optic nerve is obtained.

Retinoblastomas which do not require enucleation may be treated with chemotherapy, radiotherapy, laser or cryotherapy. Retinoblastoma is very radiosensitive and radiotherapy has been the mainstay of treatment over the last thirty years. Radiotherapy may be given as external beam or delivered focally to the tumour via radioactive plaques. External beam treatment is indicated for moderate-to-large tumours that are involving the macula or are close to the optic nerve (Figure 11.2a,b). A total of 3500 cGy is given in divided doses over a 3–4-week period using a temporal lens-sparing technique where possible.[5] Radioactive plaques may be used for solitary smaller (<15 mm) tumours

away from the disc and macula. More recently, systemic chemotherapy has been used to treat retinoblastoma (Figure 11.3a–c), but it is not yet clear whether the treatment regimes are as effective as radiotherapy or are associated with reduced side effects.[6] Smaller tumours or residual tumours remaining after chemotherapy may be treated with cryotherapy or laser photo-

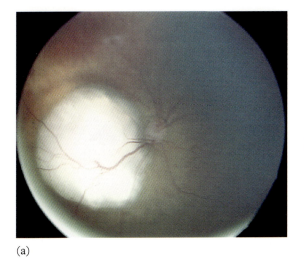

(a)

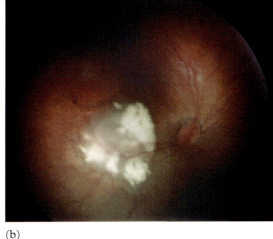

(b)

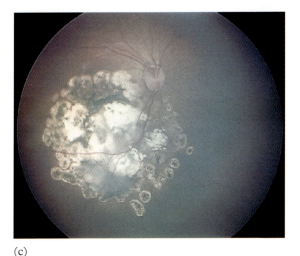

(c)

Figure 11.3   This large retinoblastoma involving the macular region of the right eye (a) was successfully treated with chemotherapy (b) and laser photocoagulation (c). (Courtesy of Mr M O'Keefe)

coagulation. Once retinoblastoma has spread outside the globe, the prognosis is very poor. Orbital extension of retinoblastoma may be treated with radiotherapy and intracranial spread with intrathecal chemotherapy, but the results of treatment are generally poor[7].

After treatment, children need careful follow up EUAs, firstly to assess the response to treatment and secondly to screen for new tumours or recurrences which can be promptly treated. Tumours which are treated with radiotherapy show a response about three weeks after starting treatment (Figure 11.4a,b) and three different types of regression pattern are recognised[4] (Table 11.3). It is often difficult initially to be sure that complete regression has occurred and close observation is necessary following treatment.

Infants with a close relative with retinoblastoma are examined at regular intervals (initially three monthly and later six monthly) under anaesthetic until the age of 3½ to 4 years when examinations are continued on an outpatient basis.

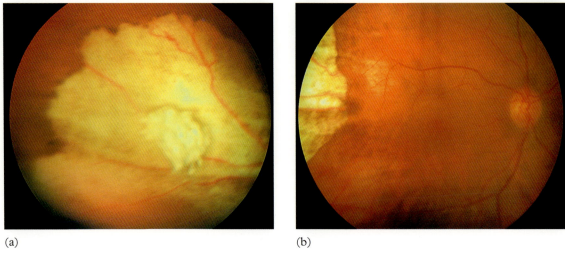

(a)                                                           (b)

Figure 11.4    (a, b) Regressed retinoblastoma in the right eye which responded well to external beam radiotherapy

## Prognosis

When treatment is undertaken in a specialist centre most children with retinoblastoma show a good response to treatment; there is a cure rate for the primary tumour in excess of 95%. However, there is still a significant mortality from pinealoblastoma and other secondary non-ocular tumours. These tumours are the leading cause of mortality in children with *RB1* mutations and the prevention and effective treatment of these tumours remains a major challenge.

## Genetic counselling

All individuals with bilateral or multifocal retinoblastoma and those with a family history have the genetic form of retinoblastoma.

Table 11.3  Regression patterns after radiotherapy for retinoblastoma[4]

| Type I | The tumours regress to a calcified mass resembling cottage cheese. |
|---|---|
| Type II | Reduction in size of the tumour which takes on a fish-flesh appearance. There is no calcification and there is often a ring of increased pigmentation around the regressed tumour. |
| Type III | In this regression pattern a combination of features in type I and type II are seen. |

Children of such affected individuals have a 50% chance of inheriting the *RB1* mutation and a 45% chance of developing retinoblastoma (the gene has a penetrance of 90%). About 15% of unilateral retinoblastoma is associated with germ line mutations of *RB1* and children of patients with sporadic unilateral retinoblastoma have a 7.5% risk of inheriting the *RB1* mutation. The risk of other relatives developing retinoblastoma can be calculated and Musarella and Gallie have published useful tables documenting the risk of developing retinoblastoma for relatives of patients with unilateral and bilateral retinoblastoma.[8] The identification of the *RB1* mutation allows precise molecular genetic diagnosis and molecular genetic investigations are cost effective as they reduce the number of screening examinations that need to be performed in at-risk family members.

## Ocular manifestations of leukaemia

Ophthalmological abnormalities in leukaemia usually occur as a result of infiltration of ocular or orbital tissues with leukaemia cells but may develop secondarily to other associated haematological abnormalities such as anaemia and hyperviscosity syndrome.[9,10] They may also occur as a complication of treatment or associated immunosuppression.[10] The eye may act as a sanctuary site for leukaemia cells during chemotherapy as the drugs may be prevented from access to the eye by the blood–ocular barriers and CNS irradiation spares the anterior segment of the eye to avoid inducing cataract. Subsequent relapse in thc anterior segment may be seen particularly in acute lymphoblastic leukaemia.

## Leukaemia infiltration

Leukaemia infiltration may affect the orbit and almost all the ocular tissues. Although post-mortem studies have shown that the choroid is the commonest site of involvement, this is rarely evident clinically. The retina is most often involved clinically as the retinopathy is usually identified as a result of routine fundus examination. Involvement of the optic nerve is uncommon but is usually associated with profound visual loss.

### Retinal involvement

Leukaemia retinopathy is seen in both acute and chronic forms of leukaemia but is more common in the former. The commonest finding is retinal haemorrhages which may occur in the nerve fibre layer or deeper in the retina (Figure 11.5a,b); subhyaloid haemorrhages are also common. Flame-shaped superficial haemorrhages may have a white centre which may represent fibrin, focal infarction or leukaemia deposit. Cotton-wool spots may also occur and are more common if there is associated anaemia or hyperviscosity. Nodular leukaemia infiltrates were common in the era before successful chemotherapy when they were usually seen at the late stage; they are rarely seen today (Figure 11.6a,b). Other findings which are more common in chromic leukaemias include vascular tortuosity, capillary closure, and microaneurysms.

### Orbital and optic nerve involvement

Orbital involvement in leukaemia may be due to infiltration of the soft tissues with leukaemia cells or to haemorrhage. It is more commonly seen in acute than chronic leukaemia. The usual presenting signs of leukaemia infiltration are proptosis, lid oedema, and conjunctival chemosis. Orbital involvement usually occurs in children with known leukaemia but may rarely be the presenting sign. Granulocytic sarcoma is a variant of myelogenous leukaemia in which the orbital deposit has a green discoloration (due to

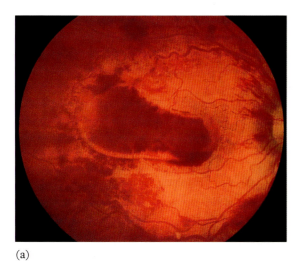
(a)

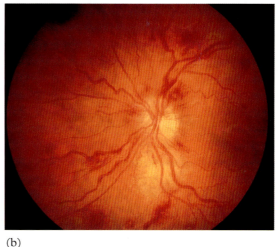
(b)

Figure 11.5   Right (a) and left (b) fundus of a young girl undergoing treatment for acute myeloid leukaemia showing multiple retinal and subhyaloid haemorrhages

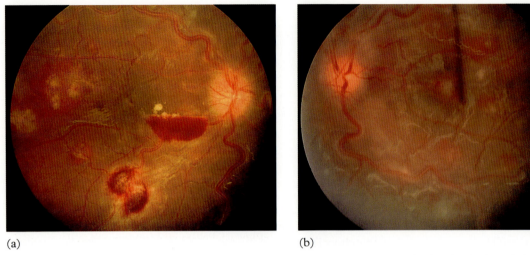

(a)                                                          (b)

Figure 11.6   Right (a) and left (b) fundus in a child with chronic myeloid leukaemia showing leukaemic infiltrates and retinal haemorrhages

the presence of a myeloperoxidase enzyme) on gross histopathological examination. The orbital tumour may be the first presenting sign of leukaemia.

Optic nerve involvement in leukaemia is seen mainly in children with acute lymphoblastic leukaemia and is now very uncommon. It occurs in two forms:

- If there is involvement of the optic nerve head, there is variable visual loss, optic disc swelling and peripapillary infiltrate and haemorrhage. The optic nerve head often has a thickened appearance.

- If the optic nerve involvement is predominantly retrolaminar, the presentation is usually with profound visual loss and there is variable disc swelling but without obvious infiltration.

Both forms respond well to radiotherapy.[9]

### Involvement of the anterior segment

Infiltration of the iris is usually seen in children with acute lymphoblastic leukaemia but is uncommon. It may be the first and rarely the only sign of relapse. The usual presentation is of unilateral or bilateral iridocyclitis which may be associated with a hypopyon. The iris shows diffuse or nodular thickening. The diagnosis can be confirmed by iris biopsy. The symptoms may be relieved with topical steroids but the underlying relapse requires treatment with chemotherapy combined with radiotherapy of the iris if necessary.

### Complications of treatment

Cytotoxic drugs may give rise to a number of complications including cranial nerve palsies (associated with vincristine) and corneal epithelial toxicity.[10] Systemic steroids may be associated with the development of posterior subscapsular cataract. Children who undergo bone-marrow transplantation may develop graft-versus-host disease[11] and are at risk of complications from total body irradiation including cataract and bone-marrow transplant retinopathy (Figure 11.7a,b).[12] Many children with leukaemia are immunosuppressed for periods during their treatment and this leaves them at risk of opportunistic infections which may involve the eye.

### Juvenile xanthogranuloma

Juvenile xanthogranuloma is a benign disorder of unknown aetiology in which there is abnormal

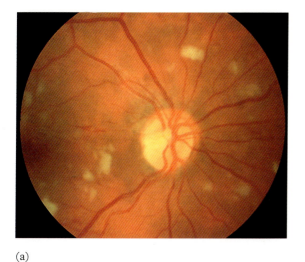
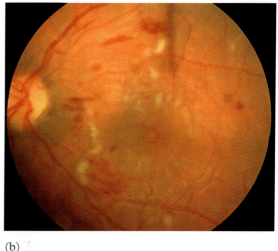

(a)                                           (b)

Figure 11.7   (a,b) Bone-marrow transplant retinopathy in a young girl given cranial irradiation including the eyes before bone-marrow transplantation. There are multiple haemorrhages and cotton-wool spots indicating an ischaemic retinopathy

proliferation of histiocytes. It usually presents as skin lesions in a young infant and these may occasionally be accompanied by ocular involvement.[13] The majority of infants with ocular involvement are less than one year of age and in most cases the involvement is confined to the iris. Ciliary body, epibulbar, orbital, and retinal involvement have been reported but are extremely rare. The usual presentation is with spontaneous hyphema (Figure 11.8) often with associated glaucoma but some infants are referred when a solitary iris tumour or heterochromia iridis is noted by the parents or on routine examination. In such

infants, a careful search should be made for skin lesions and the diagnosis may be confirmed by skin biopsy. Treatment is conservative as both the skin and eye lesions commonly undergo spontaneous regression. Ocular involvement is treated with topical or subconjunctival steroids with acetazolamide and a topical beta-blocker used if there is raised intraocular pressure. If there is no response to steroid, low-dose radiotherapy to the iris results in prompt regression.

## Vascular tumours of the retina

Two forms of vascular hamartomas, capillary haemangioma and cavernous haemangioma, may affect the retina.

### Capillary haemangioma

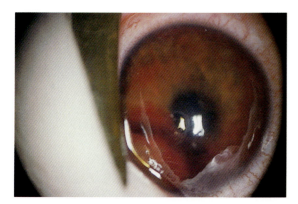

Figure 11.8   Spontaneous hyphaema in an infant caused by juvenile xanthogranuloma of the iris

Capillary haemangioma of the optic disc (Figure 11.9a,b) and peripheral retina (Figure 11.10a,b) may occur as isolated findings but are more commonly seen in association with Von Hippel–Lindau disease, an autosomal dominant cancer syndrome.[14] The angiomas are identical and their management is the same whether isolated or seen as part of this disease. This is discussed in detail in Chapter 17.

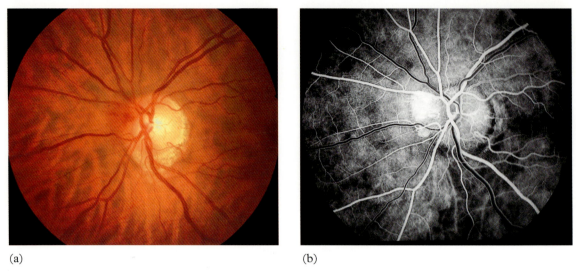

(a)                                                    (b)

Figure 11.9    Colour photograph (a) and fluorescein angiogram (b) of an optic disc angioma in a patient with von Hippel–Lindau disease

## Cavernous haemangioma

Cavernous haemangioma is a rare vascular hamartoma which is usually discovered as an incidental finding on routine fundoscopy (Figure 11.11). It is usually unilateral and seen as a grape-like cluster of dilated venous channels in the peripheral retina. Flow through the angioma is usually very slow and the angiomas fill slowly on fluorescein angiography. Most cavernous

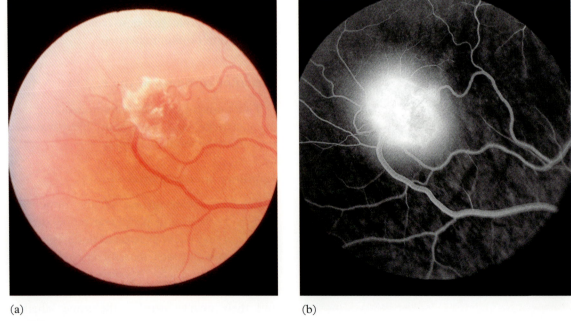

(a)                                                    (b)

Figure 11.10  Colour photograph (a) and fluorescein angiogram (b) of a peripheral retinal haemangioma in a patient with von Hippel–Lindau disease

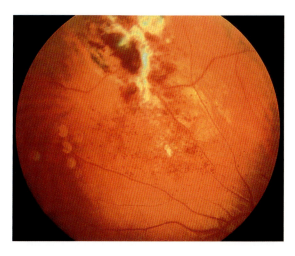

Figure 11.11 Asymptomatic cavernous haemangioma of the retina found on routine fundoscopy

angiomas do not require treatment. Occasionally there are associated cutaneous or CNS angiomas.

## Other ocular hamartomas

Iris hamartomas are a common finding in neurofibromatosis type 1 and retinal hamartomas are commonly seen in tuberose sclerosis and neurofibromatosis type 2. Retinal hamartomas may also occur in the absence of systemic disease. This subject is covered in detail in Chapter 17.

## References

1 Gallie B, Moore AT. Retinoblastoma. In: Taylor DSI, ed. Oxford: *Retinoblastoma in Paediatric Ophthalmology*, 2nd edn. Oxford: Blackwell Scientific Publications, 1997; 519–36.

2 Dunn JM, Phillips RA, Zhu X, *et al*. Mutations in the *RB1* gene and their effects on transcription. *Med Cell Biol* 1989; **9**: 4594–602.

3 Knudson AG. Mutation and cancer: statistical study of retinoblastoma. *Proc Natl Acad Science USA* 1971; **68**: 820–3.

4 Ellsworth RM. The practical management of retinoblastoma. *Trans Am Ophthalmol Soc* 1969; **67**: 462–534.

5 Hungerford J, Toma N, Plowman P, Kingston J. External beam radiotherapy for retinoblastoma: whole eye technique. *Br J Ophthalmol* 1995; **79**: 109–11.

6 Gallie BL, Budring A, De Boer G, *et al*. Chemotherapy with focal therapy can cure intraocular retinoblastoma without irradiation. *Arch Ophthalmol* 1996; **114**: 1321–30.

7 Hungerford J, Kingston J, Plowman N. Orbital recurrence of retinoblastoma. *Ophthalmic Paediatr Genet* 1987; **8**: 63–8.

8 Musarella MA, Gallie BL. A simplified scheme for genetic counselling in retinoblastoma. *J Paed Ophthalmol Strabismus* 1987; **24**: 124–5.

9 Rosenthal AR. Ocular manifestations of leukaemia. A review. *Ophthalmology* 1983; **90**: 899–905.

10 Kincaid MC, Green WR. Orbital and ocular involvement in leukaemia. *Surv Ophthalmol* 1983; **27**: 211–30.

11 Franklin RM, Kenyon K, Tutschka PJ, *et al*. Ocular manifestations of graft-vs-host disease. *Ophthalmology* 1983; **90**: 4–13.

12 Webster AR, Richards EM, Anderson JR, Moore AT. An ischemic retinopathy occurring in patients receiving bone marrow allografts and campath-IgG *Br J Ophthalmol* 1995; **79**: 687–91.

13 Zimmerman LE. Ocular lesions of juvenile xanthogranuloma. *Trans Am Acad Ophthalmol Otolaryngol* 1965; **69**: 412–42.

14 Webster AR, Maher ER, Bird AC, *et al*. A clinical and molecular genetic analysis of solitary ocular angioma. *Ophthalmology* 1999; **106**: 623–9.

# 12  Eyelid disorders

DAVID HUGHES

There are significant differences in the spectrum of diseases and disorders of the eyelids seen in children when compared to adults, i.e. there are a preponderance of congenital and developmental disorders. The situation is complicated in that disorders may be either isolated in the lid, or associated with orbital and/or systemic disease. Furthermore, eyelid disorders may affect visual development and this needs to be taken into account when managing children. The clinician must be aware that management involves the whole family in decision making. The needs of the child and the aspirations and desires of the parents must be balanced against the risks of surgery and general anaesthesia. Children may be difficult to examine, requiring considerable patience and skill.

Morphological differences between children and adults include: the wide nasal bridge which is often associated with epicanthic folds, both of which reduce with time as the face grows and develops; eyelid skin that is thicker; and lashes that are longer. From the technical point of view all the structures are smaller as will be the incisions. While local anaesthesia is the method of choice when treating conditions such as ptosis, it is not an option in most children. It is often kinder to close the skin with an adsorbable suture such as 7−0 polyglactin so avoiding the need for removal.

## Epiblepharon

This condition occurs in children and Orientals and is usually present in the lower lid. It consists of a horizontal fold of skin that rides up, pushing against the lashes such that they may rub against the cornea (Figure 12.1). The usual presenting symptom is epiphora; corneal abrasion is uncommon. It may be confused with entropion which is rare. Sometimes there are co-existent epicanthic folds and in a similar way both may resolve as the face grows. However, if this proves not to be the case or if there is significant keratitis, then surgery is indicated. Treatment consists of excising an ellipse of skin and orbicularis muscle from just below the lash line. Alternatively, and more simply, full thickness absorbable sutures can be placed through the lid from the lower fornix to the skinfold.

## Distichiasis

This is a congenital abnormality in which an additional row of lashes grows from the meibo-

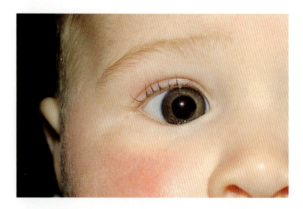

Figure 12.1   Epiblepharon. The lashes are inturning and touching the corneal epithelium

mian orifices. It occurs either as an isolated anomaly or inherited as an autosomal dominant trait. Methods of treatment include cryotherapy using a double freeze–thaw (–20°C) via a lid-splitting technique.[1,2] Alternatively, individual and occasional lash bulbs can be removed through vertical incisions in the tarsal plate.

Other conditions that affect the lashes include tarsal kink often requiring surgical correction[3] and ectopic lashes which are usually managed conservatively.

## Entropion

Congenital entropion is rare and should not be confused with epiblepharon. It may occur as a result of congenital absence of the tarsal plate or hypertrophy of the orbicularis muscle. Surgical correction includes ellipse excision of skin and orbicularis or everting sutures.

## Ectropion

Congenital ectropion usually occurs in association with other anomalies as in the blepharophimosis and Treacher Collins–Franceschetti syndromes. Rarely it occurs in isolation as the so-called Congenital Ectropion syndrome. In all of these conditions, the ectropion affects predominantly the lateral lower lid and treatment involves surgery for the associated anomalies with either skin grafting or transposition flaps to correct the ectropion. Cicatricial ectropion can occur as a result of trauma including chemical and thermal burns but also in skin diseases. In all of these situations the management is often complex with skin grafts required in all but the simplest of scars when scar excision and Z-plasty may be sufficient. In all cases of ectropion maintenance of corneal health is of paramount importance and special attention should be paid to this. Occasionally eyelids may spontaneously evert and remain in such a position resulting in discomfort and chemosis of the exposed conjunctiva. This most commonly occurs in children with Down syndrome although, rarely, it occurs after difficult childbirth. Spontaneous ectropion usually responds to lubricants and pressure pad although repositioning the lids and occasionally suture or skin grafting may be necessary.

## Epicanthic folds

These are semilunar folds of skin that stretch between the upper and lower lids in the inner canthal area. They may represent a normal racial characteristic or be a transient developmental anomaly (when they may be associated with a diagnosis of pseudoesotropia). Rarely they are pathological and inherited in an autosomal dominant manner. They may be associated with other pathology, for example blepharophimosis syndrome, telecanthus, and ptosis. Initial treatment is conservative, that is allowing time for normal facial growth to occur. There are a variety of procedures described for surgical correction from the Y-V to the more complicated double Z-plasty described by Mustarde. Telecanthus can usually be corrected at the same time.

## Telecanthus

Telecanthus describes a condition in which the distance between the two inner canthi is increased but the interpupillary distance remains within normal limits. These characteristics differentiate it from hypertelorism in which both are increased. As a simple rule of thumb the intercanthal distance is roughly half the interpupillary distance. Telecanthus may occur in isolation, with blepharophimosis or associated with developmental anomalies such as cleft palate. Rarely it results from trauma. Surgical correction involves debulking the medial canthus, which is combined with correction of any epicanthus and rarely by transnasal wiring.

## Coloboma of the eyelid

These represent developmental clefts and may occur as isolated defects or associated with cranial clefting disorders, for example Treacher

Collins syndrome. They can occur anywhere along the upper or lower lids and may be associated with dermoids and dermolipomas. Isolated colobomas are managed by excision and direct closure while complex ones are in the domain of the specialist craniofacial surgeon.

## Ptosis

### Aetiology

Ptosis in children occurs for a variety of reasons[4] and as a whole comprises about 50% of all ptosis. A classification of the causes of ptosis is given in Table 12.1. Despite the relatively long list, simple or congenital ptosis is the commonest cause and results from a dysplasia of the levator muscle. In general it occurs sporadically and is usually unilateral.

The mitochondrial myopathies may present with ptosis which is usually bilateral and associated with a slowly progressive reduction in

Table 12.1   Causes of childhood ptosis

Myogenic
    Simple (dysplastic)
    Blepharophimosis syndrome
    Myaesthenia gravis
    Mitochondrial myopathies
    Myotonic dystrophies

Aponeurotic

Neurogenic
    IIIrd nerve palsy
    Horner syndrome
    Marcus Gunn jaw wink phenomenon

Mechanical
    Inflammations
    Lid tumours
    Anophthalmia

Traumatic
    Surgery
    Foreign body
    Lid laceration or contusion
    Associated with nerve trauma

Pseudoptosis
    Hypotropia
    Microphthalmos

After Freuh.[4]

ocular excursions. Ptosis may also be the presenting feature of the infantile forms of myaesthenia.

Bilateral ptosis accompanied by limited ocular motility and strabismus is also seen in the Ocular Fibrosis syndrome. This is usually inherited as an autosomal dominant trait but sporadic cases which may represent new mutations are also seen.

Blepharophimosis syndrome describes a cluster of findings including ptosis, reduced palpebral width, epicanthus inversus, telecanthus, and lower-lid ectropion. It is inherited as an autosomal dominant trait the gene for which has recently been localised.[5] The epicanthus and telecanthus should be dealt with before the ptosis is corrected. This usually requires frontalis slings.

In contrast to the situation in adults, aponeurotic ptosis occurs only rarely in children and can be differentiated from dysplastic ptosis by the fact that the lid remains ptotic on down gaze.

IIIrd nerve palsies usually result from birth trauma and are characterised by ptosis, a variable degree of extraocular muscle weakness and an efferent pupillary abnormality. Congenital Horner syndrome is unilateral and characterised by 1–2 mm of ptosis, miosis, and iris hypochromia. The most common cause is probably brachial plexus trauma during birth. Marcus Gunn jaw winking phenomenon is caused by a synkinesis between branches of the Vth and the IIIrd cranial nerves. There is an apparent ptosis that is reduced or overcompensated during chewing or swallowing movements. This often results in a characteristic flutter of the upper lid, the so-called "winking".

Ptosis can occur with chronic conjunctivitis such as vernal conjunctivitis and has been documented after prolonged use of topical steroids. It may occur as a result of lid oedema either of inflammatory origin, for example allergy and chalazion, or from trauma. Scarring of either the anterior or posterior lamella may be associated with ptosis and often very difficult to treat. Occult foreign bodies have been the cause of ptosis that may resolve once they have been identified and removed. Ptosis has been reported after cataract surgery and there is some debate as to whether the lid speculum is the cause. Ptosis can occur in association with tumours such as capillary haemangiomas (Figure 12.2) and plexiform neurofibromas (Figure 12.3). Ptosis associated with anophthalmos or microphthalmos represents a particularly difficult surgical problem. It may result from orbital volume deficiency (Figure 12.4a,b), poor development and growth of the lids and orbit or surgical injury to the aponeurosis.

## Management

Management of ptosis includes examination to identify the particular cause. The visual acuity must be assessed to exclude amblyopia, which may occur in the absence of occlusion.[6] Measurements vital to the planning of surgery include the palpebral aperture, margin reflex distance, levator function, and skin crease height. The presence of a skin crease is an indicator of relatively good levator function.

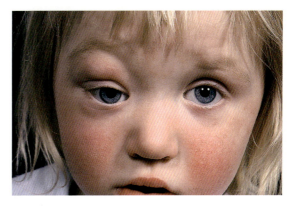

Figure 12.3   Plexiform neuroma of right upper lid resulting in a unilateral ptosis

Strabismus, aberrant regeneration of the IIIrd nerve, jaw winking and weakness of the superior rectus must be looked for and excluded. The presence of a Bell's phenomenon should be sought and if possible corneal sensation tested.

Surgical correction depends on the particular aetiology, degree of ptosis, and levator function (Table 12.2). Broadly speaking, there are three surgical methods:

- the Fasanella Servat procedure (tarso-müllerectomy),

- levator resection,

- frontalis sling procedures.

The Fasanella Servat operation is reserved for patients with Horner syndrome and frontalis slings for those with less than 5 mm of levator

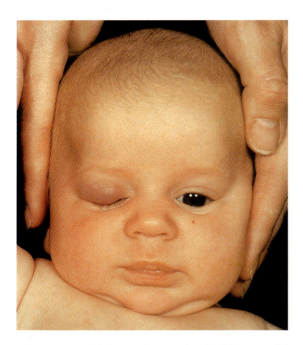

Figure 12.2   Right ptosis associated with upper-lid haemangioma

Table 12.2   Surgical correction of ptosis

| | |
|---|---|
| Fasanella Servat | Horner's syndrome only |
| Levator resection | >5 mm of levator function performed either via an anterior or posterior approach |
| Fox Pentagon | < 5 mm of levator function; very young children; synthetic materials can be used; interim measure prior to definitive procedure |
| Crawford procedure | < 5 mm of levator function; ideally performed with an autologous fascia lata |

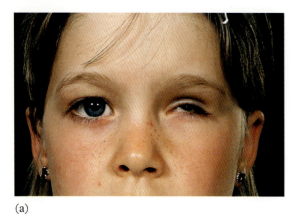
(a)

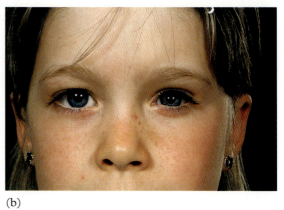
(b)

Figure 12.4  Left ptosis associated with microphthalmic eye (a). The lid position was related to a lack of orbital volume. A good result was achieved with a cosmetic shell (b)

function. The jaw winking phenomenon is usually managed either conservatively or by transecting both levator muscles and performing bilateral frontalis slings. The Fasanella Servat procedure is relatively simple and thus the temptation to perform it is great. In the past it was a very popular operation but unfortunately the results were often disappointing. With time, the indications have been clarified and it is now only performed in cases with Horner syndrome.[7]

**Levator resection**

The levator aponeurosis is repaired in rare cases of childhood disinsertion but more usually resected provided there is more than 5 mm of levator muscle function. The operation can be performed via:

- the skin (*anterior approach*) (Figure 12.5a,b)

  or

- the conjunctiva (*posterior approach*).

Both approaches give satisfactory results and the choice depends on the preference of the surgeon. Theoretically, the anterior approach allows the surgeon to perform a blepharoplasty but this is rarely required in children. The posterior approach allows for adjustment through early suture removal. The degree of resection depends on levator function; a simple rule of thumb is that

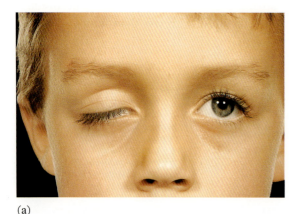
(a)

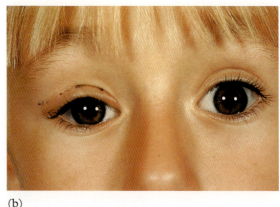
(b)

Figure 12.5  Severe right congenital ptosis treated with anterior levator resection. Preoperative appearance (a) and 10 days postoperatively (b)

if levator function is greater than 7 mm, the lid will rise after operation, less and it will fall. The aim therefore is to set the lid at the desired height (1–2 mm below the limbus) in cases with 7 mm of levator function, above this in those with less and below it in those with more. Table 12.3 gives a guide to resections after Beard.[8] Greater degrees of resection are required in cases with superior rectus weakness. An enhanced effect is gained by suturing the levator lower down the tarsal plate – although too low and the lid will pull away from the globe – and also by bringing the levator over Whitnall's ligament. The pitfalls of levator resection include overcorrection, undercorrection, asymmetrical lid crease, poor lid contour, and lash ptosis. Minor degrees of overcorrection may resolve, but if significant, a combination of suture removal and lid traction may be required. In most cases the complications are best dealt with by reoperation after healing has occurred.

**Frontalis sling**

The frontalis sling is a procedure in which the lid is attached to the brow using one of a variety of materials – synthetic,[9–12] stored human and, most satisfactorily, autologous material such as fascia lata.[13] The best results are achieved when there is preoperative evidence of frontalis overaction and with bilateral surgery. While autologous fascia lata is ideal, there is insufficient in the very young child. If there is a large abnormal head posture or risk of amblyopia, surgery can be carried out using a synthetic material such as 2/0 monofilament nylon suture (Figure 12.6a,b). Merselene mesh can be used but is associated with granuloma formation and due to its integrated is difficult to remove. While different

Table 12.3  Degrees of levator resection

| Degree of ptosis | Levator function | Degree of resection |
| --- | --- | --- |
| < 2 mm | > 10 mm | 10–13 mm |
| 3 mm | > 8 mm | 14–17 mm |
| | < 8 mm | 18–22 mm |
| > 4 mm | 5 mm | > 25 mm |

techniques have been described, the two that remain in current use are:

- Fox Pentagon procedure

- Crawford procedure

The Crawford procedure, using autologous fascia lata, probably gives the better results and the Fox Pentagon is reserved for younger children as it does not interfere with later surgery.

It is almost impossible to overcorrect a sling. However, care is needed with the siting of the skin crease incisions to avoid peaking, drooping and distraction of the lid from the globe. Minor degrees of asymmetry may resolve. If after a few months the lid is markedly overcorrected, the sling is cut, while the sling may need repeating for undercorrections. Before the operation, the parents and the patient need to be informed that there will be lid lag on down-gaze and that this is unavoidable.

## Infections and inflammations

### Chalazions

Chalazions and styes are fairly common in children and may indicate the presence of blepharitis. Chalazions are lipogranulomatous inflammations of the meibomian glands. In the acute phase there may be a considerable degree of surrounding inflammation. The chalazion may resolve, either partially or completely, with conservative measures such as hot compresses and topical antibiotics to prevent secondary infection. If a lump is persistent, or if there is an effect on vision, for example astigmatism, incision and curettage may be indicated, although in the young this requires a general anaesthetic.

### Styes

Styes represent acute infection of an eyelash follicle. There is acute discomfort but the stye usually points and discharges leading to resolution This may be accelerated by the epilation of the affected lash.

159

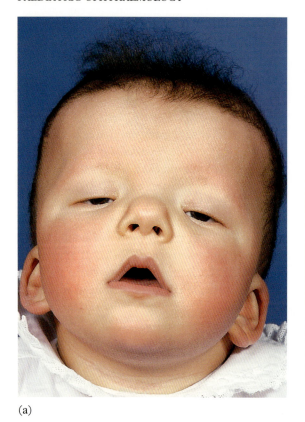

(a)

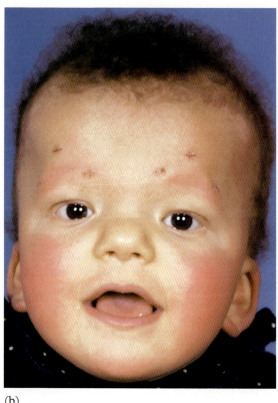

(b)

Figure 12.6  Young infant with chin-up head posture caused by bilateral ptosis (a). Her ptosis was corrected with a Crawford sling using merselene mesh (b)

## Viral warts

Viral warts may occur on the lids, as can the lesions of molluscum contagiosum (Figure 12.7). Both can be associated with a chronic follicular conjunctivitis. Viral warts can be excised, whereas the typical umbilicated lesions of molluscum should be curetted with diathermy to the core.

## Blepharochalasis

Blepharochalasis syndrome is a rare inflammatory condition of unknown aetiology. It is characterised by bouts of severe oedema over a period of years and may result in ptosis. This is caused by stretching and thinning of the aponeurosis. There is also associated dermatochalasis. Blepharoplasty and ptosis surgery may be required.

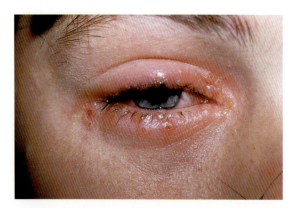

Figure 12.7    Molluscum lesions of upper and lower eye lids

## Tumours (see Chapter 13)

Tumours are rare in children. The most common are angiomas, dermoids and naevi.

## Angiomas

Capillary haemangiomas may be cutaneous, orbital or mixed. The cutaneous aspect is the characteristic strawberry naevus. Capillary haemangiomas usually undergo initial rapid expansion and, although the tumour is benign, there is often considerable parental anxiety. Most subsequently undergo complete regression. However, lid angiomas are commonly associated with astigmatic refractive errors and may give rise to anisometropic amblyopia. The main reasons for intervention are very large lesions associated with disfigurement and stimulus deprivation amblyopia. Treatment includes either perilesional depot steroid injections[14] or short courses of systemic steroids and occasionally, surgery.[15]

## Dermoids

Dermoid cysts are congenital inclusion cysts and often present as lid swelling related to the orbital rim. They occur most frequently in the upper outer quadrant and slowly increase in size with time (Figure 12.8). They should always be excised as they do not regress but can leak either spontaneously or following trauma. Rupture is associated with acute inflammation and possible sinus formation. Surgery at this stage is generally difficult.

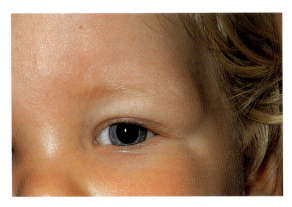

Figure 12.8    Dermoid cyst outer aspect left orbit

## Naevi

Pigmented naevi are flat or very slightly raised. Although usually small, they may slowly increase in size, showing some acceleration during puberty. Occasionally highly pigmented so-called "blue naevi" undergo fairly rapid growth over a few months. Management includes photographic documentation and observation. Surgical excision is usually only warranted to relieve anxiety and for cosmetic reasons.

## References

1 Anderson RL, Harvey JT. Lid splitting and posterior lamellar cryosurgery for congenital and acquired distichiasis. *Arch Ophthalmol* 1981; **99**: 631.
2 O'Donnell BA, Collin JRO. Distichiasis: management with cryotherapy to the posterior lamella. *Br J Ophthalmol* 1993; **77**: 289–92.
3 Price NC, Collin JRO. Congenital horizontal tarsal kink: a simple surgical correction. *Br J Ophthalmol* 1987; **71**: 204–6.
4 Freuh BR. The mechanistic classification of ptosis. *Ophthalmology* 1980; **87**: 1019.
5 Amati P, Chomel JC, Nivelon Cheavlier A, *et al*. A gene for blepharophimosis potosis epicanthus inversus syndrome maps to chromosome 3q23. *Hum Genet* 1995; **96**: 213–15.
6 Harrad RA, Graham CM, Collin JRO. Amblyopia and strabismus in congenital ptosis. *Eye* 1988; **2**: 625–7.
7 Sampath R, Saunders DC, Leatherbarrow B. The Fasanella Servat procedure: a retrospective study. *Eye* 1995; **9**: 124–5.
8 Beard C. *Ptosis*. St Louis: CV Mosby, 1981: 86–7.
9 Carter SR, Meecham WJ, Sieff SR. Silicone frontalis slings for the correction of blepharoptosis: indications and efficiency. *Ophthalmology* 1996; **103**: 623–30.
10 Sanders RA, Grice CM. Early correction of severe congenital ptosis. *J Pediatric Ophthalmol Strabismus* 1991; **28**: 271–3.
11 Manners RM, Tyers AG, Morris RJ. The use of Prolene as a temporary suspensory material for brow suspension in young children. *Eye* 1994; **8**: 346–8.
12 Downes RN, Collin JRO. The merselene mesh sling – a new concept in ptosis surgery. *Br J Ophthalmol* 1989; **73**: 1498.
13 Crawford JS. Repair of ptosis using frontalis muscle and fascia lata: a 20 year review. *Ophthalmol Surg* 1977; **8**: 31.
14 Kushner BJ. Local steroid therapy in adnexal haemangioma. *Ann Ophthalmol* 1979; **11**: 1005–9.
15 Walker RS, Custer PL, Nerad JA. Surgical excision of periorbital capillary haemangiomas. *Ophthalmology* 1994; **101**: 1333–40.

# 13  Paediatric lacrimal and orbital disease

GEOFFREY E ROSE

## Lacrimal disorders

In childhood, anomalies of the lacrimal system are almost exclusively those of lacrimal drainage and abnormalities of tear secretion, such as congenital alacrimia, need be considered only in children with persistent ocular surface disorders. Crocodile tears, in which epiphora occurs during eating is caused by aberrant innervation between the Vth and VIIth cranial nerves; in childhood it may be seen in association with other "miswiring" syndromes such as Duane's retraction syndrome and the Marcus Gunn jaw winking phenomenon.

## Congenital epiphora

The lacrimal drainage system forms from a cellular cord (the lacrimal anlage) lying in a paranasal facial cleft, this cord becoming a patent passage late in uterine life. Functional tear drainage is absent in about one-fifth of newborn children, this being assumed to be due to membranous obstruction at the lower end of the nasolacrimal duct. Such children commonly present soon after birth with a watering eye (Figure 13.1) with adherence of the lashes and with a mucoid discharge, this latter being frequently misinterpreted as infective conjunctivitis; true conjunctivitis, as opposed to a minor bacterial overgrowth in ocular debris, is uncommon. Nasolacrimal duct obstruction may occasionally be complicated by dacryocystitis. Rarely, a child is born with a lacrimal sac visibly

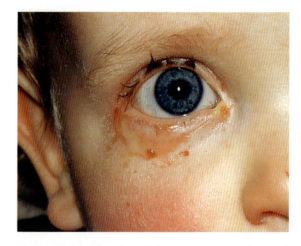

Figure 13.1    Watering sticky eye due to nasolacrimal duct obstruction

distended with blue-green fluid and mucus debris, a so-called "amniotocoele" (Figure 13.2).

Most children with nasolacrimal duct obstruction will spontaneously establish lacrimal drainage.[1] The parents should clean the lids and apply sac massage three or four times daily, both to empty any reservoir of tears and to encourage hydrodissection of the lumen of the duct; to be effective, massage must be firm and should indent the medial canthus onto the side of the nose. Massage is readily achieved whilst a baby is feeding and accelerates the natural resolution of the obstruction. Topical antibiotics are required only when a marked purulent discharge (not mucus) is accompanied by the ocular redness of conjunctivitis. Neonatal amniotocele almost always settles within a few days of birth, especially if massage is instituted.

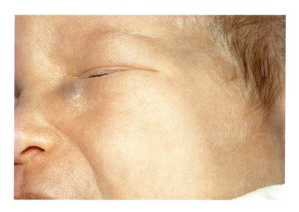

Figure 13.2    Amniotocele in a newborn infant

Although infantile dacryocystitis may cause surprisingly little systemic malaise, spreading infection necessitates a systemic antibiotic active against the common pathogens (streptococci, staphylococci, and *Haemophilus* species) (Figure 13.3). Early probing of the nasolacrimal duct is usually required once the infection has settled.

Probing of the nasolacrimal duct can be considered where symptoms of obstruction persist beyond 12–18 months of age and in the very rare cases of recurrent dacryocystitis before this time. The procedure should be carried out under general anaesthesia, care being taken to prevent infected material being washed into the airways. After examination for tarsal or corneal disease, a "0" probe should be passed gently into a canaliculus and advanced medially whilst

keeping the eyelid tight (Figure 13.4a,b); if the lid is not kept taut, the canaliculus buckles at the tip of the probe and canalicular damage, with later occlusion, may result. Near the sac, the probe should be redirected slightly anteriorly to follow the angulation of the common canaliculus as it passes through the lacrimal sac fascia; this alteration of canalicular direction is largely unrecognised and, because of this, most infantile common canalicular obstruction may be iatrogenic. The passage of a probe along a taut canaliculus should be effortless and, under no circumstances, should the probe be forced. Once in the sac, the bony stop of the medial wall of the lacrimal sac fossa can be felt and the probe should be redirected inferiorly into the nasolacrimal canal; passage through a membranous obstruction is often accompanied by a palpable "pop". Patency may be confirmed, by contact with the probe tip under the inferior turbinate or by irrigation of a small quantity of fluid through the lacrimal system, and a topical antibiotic administered.

Persistent symptoms may be treated by repeated probings and, if these fail, dacryocystorhinostomy by an experienced paediatric lacrimal surgeon will cure almost all cases. Although silicone intubation, with or without infracture of the inferior turbinate, is widely advocated, there is little or no evidence that it has a greater success rate than repeated probing alone and may also carry a greater risk of canalicular injury.

## Lacrimal drainage anomalies

Anomalies arise from a failure of the lacrimal anlage to develop or from the development of accessory structures; such anomalies may very rarely be accompanied by other developmental abnormalities, particularly those involving the cranium or the facial midline. Lacrimal drainage agenesis typically occurs in the proximal canaliculus or the nasolacrimal canal and solitary agenesis of the common canaliculus is almost unknown. If symptomatic, canalicular agenesis

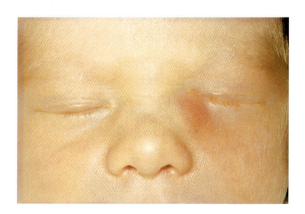

Figure 13.3    Six-week-old infant with acute dacrocystitis

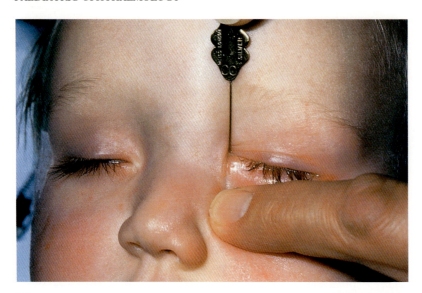

(a)

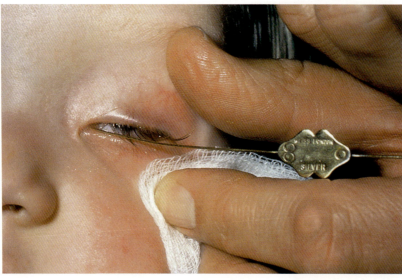

(b)

Figure 13.4   Probing of the nasolacrimal duct (a). To prevent damage to the canaliculus, the eyelid should be held taut whilst the probe is advanced along the lower canaliculus (b). (Courtesy of Mr G Rose)

warrants dacryocystorhinostomy with retrograde exploration of the canalicular system and canaliculostomy at preschool age; if this does not control symptoms, placement of a Lester Jones canalicular bypass tube may be required in the teenage years.[2] Agenesis of the nasolacrimal canal is very effectively treated by dacryocystorhinostomy.

Congenital lacrimal fistula, often arising from the common canaliculus and sited below the medial canthal tendon (Figure 13.5a,b), is an accessory epithelial-lined duct developing from the lacrimal anlage. If draining tears, the child should have the nasolacrimal duct probed; if symptoms persist, dacryocystorhinostomy with excision of the fistula should be considered.[3] Under no circumstances should cautery be applied to a fistula, as this may damage the common canaliculus.

## Orbital disease

Paediatric orbital disease is rare. It may be due to developmental abnormalities of the orbit or,

164

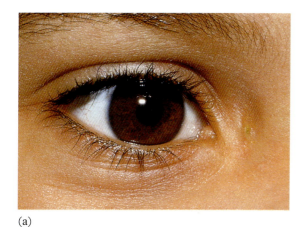

(a)

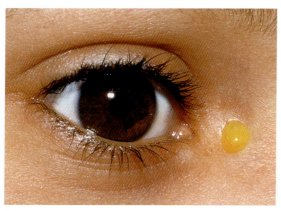

(b)

Figure 13.5   (a) Congenital lacrimal fistula (arrow), (b) with spontaneous drainage of fluorescein-stained tears. (Courtesy of Mr G Rose)

less commonly, acquired as a result of tumour, infection or orbital inflammation. Developmental abnormalities may be confined to the orbit or form part of a more widespread craniofacial malformation, when the orbital abnormalities are usually bilateral. In this latter group, there may be shallow orbits giving rise to proptosis or a disturbance in the relationship between the two orbits. The orbits may be widely separated (hypertelorism) or too close together (hypotelorism). Acquired orbital disease presents either with a periorbital swelling or with signs of an intraorbital orbital mass – proptosis, limited ocular motility, and visual loss. Most acquired disease in childhood is unilateral and

needs urgent investigation and management, preferably in a specialised unit.

The causes of proptosis and orbital disease in childhood vary in the different published series and in general reflects bias in the patient selection. For example, series based on pathological specimens will underestimate the importance of infectious causes and benign tumours, such as haemangioma, which rarely require biopsy. Furthermore series from large eye hospitals will have a different spectrum of disease from those from paediatric hospitals or neurological centres. It is, however, evident from the published data that the commonest causes of orbital disease in childhood are infection (preseptal and orbital cellulitis) and developmental abnormalities of the orbit (Table 13.1). Tumours are a less common cause and most are benign. Malignant tumours of the orbit are fortunately rare. Most children present with unilateral disease, but bilateral proptosis is common in the craniofacial malformations and may also be seen in inflammatory or, less commonly, neoplastic disease (Table 13.2).

## Developmental anomalies of the orbit

Anomalies of orbital development generally arise from aberrations in the embryonic craniofacial folding and present as clefts, choristomas, hamartomas or as craniofacial syndromes. Development of the orbital bones is also abnormal in congenital anophthalmia (see Chapter 5) and after orbital radiotherapy or enucleation in infancy.

Table 13.1   Common causes of orbital disease in childhood

Inflammatory disease
  Preseptal and orbital cellulitis
  Non-specific inflammatory disease
  Langerhans cell histiocytosis
  Thyroid eye disease

Vascular hamartomas
  Capillary haemangioma
  Lymphangioma

Dermoid cysts

Developmental abnormalities

Table 13.2 Causes of bilateral proptosis in childhood

Developmental abnormalities (shallow orbits)
  Crouzon syndrome
  Apert syndrome
  Pfeiffer syndrome
  Oxycephaly

Inflammation
  Dysthyroid eye disease
  Langerhans cell histiocytosis

Optic nerve glioma

Metastatic disease
  Neuroblastoma
  Leukaemia

## Orbital choristomas

Orbital or periorbital dermoids are the commonest anomaly and are often noted in early infancy as a rounded mass in the vicinity of the superotemporal rim of the orbit[4,5] (Figure 13.6). If readily mobile, further investigation is unwarranted and intact excision, through a small brow or eyelid incision at preschool age, is curative. If a lesion unexpectedly extends beyond the scope of a surgeon's experience, exploration should be abandoned rather than performing partial excision with the disastrous consequences of severe recurrent inflammation and fistula formation. Fixed dermoids should be explored by a surgeon experienced in surgery of the orbit and temporalis fossa, as many of these lesions extend through the lateral orbital wall[4] (Figure 13.7). Preoperative neuroradiologic imaging allows the true extent of the dermoid to be identified and allows the appropriate surgical approach to be planned.

Dermolipomas, like dermoids, are choristomas often noted in infancy which present as a mass at the lateral palpebral aperture or with irritation and discharge, due to hairs on the lesion (Figure 13.8). If symptomatic, microsurgical removal of dysplastic (dermal) conjunctiva and debulking of the lipoma anterior to the orbital rim is indicated; excessive surgery may lead to diplopia, ptosis or dry-eye – with considerable medico-legal implications.

## Orbital hamartomas

Paediatric orbital vascular hamartomas are common, and may present at any time from birth to adulthood. Two main types are recognised:

- Capillary haemangiomas

- Lymphangiomas

They are readily distinguished by their clinical appearance and natural history.

## Capillary haemangioma

Capillary haemangioma, or "strawberry naevus", usually presents as a rapidly enlarging

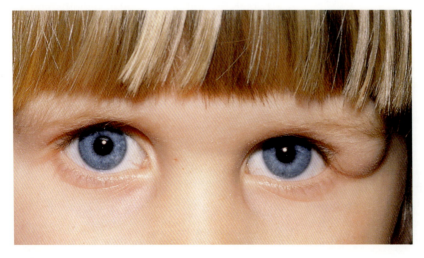

Figure 13.6 Left orbital dermoid, as commonly sited at the superotemporal rim. (Courtesy of Mr G Rose)

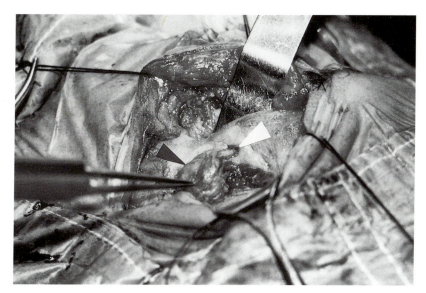

Figure 13.7 The intraorbital and extraorbital (dark arrow) components of a complex dermoid are in continuity through a hole in the lateral orbital rim (light arrow). (Courtesy of Mr G Rose)

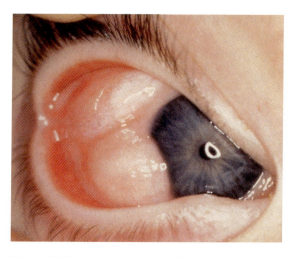

Figure 13.8 Congenital dermolipoma, in a typical location. (Courtesy of Mr G Rose)

orbital or preseptal mass in early infancy. In some cases, the vascular abnormality is present at birth, but in the majority the haemangioma will appear during the first 3–6 months of life. There is usually a rapid growth phase followed by a slowing of growth and then stabilisation before subsequent slow regression. The haemangioma typically has a high blood flow and most commonly involves the upper lid (Figure 13.9a,b). It can cause amblyopia either as a result of pupillary-occluding ptosis or, more

commonly, due to anisometropia related to astigmatism caused by distortion of the globe.[6] In this age group, it is important to exclude rhabdomyosarcoma as another, more serious, cause of a rapidly expanding mass. Neuroradiologic imaging and blood-flow measurements by Doppler ultrasonography are useful in cases where the distinction cannot be made clinically and biopsy of the lesion is rarely necessary. Extensive haemangioma may rarely be associated with a coagulation deficit caused by entrapment of platelets in the extensive vascular lesion (Kasabach Merritt syndrome).

Although capillary haemangiomas undergo spontaneous involution, this is in general slow and active treatment is required if visual development is compromised. It is very important that the visual acuity and refraction are carefully monitored. Corneal astigmatism, often with an oblique axis, is common with orbital haemangiomas, with the steeper meridian in the direction of the haemangioma. Any significant anisometropia and astigmatic refractive error should be corrected and occlusion therapy started if there is evidence of amblyopia. If there is a high degree of refractive error, or if the angioma prevents the wearing of spectacles or occludes the pupil, treatment to hasten

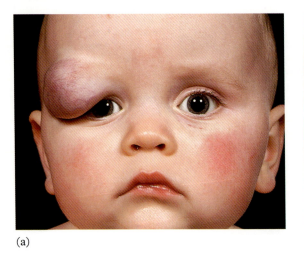
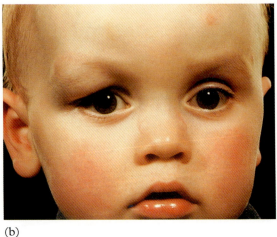

(a)                                                                                                    (b)

Figure 13.9    Large haemangioma of right upper lid (a) which was associated with astigmatism and amblyopia. The angioma was treated with intralesional steroid with a good result (b)

regression is indicated. Injection of steroids into the angioma (for example, 40 mg depot methylprednisolone) and around it (for example, 4 mg of soluble dexamethasone) will slow the growth, or induce regression, of most lesions (Figure 13.9a,b). This regime may be repeated every six weeks for two or three sessions and is associated with relatively few complications. Children with extensive haemangiomata with orbital involvement may be treated with a short course of systemic steroid, which similarly hastens regression. In rare circumstances, consideration might be given to treatment with systemic interferon or to early surgery, although there is a risk of severe haemorrhage with surgery. Surgery is unnecessary in the majority of children with haemangioma and, if indicated, is usually delayed until after the age of 8 years when any residual haemangioma that has failed to regress can be excised, together with excess skin, to improve the cosmetic appearance.

**Orbital varices (lymphangioma)**

Primary varices of the orbit have a very slow flow and may not present until adulthood. Childhood presentations include intermittent proptosis during crying or straining and sudden onset proptosis due to spontaneous orbital haemorrhage; venous anomalies may rarely extend to involve the ipsilateral half of the face, the palate or the intracranial vasculature (Figures 13.10 and 13.11). "Lymphangioma" is part of a spectrum of venous anomalies, in which some channels are isolated from a blood supply and accumulate lymph-like, protein-filled cysts; haemorrhage into these cysts may occur causing worsening proptosis and, in some cases, cause compressive optic neuropathy.[7,8] Histopathologically, the lesion is seen to be composed of endothelial lined channels filled with fluid; lymphoid tissue is also present and this may explain why some patients with orbital involvement complain of worsening proptosis during periods of upper respiratory-tract infections.

The diagnosis of orbital lymphangioma is usually evident after careful assessment of the clinical findings in those lesions with a superficial component. It may be more problematic in children who present with sudden onset proptosis in whom the lymphangioma is confined to the orbit. The presence of a soft-tissue mass, the lack of bone destruction and the demonstration of blood filled cysts on computed tomography (CT) scan and magnetic resonance imaging (MRI) should allow the diagnosis to be made.

Superficial venous anomalies are relatively readily excised, but the deeper lesions are inter-mixed with normal orbital vasculature and their excision is difficult and carries significant risk. Compressive optic neuropathy necessitates urgent surgical exploration and release of blood from tense intraorbital "chocolate" cysts.

### Orbital structural anomalies

The configuration of the orbit may be affected by facial clefting, due to arrested development or amniotic bands, or by anomalies of cranial development; with these diverse anomalies, it should be recognised that abnormalities are not only in the orbital bones, but also in the soft tissues.[9] Although there are a very large number of different disorders resulting in abnormal craniofacial and orbital development, they have in common a number of ophthalmological abnormalities including strabismus, high refractive errors, amblyopia, and exophthalmos due to shallow orbits. Optic atrophy is relatively common and may be caused by chronically raised intracranial pressure or occur as a result of abnormalities of optic canal structure; in many cases the cause is unknown. When there is marked orbital shallowing and the proptosis is extreme, corneal exposure keratitis may occur.

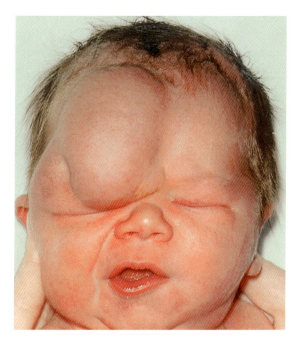

Figure 13.10   Young infant with large periorbital lymphangioma. It was partially excised through a bicoronal scalp incision in infancy to allow normal visual development

Recent trends are towards the earlier correction of osseous abnormalities by craniofacial surgery, this encouraging a better soft-tissue modelling during childhood growth. The ophthalmologist should monitor visual development and ensure that any refractive errors are corrected and amblyopia treated with occlusion therapy. Strabismus is common and is often complex; extraocular muscle surgery should be deferred until all craniofacial surgery has been completed.

Lacrimal and eyelid anomalies are often present with facial clefts and necessitate staged, or combined, reconstruction of the eyelids or lacrimal drainage systems. Clefts may also be associated with intraorbital encephalocele or nasal midline dermoids or encephaloceles.

### Orbital tumours

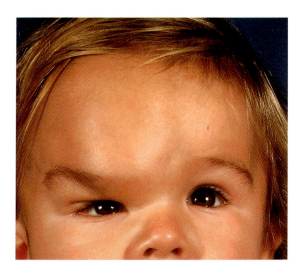

Figure 13.11   The same child aged 4 years. Further surgery will be needed

Childhood orbital tumours are very rare, but should be recognised and referred early for specialist management, as even benign tumours may lead to severe and life-threatening problems.

**Benign tumours**

Benign orbital tumours in children are commonly those of the optic nerve:

• Glioma

• Meningioma

The clinical behaviour of these two types of primary optic nerve tumour are, however, very different. Optic nerve glioma behaves very much like a slowly-growing hamartoma, with stable or only slowly progressive visual loss and does not require active management in the majority of cases.[10] Optic nerve sheath meningioma, in contrast, is associated with progressive loss of vision and has a worse visual prognosis; it is fortunately rare.

**Optic nerve glioma** Anterior visual pathway gliomas are a common finding in neurofibromatosis type 1 (NF1) and are also seen in otherwise normal children. In NF1, the gliomas are often bilateral and multifocal and are thought to have a more benign biological behaviour with a better visual prognosis. This may, in part, reflect the fact that gliomas in NF1 are often identified at an early stage by routine neuroradiological imaging, whereas in children without NF1 gliomas are only detected once proptosis or reduced vision is apparent. Since gliomas are common in NF1, it is important that a careful search is made for other evidence of NF1 in children with gliomas (see Chapter 17).

The clinical presentation of optic nerve gliomas is with proptosis, strabismus or visual failure;[10] visual loss is often mild and many children are discovered to have an optic neuropathy after the detection of reduced vision at a routine eye test. Other signs of optic neuropathy including reduced colour vision, central scotoma and optic disc swelling or more commonly atrophy, are also seen. MRI or CT scanning shows a typical fusiform swelling of the nerve (Figure 13.12).[11]

Most children will not require active treatment. Visual function (including testing of visual fields and colour vision) should be carefully monitored on a regular basis. In infants and young children, where tests of visual acuity may be unreliable, visual evoked potential (VEP) studies are helpful in monitoring optic nerve function. Magnetic resonance imaging is particularly suited to showing the expanded optic nerve, chiasm or tracts, and serial MRI scans should be used to follow the course of the disease.[11]

The management of the small minority of children who show progression is problematic. Chemotherapy and radiotherapy may be used, but at present there is no evidence to suggest which approach is better. Surgical excision is rarely necessary, but may be indicated when there is marked proptosis in a blind eye. Surgery may also need to be considered in progressive disease when there is an isolated optic nerve glioma which threatens to involve the chiasm with further progression. It is usually possible to spare the globe to give a better cosmetic result.

**Optic nerve sheath meningioma** Primary optic nerve meningioma of childhood is a sight-threatening disease with a marked tumour-related morbidity and mortality. In contrast to childhood glioma, it causes a progressive loss of vision by

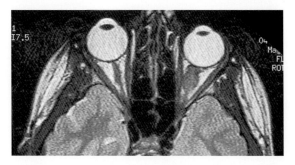

Figure 13.12 MRI scan showing left optic nerve glioma

compression of the optic nerve within its sheath and may extend, *en plaque* through the optic canal or superior orbital fissure, onto the meninges of the middle-cranial fossa and sphenoid. Radiological investigation generally shows a fairly uniform thickening of the optic nerve on the affected side, with flecks of calcification in many lesions; MRI is particularly helpful, often showing an optic nerve of normal calibre (in contrast to glioma) and the extent of intracranial extension along the surface of the bone. Optic nerve meningiomas in childhood have a propensity for intracranial spread, at which site the *en plaque* spread of tumour along the meninges is hard to eradicate and may lead to fatal intracranial disease. Paediatric primary optic nerve meningioma should, if progressive, be considered for treatment by complete removal of the affected optic nerve through a neurosurgical approach, with ablation of all affected tissue on the sphenoid surface, including that in the optic canal.

**Benign bony tumours of the orbit** A number of rare benign tumours of bone may affect the orbit and may give rise to cosmetic deformity or affect visual function if there is involvement of the bony foramina.

Fibrous dysplasia is an uncommon disorder of unknown aetiology in which normal bone is replaced by a cellular fibrous stroma containing islands of immature woven bone.[12] The disease may be confined to the orbit or involve other bones of the skull; it usually remains unilateral. The usual presentation is with involvement of the orbital roof, which gives rise to proptosis and downward displacement of the globe. Maxillary involvement causes upward displacement of the globe and epiphora due to occlusion of the nasolacrimal duct. Visual loss due to optic nerve compression may complicate sphenoidal involvement. CT scan usually shows sclerotic bone lesions, but occasionally there may be a significant cystic component. The management of this disorder is initially conservative but if there is evidence of progression then radical

surgery with craniofacial reconstruction, performed in a specialist craniofacial unit, is the treatment of choice.

A number of other rare benign disorders including aneurysmal bone cyst, osteopetrosis and osteoblastoma may involve the orbital walls in childhood. These have recently been reviewed by Lyons and Rootman.[13]

### Malignant tumours

Newer regimes for chemotherapy and radiotherapy have greatly improved the prognosis for paediatric malignant disease which, in the past, carried a very poor prognosis. The prognosis for malignant orbital tumours had shown a similar improvement but to achieve the optimum result, it is important that children are referred early to a specialist centre where a multidisciplinary approach involving a paediatric oncologist, radiotherapist, ophthalmologist and other specialists can be followed.

**Rhabdomyosarcoma** Rhabdomyosarcoma is the commonest childhood primary orbital malignancy and presents as a rapidly progressive proptosis or as an "orbital cellulitis" that does not settle on treatment; such an "inflammatory" pattern of presentation must be recognised, as it is a common cause for delay in treatment. In infancy, both rhabdomyosarcoma and capillary haemangioma may present with rapidly increasing proptosis, but may be differentiated by the clinical and radiological characteristics and by blood-flow studies. If any doubt about the diagnosis persists, surgical exploration and biopsy is indicated. In most cases, orbital rhabdomyosarcoma presents in later childhood and unless there is an atypical presentation, the clinical picture and radiological abnormalities allow the diagnosis to be made quickly (Figure 13.13a,b). A CT scan of the orbit allows the extent of the tumour to be defined; the tumour is usually confined to the orbit in early disease but may later show local spread to involve anterior or middle-cranial fossa. Once the extent of the tumour has been localised on a CT scan, it is

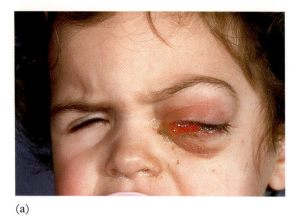

(a)

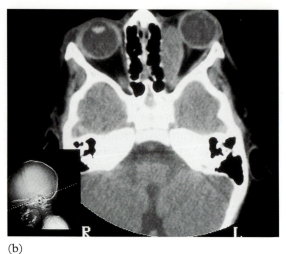

(b)

Figure 13.13  Left orbital rhabdomyosarcoma (a). CT scan (b) showed left medial orbital mass

important to perform a biopsy so that a histological diagnosis can be made.

The aim of the treatment is to achieve cure with minimum morbidity. For this reason chemotherapy has become the first-line treatment, with radiotherapy and surgery used for tumours that fail to respond.[14] Radiotherapy is associated with a significant risk of complications including reduced orbital growth, radiation keratitis, dry-eye syndrome, cataract, and radiation retinopathy.

**Langerhans cell histiocytosis (Histiocytosis X)**  Langerhans cell histiocytosis, a rare disorder characterised by proliferation of abnormal histiocytes, may also involve the orbit. It is not, strictly speaking, a malignant disorder, but is due to a clonal proliferation of Langerhans cells which then infiltrate a variety of different tissues. Historically, three forms of the disorder have been recognised.

- *Eosinophilic granuloma* is a disease confined to a single tissue, usually bone, and has a good prognosis.

- *Hands–Schuller–Christian disease* is a chronic form of the disorder in which there is a characteristic triad of diabetes insipidus (due to

pituitary involvement), proptosis and lytic lesions of the skull.

- *Letterer–Siwe disease* involves infantile onset of a multisystem disease.

It is now evident that these three disorders form part of a spectrum of the same disease.

Orbital involvement occurs in 20% of cases of Langerhans cell histiocystosis; the usual presentation is with proptosis in a child with known Langerhans cell histiocystosis but may occur as isolated orbital involvement.[15] There is almost always bony involvement and lytic lesions are commonly seen on a CT scan. In children with systemic involvement, the diagnosis can be made by biopsy of another more accessible site, but orbital biopsy is necessary in isolated orbital disease. Children with isolated orbital disease have a good prognosis; the disease may regress spontaneously or following biopsy or may respond to intralesional steroids. The prognosis in those children with systemic disease is poorer.

**Other malignant diseases**  Other primary malignancies of the orbit are extremely rare, although sarcomas may present as young as infancy and some haematological malignancies may present solely within the orbit. Secondary orbital malignant disease may arise by direct spread from nasosinus tumours (such as olfactory neuroblastoma or sinus sarcomas), from orbital spread of retinoblastoma or by metastasis, as with neuroblastoma or the leukaemias. Almost all such tumours present with proptosis increasing over a few weeks, often in a child that is systemically unwell. The mainstay of treatment is chemotherapy once a biopsy has confirmed the correct diagnosis.

## Orbital inflammation

### Infective orbital inflammation

Inflammation within the childhood orbit is generally due to the spread of infection from the neighbouring sinuses, although rare causes include leakage of lipid contents from dermoid cysts, paraneoplastic inflammation, orbital manifestation of systemic vasculitides or target-specific orbital inflammation, such as myositis. Idiopathic orbital inflammatory disease is extremely rare in children and should never be assumed to be the cause of inflammatory signs, without full and appropriate investigation of the child.

**Preseptal cellulitis** Bacterial infection in the tissues anterior to the orbital septum (preseptal cellulitis) is more common than true orbital cellulitis; it may be associated with lid trauma, upper respiratory tract and sinus infections or occur secondarily to localised lid or lacrimal sac infection.[16] The commonest organisms involved are *Staphylococcus aureus* and beta-haemolytic streptococci. *Haemophilus infuenzae* was a common cause in young children until the introduction of the *Haemophilus influenzae* type-B (HiB) vaccine; it is now rarely seen as a cause of preseptal cellulitis.[17]

The usual clinical presentation of preseptal cellulitis is with lid oedema in a child with a recent upper respiratory-tract infection. There is often a high temperature and the child is generally unwell. In contrast to orbital cellulitis, there is no proptosis, the vision is normal, and ocular motility is normal.[16] Young infants with preseptal

cellulitis should be admitted, cultures taken from blood, upper respiratory tract and conjunctiva, and treatment started with a systemic broad-spectrum antibiotic such as a third-generation cephalosporin. Older children who are not systemically unwell can usually be managed on an outpatient basis with oral antibiotics.

**Infective orbital cellulitis** Infective orbital cellulitis arises almost exclusively by the spread of preceding bacterial infection from the paranasal sinuses; the ethmoidal sinuses are the commonest source, the maxillary sinuses less so and almost never the sphenoidal or frontal sinuses.[18] Due to the preceding sinusitis, children with orbital cellulitis generally have a history and signs of coryza, nasal discharge, systemic malaise, and fever. Mild swelling of the eyelids and slight conjunctival redness are the first signs of impending orbital infection; without prompt treatment, these signs progress rapidly to marked eyelid swelling, conjunctival chemosis, tense proptosis with global restriction of eye movement and impairment of optic nerve function, with a reduced acuity and development of a relative afferent pupillary defect (Figure 13.14).

If a child with a history of coryza presents with mildly swollen eyelids and ocular redness, it is prudent to immediately treat the child with high doses of an oral antibiotic of appropriate spectrum for respiratory pathogens (such as a second-generation cephalosporin). A single radiograph of the sinuses will generally show opacification of the ethmoid sinuses and confirms the likely diagnosis, although under no circumstances should acquisition of a radiograph delay the start of treatment. The child should be reviewed within 24 hours, at which time the symptoms and the signs of orbital involvement should be improving.

Whenever there is major systemic illness or marked eyelid swelling, conjunctival chemosis, proptosis, reduced ocular motility or optic nerve impairment, the child should receive immediate intravenous antibiotic therapy and possibly rehydration; a third-generation cephalosporin at high

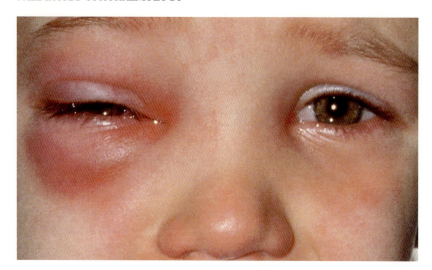

Figure 13.14 A child with infectious orbital cellulitis presenting with pain, redness and swelling of the eyelids, conjunctival chemosis and restricted eye movements. (Courtesy of Mr G Rose)

dosage is generally sufficient to give rapid improvement. An antibiotic directed specifically against anaerobes, such as metronidazole, is not usually required in children. Prompt treatment is essential if the complications of orbital cellulitis are to be avoided (Table 13.3). The possibility of undetected diabetes mellitus should be excluded on admission and the child later screened for underlying diseases. Clinical signs should be monitored several times daily until a definite improvement is observed. Where raised orbital pressure causes significant impairment of vision (with a relative afferent pupillary defect) or worsening vision, the orbit must be explored for release of pus or gas (Figure 13.15).

Orbital exploration in children with infective cellulitis and visual failure, whilst preferably performed by an orbital surgeon, should never be delayed as recovery of vision is rare after neglected profound visual impairment. Where rapidly deteriorating vision necessitates urgent surgery, the direction of globe displacement can give a valuable indication of the site for primary

Table 13.3  Complications of orbital cellulitis

Subperiosteal or orbital abscess
Meningitis
Brain abscess
Cavernous sinus thrombosis
Optic neuropathy
Central retinal artery occlusion
Septicaemia

exploration. The medial extraperiosteal space should, in general, be the first site, with the inferior extraperiosteal and intraperiosteal spaces being examined if medial orbitotomy does not lead to release of infected material and a reduced intraorbital pressure; after surgery, free drainage of the spaces should be maintained with appropriate surgical drains. Otolaryngological surgeons are generally familiar with exploration of the medial extraperiosteal space and the assistance of such a colleague not only increases the likelihood of successful exploration, but also allows definitive sinus surgery to be performed. Through an incision based in eyelid skin folds, the normal orbital tissues should be separated by blunt dissection until the collections of abnormal fluid are reached and released; the extraperiosteal space should be opened at a point close to the arcus marginalis.

The surgical exploration of a tense orbit in a child with significant, or increasing, visual impairment should not be delayed unduly to await a CT scan or the services of an otolaryngological surgeon. An orbitotomy that subsequently proves unnecessary is unlikely to cause long-term morbidity and is preferable to a complete loss of vision, which can occur with devastating rapidity if rising orbital pressure is neglected or inadequately treated.

With treatment, there should be a rapid improvement in clinical signs and both the

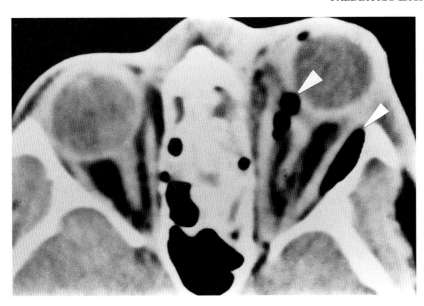

Figure 13.15 CT scan demonstrating intraorbital gas (arrows), in a child with orbital cellulitis. (Courtesy of Mr G Rose)

medications and the frequency of review may be modified accordingly. If not already under the care of an otolaryngologist, the child's airways should be assessed as soon as the orbital infection has been shown to be responding to systemic therapy.

An orbital CT scan should be performed where there is a persistence or a relapse of symptoms. Continued symptoms may be due to organisms resistant to therapy or, more commonly, due to loculated infection within the orbit or sinuses; drainage of an abscess, with microbiological investigation to direct further therapy, will generally result in rapid cure. The possibility of underlying orbital tumour must be considered in all children in whom orbital cellulitis does not respond appropriately.

Chronic infection due to unusual organisms, such as *Myco tuberculosis* or fungi, are rare but should be considered in children predisposed to such bacterium.

### Non-infective orbital inflammation

Non-infective orbital inflammation is rare in children and the possibility of an underlying tumour (particularly haematological malignancy, or rhabdomyosarcoma) or an occult dermoid cyst must be considered. Inflammation specific to one orbital tissue, such as orbital myositis or scleritis, typically presents a very characteristic clinical picture and should respond to therapy with non-steroidal antiinflammatory drugs or in those with more advanced disease — systemic steroids. Although uncommon in childhood, dysthyroid eye disease should also be considered as a cause of proptosis or orbital inflammation in older children, particularly if there is family history of thyroid hormone dysfunction; the symptoms and signs and radiological abnormalities are similar to those seen in adults but are generally milder. In those children thought to have orbital inflammatory disease, persistence of the inflammation, or a relapse, should prompt a search for an alternative diagnosis or for an underlying systemic disease or orbital tumour.

Most children with non-infective orbital inflammations require orbital imaging, most usefully a CT scan, and incisional or excisional biopsy; contrary to popular belief, neither the ultrasonographic nor the magnetic resonance characteristics of a tissue adequately define an orbital disease and do not, therefore, obviate the need for biopsy. Although orbital sarcoidosis is rare in childhood, the presence of non-caseating granulomata in an orbital biopsy specimen should be further investigated. Likewise, perivascular inflammation should prompt an investigation for systemic disease, such as "collagen disease" (particularly rheumatoid arthritis, polyarteritis nodosa and systemic lupus erythematosus) or Wegener's granulomatosis.

## References

1 MacEwen CJ, Young JD. Epiphora in the first year of life. *Eye* 1991; **5**: 596–600.
2 Lyons C, Rosser P, Welham R. The management of punctal agenesis. *Ophthalmology* 1993; **100**: 1851–5.
3 Welham R, Bates A, Stasior G. Congenital lacrimal fistula. *Eye* 1992; **6**: 211–14.
4 Sathananthan N, Moseley IF, Rose GE, Wright JE. The frequency and clinical significance of bone involvement in outer canthus dermoid. *Br J Ophthalmol* 1993; **77**: 789–94.
5 Shields JA, Kaden IH, Eagle RC Jr, Shields CL. Orbital dermoid cysts: clinicopathologic correlations, classification, and management. The 1997 Josephine E. Schueler Lecture. *Ophthal Plast Reconstr Surg* 1997; **13**: 265–76.
6 Haik BG, Karcioglu ZA, Gordon RA, Pechous BP. Capillary haemangioma (infantile periocular haemangioma) *Surv Ophthalmol* 1994; **38**: 399–426.
7 Wright JE, Sullivan TJ, Garner A, *et al*. Orbital venous anomalies. *Ophthalmology* 1997; **104**: 905–13.
8 Harris GJ, Sakol PJ, Bonavolonta G, de Concillis C. An analysis of 30 cases of orbital lymphangioma. Pathologic considerations and management recommendations. *Ophthalmology* 1990; **97**: 1583–92.
9 Lyons C. Craniofacial abnormalities. In: Taylor DSI, ed. *Paediatric Ophthalmology*, 2nd edn. Oxford: Blackwell Scientific Publications, 1997: 366–81.
10 Hoyt WF, Baghdassarian SA. Optic nerve glioma of childhood. Natural history and rationale for conservative management. *Br J Ophthalmol* 1969; **53**: 793–8.
11 Hollander MD, FitzPatrick M, O'Connor SG, *et al*. Optic gliomas. *Radiol Clin North Am* 1999; **37**: 59–71.
12 Moore AT, Buncic JR, Munro I. Fibrous dysplasia of the orbit in childhood clinical features and management. *Ophthalmology* 1985; **92**: 12–20.
13 Lyons C, Rootman J. Other mesenchymal abnormalities. In: Taylor DSI, ed. *Pediatric Ophthalmology*, 2nd edn. Oxford: Blackwell Scientific Publications, 1997: 342–9.
14 Mannor GE, Rose GE, Plowman PN, *et al*. Multidisciplinary management of refractory orbital rhabdomyosarcoma. *Ophthalmology* 1997; **104**: 1198–201.
15 Moore AT, Pritchard J, Taylor DSI. Histiocytosis X, an ophthalmological review. *Br J Ophthalmol* 1985; **69**: 7–14.
16 Weiss A, Friendly D, Eglin K, *et al*. Bacterial periorbital and orbital cellulitis in childhood. *Ophthalmology* 1983; **90**: 195–203.
17 Donahue SP, Schwartz G. Preseptal and orbital cellulitis in childhood. A changing microbiologic spectrum. *Ophthalmology* 1998; **105**: 1902–5.
18 Bergin DJ, Wright JE. Orbital cellulitis. *Br J Ophthalmol* 1986; **70**: 174–8.

# 14 The management of childhood strabismus

ANTHONY VIVIAN

Strabismus is a common disorder of childhood having a prevalence of 3–5% of the population. As a consequence, the management of childhood strabismus and associated amblyopia accounts for a large proportion of the ophthalmological workload. This chapter deals with some of the basic concepts of management of strabismus in children, rather than detailed management which is covered in several excellent textbooks of strabismus.[1–4]

## Horizontal strabismus

Horizontal strabismus is common in childhood and may be broadly subdivided into convergent (eso-) or divergent (exo-) deviations (Table 14.1).

Table 14.1   Classification of horizontal strabismus

*Esodeviations*
Infantile esotropia
Accommodative esotropia
Partially accommodative and non-accommodative esotropia
   Without distance/near disparity
   With distance near/disparity (convergence excess)
Secondary esodeviations

*Exodeviations*
Infantile exodeviations
Latent, intermittent and manifest exotropia
   Without distance/near disparity
   With distance near/disparity
     Near exotropia
     Distance exotropia
   Secondary exotropia

## Esodeviations (convergent strabismus)

### Infantile esotropia

Infantile esotropia (Figure 14.1) develops before the age of six months and in addition to the convergent strabismus there is often associated latent nystagmus, inferior oblique overaction and dissociated vertical deviation (DVD).[5,6] The differential diagnosis includes bilateral VIth nerve palsy, esotropia associated with congenital nystagmus, accommodative esotropia, Duane's retraction syndrome and esotropia associated with other disorders such as albinism, Down syndrome, developmental delay or hydrocephalus. Infants with broad epicanthus can look as if they have an esotropia but have a normal cover test (Figure 14.2).

**Sensory assessment**   Amblyopia is unusual in infantile esotropia. Visual acuity usually

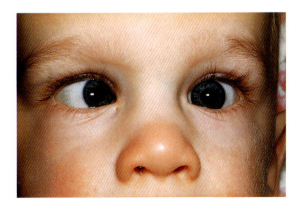

Figure 14.1   Large infantile esotropia

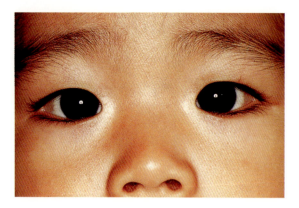

Figure 14.2   A broad epicanthus giving the appearance of esotropia. The corneal reflections are symmetrical. (Courtesy of Mr A Vivian)

remains equal in each eye because these infants cross-fixate, that is they use the left eye to look to the right and their right eye to look to the left. Because they tend to be young when assessed, an estimate of acuity can be achieved using fixation patterns and preferential-looking acuity cards (see Chapter 2). Uniocular acuity testing may be complicated by latent nystagmus which occurs when the eye not being tested is covered. As the esotropia tends to be large, testing for binocular single vision potential is difficult and it is doubtful whether true bifoveal fixation is an achievable aim in these children even after their eyes are aligned. However, some degree of binocular cooperation is demonstrable postoperatively in a majority of cases and so surgery is more than just cosmetic. As with all strabismus patients, refraction is essential and any significant hypermetropia should be corrected before a decision about surgery is made.

**Motor assessment**   Determining the angle of deviation in the primary position often requires two prisms, one held in front of each eye, because the angles are large (up to 70–80 dioptres) (Figure 14.3a,b). Using single prisms, it is possible to hold two prisms in one hand, leaving the other hand free to hold a light or perform a cover test. If the patient is very young, it may only be possible to assess the angle using corneal reflections. Bilateral VIth nerve palsy is a rare entity, but it can present like infantile esotropia. It is thus important to ensure that each eye abducts fully and this can be achieved by testing eye movements with one eye occluded to prevent cross-fixation. Some idea about lateral rectus function can be obtained by rotating the child to induce a vestibulo-ocular reflex or testing doll's eye movements.

Inferior oblique overaction and DVD are both features of infantile esotropia, although they may not become obvious until later in the course of the condition. It is often difficult to differentiate between the two, and they may co-exist, further complicating assessment. It is however an important differentiation to make as the treatments for inferior oblique overaction and DVD

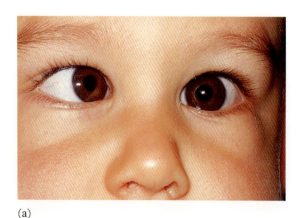

(a)

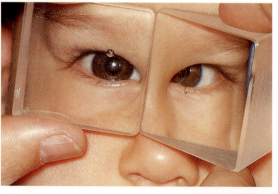

(b)

Figure 14.3   Infant with large esotropia (a). Loose prisms are used to measure the angle of deviation (b)

are different and if the conditions co-exist surgery to treat both simultaneously can be considered. There are several features of inferior oblique overaction and DVD which can help differentiate the two and these are discussed in the section on vertical strabismus. Latent nystagmus may be truly latent (only evident when one eye is occluded) or it may be present with both eyes open but becomes worse when one eye is occluded (manifest-latent nystagmus). It is important, although often difficult, to differentiate between infantile esotropia with manifest-latent nystagmus and congenital nystagmus with esotropia employed to dampen the nystagmus (nystagmus blockage syndrome).

**Management** A majority of infants with infantile esotropia require surgery to obtain alignment. To obtain the best surgical results, however, amblyopia and refractive errors must be managed preoperatively. Refractive errors should be fully corrected as with other esotropias. Bimedial recession is the surgical treatment of choice for correcting the horizontal deviation in infantile esotropia. Recessions of up to 8 mm from the original insertion have been reported to be successful without limiting abduction.[7] If the deviation is very large, additional unilateral or bilateral lateral rectus resection may be unavoidable. After horizontal muscle surgery for infantile esotropia, the most satisfactory postoperative position for the eyes is between 0–10 prism dioptres of esotropia (Figure 14.4). A small exotropia (less than 10 prism dioptres) is a less satisfactory result but does not warrant further surgery unless it is cosmetically unacceptable. Eso- or exodeviations of greater than 10 prism dioptres at the three months' postoperative visit should be corrected by further surgery. Once alignment to a small residual angle is achieved it is more likely that an infant will adopt a preferred eye for fixation and amblyopia is more likely to develop. Further careful follow-up with occlusion, if needed, is necessary to maintain equal vision in each eye.

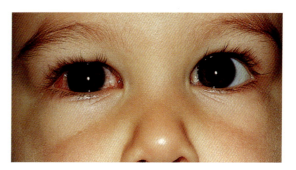

Figure 14.4 Same patient as in Figure 14.3 one week after three horizontal muscle surgery showing good alignment

### Accommodative and non-accommodative esotropia

A hypermetropic child has to accommodate in order to focus an image on the retina. With excessive hypermetropia, excessive accommodation is required and consequently excessive convergence. Childhood esotropia may be due entirely or in part to excessive accommodative convergence. It is important to correct this with a full hypermetropic correction before considering surgery. After refraction and full hypermetropic correction, children with esotropia can be classified into three groups:

• Fully accommodative esotropia: the convergent squint is completely corrected by the hypermetropic correction, and no further treatment is needed (Figure 14.5a,b).

• Partially accommodative esotropia: full hypermetropic correction decreases the angle of the squint, but there remains a significant esotropia which may require surgery.

• Non-accommodative esotropia: full hypermetropic correction has no effect on the angle of the squint, and strabismus surgery is usually required.

Most patients who require surgery for partially or non-accommodative esotropia can be treated with bimedial recessions. The amount of surgery will depend upon the size of the squint. A more predictable outcome can be obtained by using a prism adaptation test preoperatively.[8]

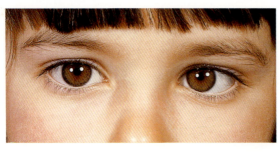

(a)

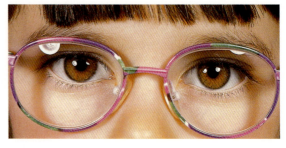

(b)

Figure 14.5    Child with left esotropia (a) which is fully controlled when she wears her full hyperopic correction (b)

**Micro-esotropia (monofixation syndrome)**

The best results from surgery for esotropia is a complete cure with bifoveal fixation. In children who have well-established squints, this is rarely possible. The next best result is a microtropia (or monofixation syndrome). The child is left with a very small, cosmetically acceptable, esotropia (less than 10 prism dioptres). Diplopia is avoided by suppressing the non-fixing eye, but peripheral fusion is good, ensuring long-term stability of the deviation. The non-fixing eye will be amblyopic, but the vision may be very good if occlusion treatment was successful preoperatively. If a child with a well-established microtropia has an increase in the angle of the esotropia at a later date, diplopia can occur. In this instance modification of the glasses may be necessary, or further surgery to reduce the deviation to less than 10 prism dioptres, which will eliminate the diplopia.

Micro-esotropia may also be seen as a primary form of strabismus in children who have had no previous surgery. The diagnosis is usually made at visual screening or when the monocular visual acuity or stereopsis is tested for some other reason. It is often associated with anisometropic refractive errors. The management is correction of any significant refractive error and occlusion therapy for amblyopia.

**Convergence excess esotropia**

Convergence excess esotropia is an esodeviation which is at least 10 prism dioptres greater for near fixation than distance fixation (after full hypermetropic correction). Assessment of patients with convergence excess esotropia should include measurement of the binocular visual acuity for near. One of the most troublesome effects of convergence excess esotropia is loss of binocularity for near. Most children with convergence excess esotropia have reasonable binocular single vision for distance, but as they attempt to accommodate on a near target, they become esotropic and thus lose binocular single vision. This is why it is important to measure this function in the initial assessment of these patients and it is a useful measurement when monitoring the effect of treatment.

There are two objectives in the management of convergence excess esotropia:

- To encourage binocular single vision for both distance and near.

- To produce cosmetically acceptable ocular alignment for both near and distance.

Although it may be possible to achieve this using bifocals, most patients benefit from surgery. There is no longer a place for using miotics in the long-term management of convergence excess esotropia and surgery is the treatment of choice. The distance-near deviation is reduced in most patients by bimedial recessions, but additional posterior fixation sutures (Faden procedure) may be necessary for large deviations.

180

## Exodeviations (divergent strabismus)

### Infantile exotropia

Infantile exotropia is much rarer than infantile esotropia, but is probably a distinct condition that should be treated differently from acquired exotropia. The condition is usually present at birth or within the first three months of life; it is often associated with other ocular or neurological abnormality.[9] Characteristically there is a large-angle exotropia (30–60 dioptres) which is equal for near and distance and in all positions of gaze. The strabismus usually alternates freely and amblyopia is rare. Associated inferior oblique overaction and DVD are common.

**Management** Although amblyopia is unusual because these infants tend to alternate, if it is present it should be treated prior to surgery by occlusion therapy. Refractive errors of greater than 3 dioptres of hypermetropia or myopia should be treated prior to surgery. Most patients with infantile exotropia require surgery which should be carried out before two years of age. The operation of choice is bilateral lateral rectus recessions and the aim of surgery is alignment to within 10 prism dioptres of straight. These patients seem to do well if they are slightly esotropic or slightly exotropic, and so, if they are within 10 prism dioptres of being straight, further surgery should be resisted. If the deviation is large, additional resection of one or both medial recti may be necessary. The parents should be warned about the risks of overcorrection which are common following this. Stereopsis is not a realistic achievement, although some degree of peripheral fusion is achievable.

### Exophoria

The hallmark of exophoria is that affected individuals become diplopic if their eyes are dissociated. They control the tendency of their eyes to diverge by employing their large fusional amplitudes and using bifoveal fusion as a feedback. If bifoveal fusion is disrupted (for instance by performing an alternate cover test) the eyes become divergent, and when they are divergent they experience diplopia. The latent deviation is usually equal for near and distance and stereopsis is normal. Aesthenopia (eye strain) is the most common presenting symptom, and is usually worse for reading. Intermittent diplopia may also occur infrequently (i.e. when the child is ill), or may occur whenever the child is tired. Individuals who are exophoric have no facility to suppress; if they develop suppression they are unable to control the exotropic tendency and become intermittent exotropes.

**Non-surgical management** Orthoptic exercises are the mainstay of treatment for pure exophoria. By increasing motor fusion potential by performing exercises, aesthenopia can be reduced. Near-point of convergence exercises, and overcoming base-out prisms or minus lenses can improve symptoms. Prisms are rarely helpful.

**Surgical management** Surgery should be avoided in exophoria (as distinct from intermittent exotropia). It is often complicated by overcorrection and the development of diplopia. Persistence of aesthenopic symptoms or the presence of diplopia for significant proportions of the day may, however, make surgery unavoidable. Unilateral lateral rectus recession is the surgical treatment of choice. It may be necessary to operate on the other lateral rectus if the symptoms remain.

### Intermittent and manifest exotropia

It is useful to divide the acquired exotropias into two groups: those with distance/near disparity (where the difference between the distance and near deviation is greater than 10 prism dioptres), and those without distance/near disparity.[10] Those patients with distance/near disparity in whom the near exotropia exceeds the distance exotropia are termed "near exotropia" and those patients in whom the distance exotropia exceeds the near exotropia are termed "distance exotropia". It is useful to differentiate between these different groups because their management is different.

**Exotropia without distance near disparity**  Most patients with distance exotropia measure more for distance than near because of the influence of accommodative convergence. The effect of accommodative convergence can be neutralised by measuring the near deviation through +3 lenses, or by dissociating the eyes with patching for 45 min (and performing the alternate cover test to an accommodative target without allowing the eyes to reassociate). In a majority of cases the distance/near disparity will be eliminated. For patients with no distance/near disparity, bilateral lateral rectus recession is the treatment of choice.[10]

**Near exotropia**  In near exotropia there is a distance/near disparity with a near deviation greater than the distance deviation (after eliminating the effect of accommodation). This is uncommon and when seen is usually in adults rather than children. Affected individuals usually have a remote point of convergence and the surgery of choice is bilateral medial rectus resection. As it tends to occur in adults, adjustable sutures can be used.

**Distance exotropia**  In distance exotropia where the deviation is greater for distance than for near, the surgery of choice is bilateral lateral rectus recessions.[10]

### A and V patterns

It is common for the amount of horizontal deviation to be different in upgaze or downgaze. This difference is often eliminated with conventional horizontal squint surgery. Occasionally, however, the deviation is significantly more in up or downgaze and needs to be corrected. In general, A and V patterns are more troublesome when the maximum deviation is in downgaze, for instance a V esotropia or an A exotropia.

A and V patterns are often caused by oblique muscle overaction. Inferior oblique overaction results in a V pattern and superior oblique overaction causes an A pattern. Occasionally A and V patterns are present without any obvious oblique overaction. In a proportion of these patients, the extraocular muscle insertions are abnormal.

**Management**  Surgical management of A and V patterns requires either surgery to the obliques or transposition of the horizontal muscle insertions up or down. Weakening (myectomy or recession) of overacting inferior oblique muscles will reduce a V pattern. An A pattern caused by overacting superior oblique muscles can be treated by performing a posterior tenotomy of the superior obliques (leaving the anterior fibres to perform cycloversional movements). If there is no oblique overaction, A and V deviations can be reduced by moving the medial and lateral rectus insertions either up or down, usually while performing recession or resection of the horizontal muscles.

## Vertical deviations

### Inferior oblique overaction and dissociated vertical deviation

Primary overaction of the inferior oblique is usually associated with horizontal strabismus. (Figure 14.6) Although most commonly associated with infantile esotropia (along with latent nystagmus and dissociated vertical deviation) it also occurs in association with acquired esotropia

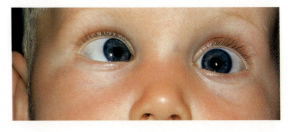

Figure 14.6  Infantile esotropia with associated right hypertropia due to inferior oblique overaction

and exotropia. Inferior oblique overaction also occurs secondary to ipsilateral superior oblique paresis (either congenital or acquired).

Primary inferior oblique overaction is associated with upshoot of the affected eye in abduction and a V-pattern strabismus (Figure 14.7a,b). Occasionally there is a hypertropia in the primary position if the oblique muscle dysfunction is asymmetric. The differential diagnosis includes superior oblique paresis, contralateral superior rectus paresis, and Duane's syndrome. Duane's syndrome is occasionally associated with an upshoot in adduction but other ocular motor abnormalities allow this syndrome to be distinguished from primary inferior oblique overaction.

Dissociated vertical deviation (DVD) is usually seen in association with infantile esotropia or exotropia. It is characterised by an updrift of one or both eyes when the two eyes are dissociated. Inferior oblique overaction and DVD often co-exist especially in association with infantile esotropia. There are several features of inferior oblique overaction and DVD which can help differentiate the two:

- Inferior oblique overaction is often associated with a V-pattern.

- When the affected eye elevates in DVD it is associated with excyclotorsion and when the eye returns to the primary position it is a slow recovery associated with incyclotorsion of the eye.

- When one eye is fixing in adduction the fellow eye is hypotropic in inferior oblique overaction and hypertropic in DVD.

**Management**

Inferior oblique overaction should be treated surgically if it is cosmetically unacceptable, or causes a significant V-pattern. The three commonly used weakening procedures are inferior oblique disinsertion, myectomy or recession. They are all equally effective. Surgical management of DVD is more difficult. DVD is hardly ever symptomatic and so the surgery is usually undertaken for cosmetic reasons. Surgery is more successful if performed bilaterally, and the choice of operations includes superior rectus recession (with or without a Faden procedure) or inferior oblique anterior transposition.[11]

**Double elevator palsy**

Double elevator palsy refers to a group of conditions characterised by limitation of elevation in both abduction and adduction. It was thought to be due to a paresis of both the superior rectus and inferior oblique, hence the name. In fact there are several causes of this condition including superior rectus paresis, inferior rectus contracture and supranuclear abnormality of upgaze. It is almost always unilateral and may be associated with ptosis (Figure 14.8).

The diagnosis is made by showing that the eye fails to elevate in both adduction and abduction.

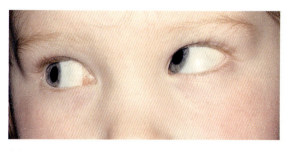

(a)

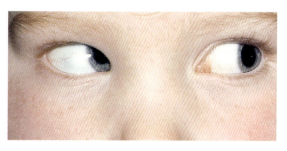

(b)

Figure 14.7   Horizontal versions showing bilateral inferior oblique overaction causing a vertical deviation on side gaze

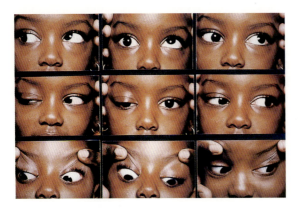

Figure 14.8   Right double elevator palsy with right ptosis. (Courtesy of Mr A Vivian)

There is usually no abnormality in the primary position although occasionally the child has to adopt a chin-up head posture. A forced duction test will differentiate between inferior rectus tethering and superior rectus paresis or a supranuclear paresis. In a supranuclear paresis the eye may elevate during a Bell's reflex but not voluntarily. The differential diagnosis includes Brown's syndrome, orbital floor blow out fracture and thyroid eye disease (which is exceedingly rare in childhood).

**Management**

Surgery is the only effective treatment of double elevator palsy. It is only indicated if there is a deviation in the primary position or if a chin-up head posture is necessary to obtain single vision. The choice of surgical procedure depends on the findings at operation. If the forced duction test suggests that the inferior rectus muscle is tight, an inferior rectus recession is performed as the primary procedure. If the forced duction test shows that there is no restriction of passive elevation then a Knapp procedure is indicated. This involves transposing the medial and lateral rectus insertions upwards to the side of the superior rectus insertion. Ptosis surgery should only be considered after squint surgery is completed as the ptosis is often much improved once the eye is moved from its hypotropic position (pseudoptosis).

# Neurological strabismus

## IVth nerve paresis

Most cases of childhood superior oblique palsy are assumed to be congenital, and this diagnosis may be confirmed by the finding of a head posture in early photographs. Other causes include closed head and posterior fossa tumours. The usual presentation is with an abnormal head posture, but some children present when they develop diplopia later in childhood. In acquired paresis, diplopia is more common. Traumatic cases are often bilateral and vertical diplopia may be complicated by torsional diplopia.

In unilateral IVth nerve paresis there is an ipsilateral hyperdeviation in the primary position which increases on gaze to the opposite side. The deviation usually increases on head tilt to the affected side. Assessment of ocular movements will show underaction of the ipsilateral superior oblique muscle and usually overaction of the ipsilateral inferior oblique muscle (Figure 14.9).

## Management

Congenital cases can be managed conservatively if the child can remain binocular, and the head posture is not too severe. Children with congenital IVth nerve palsies develop a large vertical fusion range which allows them to avoid

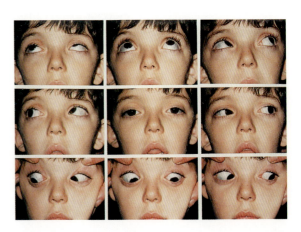

Figure 14.9   Left superior oblique palsy. Note the left superior oblique underaction and marked left inferior oblique overaction

diplopia. They may however become symptomatic later in life. Acquired cases need neurological investigation. In acquired palsies, time for spontaneous recovery must be allowed before surgery is undertaken during which time diplopia can be treated with prisms or occlusion.

Surgery for IVth nerve paresis is often necessary and the approach depends upon whether the palsy is unilateral or bilateral and the size of the deviation. Unilateral cases often respond well to an ipsilateral inferior oblique weakening procedure. If the deviation is very large, however, further vertical surgery such as an ipsilateral superior oblique tuck, ipsilateral superior rectus recession or contralateral inferior rectus recession may be necessary. In bilateral acquired palsies where torsional factors play an important part, advancing the anterior portion of both superior oblique tendons can correct the excyclotorsion effects of bilateral paresis.

## IIIrd nerve paresis

Congenital IIIrd nerve paresis is uncommon and the clinical signs are evident from birth (Figure 14.10a). It is often associated with aberrant re-innervation. Acquired IIIrd nerve palsy may complicate a number of different conditions such as closed head trauma, meningitis, intracranial tumours, and ophthalmoplegic migraine.[12] Clinically, there can be any combination of ptosis, vertical and horizontal muscle imbalance, and abnormality of pupil size (Figure 14.11). In addition, there may be signs of aberrant regeneration (oculomotor synkinesis).

## Management

In acquired IIIrd nerve paresis investigations including neuroimaging are necessary. The development of amblyopia can be prevented by correction of refractive errors and patching. If the ptosis is severe in a child at risk of developing amblyopia, a cautious brow suspension procedure may be necessary to lift the lid above the visual axis (Figure 14.10b). Prisms are rarely effective in the management of diplopia and if

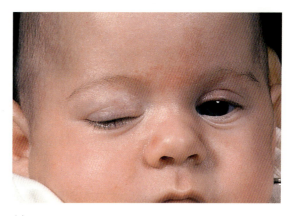

(a)

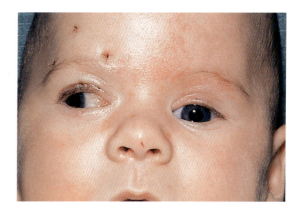

(b)

Figure 14.10   Infant with right IIIrd nerve palsy (a). A right brow suspension procedure was performed to enable treatment of amblyopia (b)

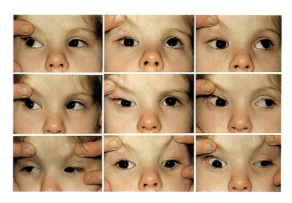

Figure 14.11   Four-year-old girl with partially recovered IIIrd nerve palsy. There is a right ptosis and limited elevation and depression of the right eye

there is not a significant ptosis, occlusion by other means may be the only relief from diplopia. In acquired paresis it is important to allow time for spontaneous recovery before contemplating surgery. Recovery can take as long as a year from the onset of paresis. In complete IIIrd nerve palsy the aims of surgery are often limited to a cosmetic improvement, or at best a small area of binocular fixation. With a partial paresis, surgery to treat diplopia is more successful. If there is reasonable residual medial rectus function, a large lateral rectus recession and medial rectus resection can be effective in the management of the horizontal deviation. There is usually an additional vertical deviation and multiple muscle surgery is often required. Surgery should be staged to avoid the risk of anterior segment ischaemia, although this is rare in childhood.

## VIth nerve paresis

Most VIth nerve palsy in childhood is idiopathic or follows a viral illness or immunisation. Other causes include trauma, hydrocephalus, and intracranial tumours, or it may complicate neurosurgical procedures.[12] Transient VIth nerve palsy in infancy is relatively common and resolves spontaneously. Spontaneously resolving VIth nerve palsy may also follow viral illnesses or immunisation or may be idiopathic. If the VIth nerve palsy fails to recover or is seen in association with other neurological signs such as nystagmus or papilloedema, further investigation is essential.

## Management

VIth nerve palsy, even if it is temporary, may cause amblyopia, and both amblyopia and diplopia can be managed by patching. Partial recovery resulting in an esotropia in the primary position with abduction beyond the midline may be treated by medial rectus recession and lateral rectus resection (Figure 14.12a–c). If there is no recovery of lateral rectus function (Figure 14.13a–c), the only surgery which is likely to be

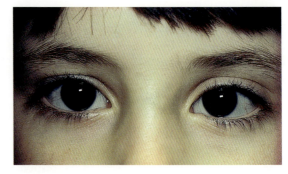

(a)

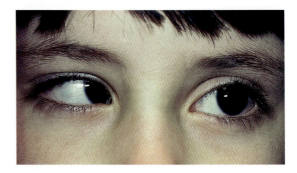

(b)

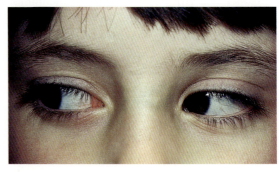

(c)

Figure 14.12 Partially recovered left VIth nerve palsy. There is a small left esotropia (a) with reduced left abduction (b) but normal right abduction (c)

successful is transposition of the vertical recti laterally combined with botulinum toxin to the medial rectus muscle or medial rectus recession (Figure 14.14a–c). Occasionally botulinum toxin to the medial rectus alone is useful.

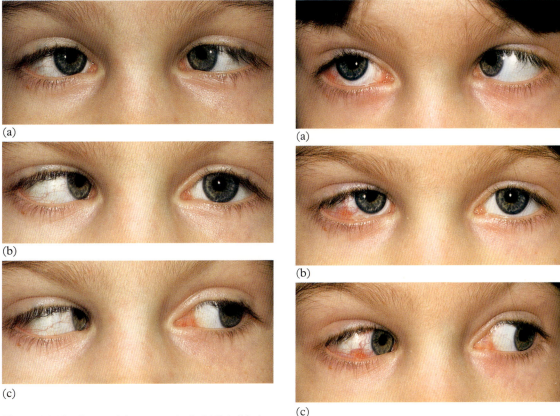

(a)

(b)

(c)

Figure 14.13  Large right esotropia (middle) (b) due to complete right VIth nerve palsy. On looking to the right there is no abduction beyond the midline (top) (a) but left abduction is normal (bottom) (c)

(a)

(b)

(c)

Figure 14.14  Same patient after vertical transposition procedure combined with botulinum toxin to right medial rectus. The primary position alignment (middle) (b) and right abduction is improved (top) (a) but further surgery will be necessary to improve the primary position alignment

## Developmental syndromes

### Brown's syndrome

In Brown's syndrome, there is a restriction of elevation of the eye in abduction which is caused by an abnormality of the superior oblique tendon sheath preventing it passing smoothly through the trochlea (Figure 14.15). It is usually idiopathic and although it may be congenital it usually presents later in infancy or childhood.[13] It is more common in boys and affects the right eye more commonly than the left. Occasionally it is associated with juvenile chronic arthritis, trauma and Marfan syndrome. Differential diagnosis includes double elevator palsy, congenital fibrosis syndrome, inferior oblique palsy and blowout fracture.

Most children with Brown's syndrome are asymptomatic, and they present because the parents have noticed the abnormal eye movements in upgaze. Some children develop a chin-up abnormal head posture to avoid having to look upwards or compensate for a hypotropia in the primary position.

187

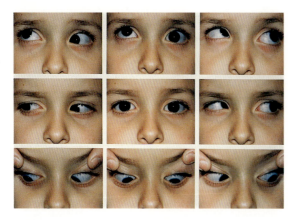

Figure 14.15 Typical left Brown's syndrome with inability to elevate the left eye in adduction and mild downdrift of the left eye on gaze to the right

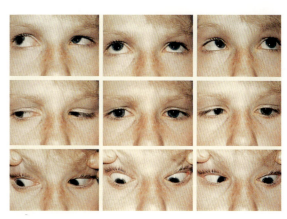

Figure 14.16 Left Duane's retraction syndrome. There is a small esotropia in the primary position, reduced left abduction and narrowing of the left palpebral fissure on adduction

## Management

In general, Brown's syndrome is self-limiting. Resolution is often preceded by a click of the tendon as it manages to pass through the trochlea on attempted upgaze. If Brown's syndrome is symptomatic and especially if it is associated with local inflammation, it may respond to local steroid injection. Surgical correction often has disappointing results and is only indicated if there is a significant hypotropia in the primary position. Best results are obtained by performing ipsilateral superior oblique tenotomy combined with an ipsilateral inferior oblique weakening procedure (to prevent a vertical deviation secondary to a surgically induced superior oblique weakness).[13,14]

## Duane's syndrome

The cardinal features of Duane's syndrome are limitation of abduction and narrowing of the palpebral aperture due to globe retraction during adduction of the affected eye[15] (Figure 14.16).

Adduction is often limited as well and upshoots and downshoots in attempted horizontal gaze may be an additional feature (Figure 14.17). The condition is congenital, is more common in girls and tends to affect the left eye more commonly than the right. It is occasionally bilateral. The cause is not known but several

cases have been found to have hypoplasia of the VIth nerve nucleus at postmortem. The oculomotor abnormalities are thought to be caused by lateral rectus weakness in abduction, and co-contraction of the medial and lateral rectus during attempted adduction resulting in globe retraction. The ocular features are occasionally accompanied by other developmental abnormalities.

## Management

A majority of patients with Duane's syndrome maintain binocular vision, are straight in the primary position, or adopt a small head posture

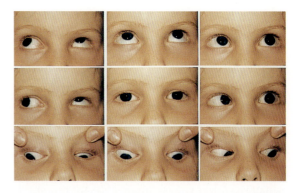

Figure 14.17 Left Duane's retraction syndrome with limited abduction of the left eye with upshoot on adduction

and this group of patients does not require intervention. The most common reason for surgery is for the management of a cosmetically unacceptable head posture. A general rule in the approach to surgery in patients with Duane's syndrome is to recess muscles but avoid resections. Many patients will benefit from bimedial recession, and if globe retraction of upshoots and downshoots are a problem, ipsilateral recession of both the lateral and medial rectus can be effective.

## Mobius syndrome

Mobius syndrome is a congenital paresis of various cranial nerves in association with systemic abnormalities including facial dysmorphism, limb abnormalities, and mild learning difficulties.[16] The most commonly affected cranial nerves are the VIth and VIIth nerves, and the condition is usually bilateral. Mobius syndrome usually presents in early childhood. VIIth nerve paresis results in a flat facial expression and occasionally poor eye closure causing corneal exposure. Bilateral VIth nerve paresis results in an esotropia, but there is often in addition, a gaze palsy. Bulbar cranial nerve palsy may result in a hypoplastic tongue.

## Management

Management of poor ocular closure by the use of lubricants should be started as early as possible to prevent corneal scarring. Amblyopia is common, and because eye movements are so limited, binocular single vision is rarely achievable. Strabismus surgery may be performed to improve cosmetically unacceptable esotropia. Large bilateral medial rectus recessions (up to 9 mm recessions) are required and the esotropia is still often undercorrected.

## Congenital ocular fibrosis syndrome

This dominantly inherited syndrome is characterised by an almost complete absence of eye movements associated with ptosis and an abnormal head posture (Figure 14.18). The head

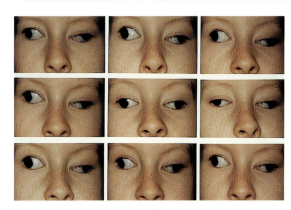

Figure 14.18    Ocular fibrosis syndrome in a young girl with left ptosis and a divergent and vertical strabismus. There is very little ocular movement in any position of gaze

posture is usually a chin-up due to the inability to elevate the eyes and because of the ptosis. It is not possible to increase eye movements by performing muscle surgery, but occasionally the dominant eye can be moved by surgery to reduce an abnormal head posture.

## References

1 Helveston EM. *Surgical Management of Strabismus*. St Louis: Mosby, 1993.
2 Good WV, Hoyt CS. *Strabismus Management*. Boston: Butterworth-Heinemann, 1996.
3 Pratt-Johnson JA, Tillson G. *Management of Strabismus and Amblyopia*. New York: Thieme, 1994.
4 Von Noorden GK. *Binocular Vision and Ocular Motility: Theory and Management of Strabismus*. St Louis: Mosby, 1990.
5 Nelson LB, Wagner RS, Simon JW, Harley RD. Congenital esotropia. *Surv Ophthalmol* 1987; **31**: 363–83.
6 Von Noorden GK. Bowman Lecture. Current concepts of infantile esotropia. *Eye* 1988; **2**: 343–57.
7 Szmyd SM, Nelson LB, Calhoun JH, *et al*. Large bimedial rectus recessions in congenital esotropia. *Br J Ophthalmol* 1985; **69**: 271–4.
8 Prism Adaptation Research Study Group. Efficacy of prism adaptation in the surgical management of acquired esotropia. *Arch Ophthalmol* 1990; **108**: 1248–56.
9 Hunter DG, Ellis FJ. Prevalence of systemic and ocular disease in infantile exotropia: comparison with infantile esotropia. *Ophthalmology* 1999; **106**: 1951–6.
10 Kushner BJ. Selective surgery for intermittent exotropia based on distance/near differences. *Arch Ophthalmol* 1998; **116**: 324–8.
11 Burke JP, Scott WE, Kutsche CO. Anterior transposition of the inferior oblique muscle for dissociated vertical deviation. *Ophthalmology* 1993; **100**: 245.
12 Kodsi S, Younge B. Acquired oculomotor, trochlea and abducens cranial nerve palsies in paediatric patients. *Am J Ophthalmol* 1992; **114**: 568–74.

13  Wilson ME, Eustis HS Jr, Parks M. Brown's syndrome. *Surv Ophthalmol* 1989; **34**: 153–72.

14  Parks MM, Eustis HS. Simultaneous superior oblique tenotomy and inferior oblique recession in Brown's syndrome *Ophthalmology* 1987; **94**: 1043–8.

15  DeRespinis PA, Caputo AR, Wagner RS, Guo S. Duane's retraction syndrome. *Surv Ophthalmol* 1993; **38**: 257–88.

16  Amaya LG, Walker J, Taylor D. Mobius syndrome: a study and report of 18 cases. *Binocular Vision* 1990; **5**: 199–32.

# 15 Paediatric eye movement disorders

PETER HODGKINS, CHRISTOPHER M HARRIS

To obtain the optimal visual acuity, images need to be focused and then held steady on the fovea. If both the observer and object were always static this could be comparatively easily achieved. However, even image motion of only a few degrees per second can lead to significant blurring. It is therefore crucial that the image is held still at all times. The visual demands of the fovea have led to the evolution of special eye movement systems, to maintain foveal registration of a visual object, and to permit new objects to be foveated. In this chapter we discuss some of these ocular movement systems, particularly in relation to children where a mixture of congenital and acquired problems are found. We also briefly summarise some clinical conditions where oculomotor disorders are prominent.

## The conjugate eye movement systems

### Saccades

Saccades are fast flicks of the eyes that redirect the fovea towards different visual targets, as well as being the fast phases of nystagmus. Abnormalities in the accuracy, timing, and speed of saccades can be caused by a wide range of disorders. However, unless the disorder is severe, saccade abnormalities tend to be difficult to detect clinically, and they are frequently overlooked or sometimes mistaken for nystagmus. Disorders of accuracy (dysmetria) are the most common.

- Hypometria
  In hypometria, saccades fall short of their target necessitating secondary saccades, which is normal in the young infant.[1] After about six months, hypometria may indicate acquired cerebellar disease, in which case it is usually associated with other cerebellar signs. Hypometria may also be associated with saccade initiation failure (SIF) ("ocular motor apraxia"; see below), even though other cerebellar signs may not be apparent. In homonymous hemianopia, saccades into the blind field are usually markedly hypometric in children and appear as a staircase of saccades.

- Hypermetria
  In saccade hypermetria, a saccade overshoots its target and requires a backward corrective saccade. Hypermetria is the hallmark of cerebellar disease and in childhood is often associated with opsoclonus. Slow saccades can occur in brainstem disease, but also in peripheral disorders such as myasthenia gravis.

### Testing

In children suddenly presenting, a large eccentric target easily seen even by those with some visual impairment, is a good method of inducing a large saccade to the patient whose head is held. The addition of sound eases the elicitation of saccades from small infants. For children with alternating esotropia, it is necessary to occlude one eye because peripheral targets may be foveated by cross-fixation with anomalous eye movements.

## The vestibulo-ocular reflex (VOR)

The VOR is a reflex in which the eyes move in the opposite direction to the head. It is stimulated by the semicircular canals and it maintains steady gaze during rapid head movements. It is not directly visually mediated and occurs in complete darkness. It is present at birth. In contrast to adults, VOR abnormalities are rare in early childhood, and unless severe, they are also difficult to detect clinically. Because of its robustness, stimulating the VOR is a useful clinical tool for testing eye movements in a preverbal or uncooperative child, and is part of the standard paediatric neuro-ophthalmological investigation.

### Testing

In the clinic there are two simple ways of stimulating the VOR: the oculocephalic or "doll's head manoeuvre" and manual spinning.

### Oculocephalic ("doll's head") manoeuvre

Passive or active rapid turns of the head are a quick test for vestibular function, and can be used to test vertical as well as horizontal VOR. In a normal child of any age, the manoeuvre will cause the eyes to rotate in the opposite direction to the head movement. In a child without spontaneous nystagmus, failure of both eyes to cross the horizontal midline indicates a nuclear gaze palsy, whereas a uniocular deficit indicates an infranuclear problem. The distinction among vertical supranuclear, nuclear, and infranuclear disorders is not always clear-cut due to the proximity of the midbrain gaze centres and the IIIrd nerve nuclei.

The presence of a normal horizontal doll's head manoeuvre in the absence of an inability of the child to make normal voluntary shifts of gaze (when the head is held still) suggests severe SIF (sometimes called "occular motor apraxial" or "supranuclear gaze palsy"). The horizontal doll's head manoeuvre may be quite abnormal in a child with early-onset nystagmus (see below), but this does not indicate additional pathology.

### Manual spinning

In the light, the examiner holds the infant at arm's length face to face and rotates themself and the infant to the examiner's right through several revolutions. This normally induces a per-rotatory large amplitude vestibular nystagmus with quick phases to the infant's right (examiner's left). If the rotation is abruptly stopped, a post-rotatory vestibular nystagmus is induced with quick phases to the infant's left. The procedure is then reversed.

In the light, the post-rotatory nystagmus should dampen within a few beats due to visual stabilisation. Sustained post-rotatory vestibular nystagmus is a sign of low vision or an abnormality of the smooth pursuit/fixation system.

Failure of nystagmus quick phases causes the eyes to deviate to the mechanical limit of gaze, which we call "locking-up". This is a useful test for SIF (see below), but it is important to note that some normal infants may exhibit this phenomenon in the first month of life.

## Optokinetic nystagmus (OKN)

OKN is a reflexive physiological nystagmus induced by movement of the whole visual field (full-field stimulation), although it can also be induced by smaller areas of the visual field (small-field stimulation). OKN is an alternating sequence of slow following and fast/quick resetting phases, and although conventionally the direction of OKN is determined by the quick phases, it is actually the slow phases that represent the optokinetic response. Clinically, the rate of OKN quick phases (beat frequency) can be used as a rough measure of OKN performance, provided SIF is not present (see below).

Note that preschool children have a lower beat frequency and higher amplitude OKN than older children.

The presence of OKN indicates some degree of vision in the apparently blind patient, although OKN is a poor way to quantify vision clinically. OKN is present from birth, and its absence to full-field stimulation (regardless of age) usually indicates either:

- very low vision;

- early-onset ("congenital") or acquired gaze-paretic nystagmus;

- intracranial lesions of the occipitoparietal cortex, the descending pathways, the cerebellum, and brainstem;

- SIF;

  or

- a gaze palsy in the plane of OKN stimulation.

## Biocular asymmetry of OKN

Asymmetrical biocular OKN (i.e. viewing with both eyes open) occurs when the speed of the slow phases (or the frequency of beats) is lower towards one side than the other. This can be caused by unilateral lesions anywhere in the optokinetic pathway, where the poorer response is for stimulus motion towards the side of the lesion. Isolated biocular asymmetry is suggestive of cortical disease, and a hemianopia is frequently present, although not always as, for example, in some cases of Sturge–Weber syndrome.

## Monocular asymmetry of OKN

Healthy neonates with both eyes open demonstrate symmetrical OKN. If either eye is occluded, monocular OKN (mOKN), slow phase speed and beat frequency are lower for stimulus motion in the nasotemporal direction than temporonasal (mOKN asymmetry).[2] The asymmetry reverses if the occlusion is reversed. This physiological asymmetry declines over the first six months for moderate stimulus speeds (about 30°/s). Disturbances of binocular vision in the first year, due to strabismus, anisometropia, or unilateral cataract may lead to a permanent mOKN asymmetry usually in both eyes. A later onset allows symmetry to develop. Asymmetrical mOKN is evidence for a uniocular deficit occurring in the first year, which can be a useful test when an older patient presents with an apparently late-onset squint with an uncertain history. However, symmetrical mOKN does not necessarily exclude an early onset.[3,4]

It must be emphasised that a mOKN asymmetry may appear as a biocular asymmetry if vision in one eye is poor or suppressed. So if a biocular asymmetry is detected, it is important to also examine the child monocularly.

### Testing

Small field OKN may be induced with a patterned drum or tape which can be rotated horizontally or vertically. No response with the drum or tape does not preclude a normal full-field OKN (see delayed visual maturation below). To test for an OKN response, the patient should look straight ahead at the stimulus since some types of gaze-evoked nystagmus can appear like OKN in lateral gaze.

## Smooth pursuit

Viewing a small smoothly moving visual target without head movement employs the smooth pursuit system. Most people are unable to generate smooth pursuit voluntarily without a moving visual target. Biocular smooth pursuit takes a few months to develop, whereas biocular OKN is present from birth. Acquired abnormalities of smooth pursuit and OKN have similar aetiologies. One major advantage of smooth pursuit over OKN is that slightly low gains lead to catch-up saccades, which are clinically easy to see since the following movement appears jerky. One major disadvantage is that smooth pursuit is not reflexive and requires active attention.

### Testing

Get the patient to follow a slowly (10–40°/s) moving target horizontally and vertically with the head held still. A common error is to move the target far too fast and not over sufficient range at constant speed. This is not a test of visual acuity, so an easily resolvable target is needed.

## Nystagmus

Nystagmus is a spontaneous rhythmic oscillation of one or both eyes. It may have an onset at any age including early infancy, and may be associated with a wide range of conditions ranging from the relatively benign to life-threatening. The distinction between "congenital" and "acquired" nystagmus (often interpreted as meaning "relatively benign" and "neurologically acute") is not always easily made in the young child. First, nystagmus may be acquired secondary to neurological disorders in the first few months of life at the same time as "congenital" nystagmus may first appear; and secondly, medical history can be uncertain. Because of the various clinical connotations of the term "congenital nystagmus", Casteels *et al.*[5] recommended that the term be avoided, and labelled nystagmus with an onset before six months as "early onset", which they subdivided into three categories:

- Sensory-defect nystagmus (SDN) and latent nystagmus.

- Congenital idiopathic nystagmus (CIN) in which no sensory or neurological defect can be established.

- Neurological nystagmus which is usually associated with a neurological disease.

This provides a rough guide for investigations, although the majority of early-onset nystagmus is secondary to a visual defect or idiopathic. Electronystagmography can be of some use in distinguishing among the different types of nystagmus, but this is available only in a few units.

**Latent nystagmus**

Latent nystagmus appears when one eye is occluded (but both eyes oscillate). It is horizontal and beats in the direction of the fixing eye, and hence reverses direction on reversing occlusion. The nystagmus intensifies on abduction and dampens on adduction of the fixing eye. Electronystagmography reveals slow phases that are decelerating (but may appear linear if the amplitude is low) (Figure 15.1). The onset is usually in the first year, although it may not be detected until much later. Latent nystagmus is most commonly associated with early-onset squint, but can occur with various uniocular disorders (cataract, anisometropia, and many others).

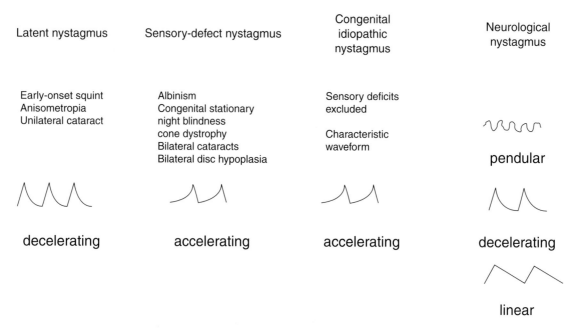

| Latent nystagmus | Sensory-defect nystagmus | Congenital idiopathic nystagmus | Neurological nystagmus |
|---|---|---|---|
| Early-onset squint<br>Anisometropia<br>Unilateral cataract | Albinism<br>Congenital stationary night blindness<br>cone dystrophy<br>Bilateral cataracts<br>Bilateral disc hypoplasia | Sensory deficits excluded<br><br>Characteristic waveform | pendular |
| decelerating | accelerating | accelerating | decelerating<br><br>linear |

Figure 15.1   Classification of early onset nystagmus

Despite its label, latent nystagmus may be unmasked with both eyes open (manifest latent nystagmus) if one eye has low vision (e.g. amblyopia). Latent nystagmus may also become manifest when gaze is deviated to one side (possibly because vision in the adducting eye is blocked by the nose). When latent nystagmus is manifest, it is important to recognize that both eyes exhibit the nystagmus, thereby degrading vision in the "good" eye. Not all infants with uniocular defects develop latent nystagmus, and the possibility of a genetic predisposition has been suggested.[6]

Truly latent nystagmus is asymptomatic and requires no management. Manifest latent nystagmus reduces vision and may lead to an abnormal head posture in which the head is turned so that the fixing eye is in full adduction, since this dampens the nystagmus. Surgery for a head turn with or without squint correction can alleviate the abnormal head posture and dampen the nystagmus.

## Sensory-defect nystagmus and congenital idiopathic nystagmus

Early-onset sensory-defect nystagmus (SDN) can be associated with a wide variety of congenital sensory disorders but does not occur secondary to cortical disease. The nystagmus typically has an onset in the first few months. In the young child, electroretinography and pattern visual evoked potentials may be needed to detect subtle defects such as in ocular albinism, cone dysfunction, and congenital stationary night blindness. The label of congenital idiopathic nystagmus (CIN) cannot be used until such disorders have been excluded. SDN is often inherited, depending on the underlying diagnosis. CIN may be inherited as an autosomal dominant trait, with other modes being less common.

SDN and CIN are conjugate and usually horizontal in all gaze directions, and head shaking may also be present. There may be a gaze direction in which the nystagmus is minimal, called the "null region", which if not in primary position, may lead to an abnormal head posture. Sometimes the nystagmus dampens on convergence. Typically the nystagmus intensifies in lateral gaze, and electronystagmography reveals accelerating horizontal slow phases, although they are not invariably present. When present, they are virtually unique to SDN and CIN, distinguishing them from neurological nystagmus. However, the waveforms do not distinguish among the various sensory defects underlying SDN or between SDN and CIN.

Visual acuity depends on the underlying sensory defect (if present), as well as the nystagmus waveform and head position. A hallmark of SDN/CIN is the enormous variability in the features of the nystagmus (waveform, null zone, sometimes head posture) that can change within minutes. The combination of these factors is difficult to control, and should always be borne in mind when assessing the visual performance of the patient with SDN and CIN.

### Management

It is important that appropriate investigations are performed to allow the correct diagnosis to be made. This will enable the parents to be given an accurate visual prognosis and will aid genetic counselling. The main aim of management is to maximise the visual performance within the constraints of the underlying diagnosis. It is important that any significant refractive errors are corrected and that low vision aids are prescribed when appropriate. The parents, child and teachers should be made aware of the importance of utilising the null zone. The child should be seated in an appropriate part of the class to aid use of the null zone and should be allowed to use an abnormal head posture or any adaptive head oscillations. Involvement of the peripatetic teaching service is helpful as they can advise teaching staff and parents of the educational and social problems encountered in children with nystagmus.

Most children with SDN and CIN do not require surgery but extraocular muscle surgery may be indicated for any associated strabismus or for correction of a very large abnormal head posture.

## Neurological nystagmus

Nystagmus that cannot be firmly identified as CIN or firmly associated with an early-onset sensory defect should be investigated for the possibility of a neurological or neuromuscular disorder. Rarely, forms of nystagmus that are identical to neurological nystagmus can be congenital idiopathic, but this can only be established by exclusion. It is also essential to realize that the presence of a sensory defect (e.g. optic atrophy, progressive retinal dystrophy) does not mean that the nystagmus is SDN, and similarly a squint does not automatically indicate that a nystagmus is latent nystagmus regardless of the age of onset. We summarise some of the more common types of latent nystagmus; for further details and types of neurological nystagmus, see Leigh and Zee[7] and Harris.[8]

### Gaze-paretic nystagmus (GPN)

Gaze-paretic nystagmus is a jerk nystagmus that becomes manifest on lateral gaze and beats in the direction of gaze, with decelerating slow phases (Figure 15.1). Unlike end-point nystagmus, GPN occurs when the eyes are not just at the extreme of gaze, and horizontal smooth pursuit is usually defective as well. Horizontal GPN may sometimes be accompanied by a small upbeat nystagmus in upgaze. GPN must be distinguished from latent nystagmus, since the latter may also become manifest on lateral gaze. Unlike latent nystagmus, GPN does not change appreciably on monocular occlusion. Oscillopsia may be present in lateral gaze, but this can be difficult to ascertain in the child. GPN is associated with a very wide range of cerebellar diseases. Other cerebellar signs may be present (ataxia, tremor, etc.), but GPN may be a presenting sign.

### Acquired pendular nystagmus (APN)

APN is a high-frequency low-amplitude pendular nystagmus. It may be purely horizontal, purely vertical, circular or elliptical; it may occur in only one eye, or be more prominent in one eye (asymmetric). Although labelled as "acquired", APN can have an onset in the first few months of life in white-matter disorders. SDN may also appear as a fine pendular nystagmus, often in association with subtle congenital sensory defects (cone dysfunction, congenital stationary night blindness). However, usually the SDN becomes jerk on lateral gaze, whereas APN remains a fine pendular nystagmus in all gaze directions.

In infancy, APN is often associated with demyelinating disease, and there may also be an associated congenital saccade initiation failure.[9] APN is also associated with demyelinating disease, and other oculomotor abnormalities may be present, such as internuclear ophthalmoplegia.

Spasmus nutans is a triad of asymmetric APN, head nodding and torticollis seen in children younger than two years with resolution over six to twelve months. A small number of these children have been found to have optic nerve or IIIrd ventricle gliomas although it has been suggested[10] that in the absence of visual or obvious neurological deficit it is reasonable to just follow.

### Vertical nystagmus

The child with vertical nystagmus (pendular, downbeat, and upbeat) should always be investigated on the suspicion of a posterior fossa disorder. Only rarely is it secondary to a congenital visual defect. In children, vertical nystagmus is often intermittent. Downbeat nystagmus is often associated with cervicomedullary malformations.

**See-saw nystagmus** In see-saw nystagmus, one eye elevates while the other depresses, and there is usually a torsional component. See-saw nystagmus is often secondary to parasellar masses, but rarely may occur in midline malformations.

### Periodic alternating nystagmus (PAN)

PAN is a rare horizontal jerk nystagmus that spontaneously reverses direction every few minutes. It can be acquired through posterior fossa lesions, or secondary to cervico-medullary malformation. PAN may also be congenital, when it is usually associated with SDN or CIN; in these children the SDN/CIN dominates investigations and any associated PAN is usually overlooked. Although PAN associated with SDN/CIN does not indicate additional pathology, it is important to recognise if surgical treatment for an AHP is being contemplated, since the AHP may also alternate.

## Other paediatric eye movement abnormalities

### Normal infant

Although not abnormal, eye movements in the healthy infant are quite different from adult eye movements. The normal infant has:

- normal biocular OKN;
- asymmetric monocular OKN;
- normal VOR;
- hypometric saccades;
- saccadic pursuit;
- no spontaneous nystagmus, although some gaze-evoked nystagmus may occur in lateral gaze in the first month.

This is a unique constellation of eye movements that occurs only in infancy, and under three months it is clinically obvious, but after about six months, infant eye movements appear adult-like clinically (although eye movement recordings will still reveal immaturity).

### Infantile esotropia (see Chapter 14)

Esotropia with an onset in the first six months of life probably represents the most common association with abnormal eye movements in young children. This includes:

- latent nystagmus;
- dissociated vertical deviation (DVD);

- persistent monocular optokinetic asymmetry;
- various incomitant deviations (A and V patterns, and inferior oblique overaction).

This constellation has sometimes been called the "infantile esotropia syndrome", but the complete repertoire is usually not present, and any combination can occur. A controversial issue has arisen over the relationship between the development of mOKN symmetry and the development of binocularity. In most children with infantile esotropia neither usually develop normally. This has led to the idea that mOKN development could be used as an index of esotropia management, where the development of symmetrical mOKN is the desired goal. However the development of mOKN and binocularity are poorly correlated[11] and symmetric mOKN may occur in children with infantile esotropia and no binocularity,[4] or even in children with only one functioning eye.[12]

### Saccade initiation failure ("ocular motor apraxia")

"Ocular motor apraxia", whether congenital or acquired, is a term that has come to mean a supranuclear problem that prevents the normal triggering of saccades. In children, there is an intermittent or total failure of reflexive optokinetic and/or vestibular nystagmus quick phases[9] and the term "saccadic initiation failure" (SIF) better describes what is happening. SIF is often thought to be rare, but is probably underreported. It is associated with myriad disorders and it may be a presenting sign of a CNS disorder.[8] The main associations for horizontal SIF include:

- Congenital malformations, often affecting midline CNS structures, including the corpus callosum, IVth ventricle, and cerebellar vermis.
- Early-onset neurometabolic conditions, such as Gaucher II (infantile), Krabbe's, Pelizaeus, and Merzbacher diseases (and others).

- Later-onset neurodegeneration, such as in ataxia telangiectasia, spinocerebellar degenerations, Wilson's disease, Gaucher III (juvenile) disease.

- Intracranial tumors (rarely).

- Usually no underlying pathology is found, and the condition is termed "idiopathic".

Vertical SIF is much rarer and usually indicates midbrain lesions, but it can be a presenting sign of Niemann–Pick type C disease.

Except in end-stage neurodegeneration, SIF is intermittent and becomes more noticeable when the child is stressed, tired, or trying very hard to look at an object. Other eye movements (including saccade speed) may or may not be abnormal depending on the underlying diagnosis. Affected children often adopt compensating strategies to shift gaze, particularly head thrusts, which have become the classic sign. In this strategy, the child shifts gaze by hypermetric headthrusts to overcome the saccade problem. However, this requires a degree of head control that may be absent in the young or developmentally delayed child. Older children may shift gaze by synkinetic blinks instead of head thrusts; this can be very difficult to detect.

Vision is usually normal in children with the idiopathic form, but poor visual evoked potentials or electroretinogram is suggestive of associated disease.[13] Posterior fossa abnormalities are not uncommon and MRI is the preferred imaging technique. Regardless of aetiology (including the idiopathic form), infants with SIF tend to be hypotonic with mild-to-moderate late sitting and walking. They tend to be clumsy with a wide-based gait, although frank cerebellar signs are uncommon. Speech development may also be slow, and reading difficulties are common, although intelligence is usually normal.

### Detection

The most reliable means of detection is to examine the quick phases of induced optokinetic and vestibular nystagmus. All affected children will show an intermittent failure of quick phases which intermittently allows the eyes to become deviated to the mechanical limit of gaze ("locking-up"). If an eye movement laboratory is not available, this can be tested by manual spinning (see VOR above).

### Delayed visual maturation (DVM)

The term "delayed visual maturation" is used to describe a young infant who has absent or very poor visual behaviour but subsequently, spontaneously develops normal or near-normal visual behaviour.

The condition has been divided into three types:

- In type 1 DVM (idiopathic or isolated DVM) there is no underlying pathology and usually between three and six months of age there is a sudden and rapid spontaneous development of visual behaviour to normal levels.[14]

- In type II, DVM there is associated systemic disease or mental retardation. The vision usually improves although this takes longer and there may be residual defects.

- In type III DVM there is an underlying ocular disease, for example cataracts or nystagmus. Despite this, the vision is much worse than expected. Subsequently the vision does improve towards a reduced final level.

During the visually unresponsive period, pattern visual evoked potentials are usually normal for age,[15] which is essential to distinguish DVM from cortical blindness in type I and II. In spite of the visual unresponsiveness, full-field OKN can be elicited from type I and usually from type II.[16]

The visual outcome in infants with DVM is usually very good, but the possibility of enduring neurological problems cannot be ruled out, and follow-up is needed.

### Opsoclonus and ocular flutter

Full-blown opsoclonus consists of bursts of high-frequency back-to-back saccades in all directions. Unlike nystagmus, it appears as an abrupt "clonic" jitter of the eyes, and once seen is never forgotten! The bursts can be almost incessant during the acute stage, but they become less frequent as the condition resolves and may become only horizontal (when they are called "ocular flutter"). Opsoclonus is usually acquired, but rarely it may be congenital.

In children, acquired opsoclonus is part of the opsoclonus–myoclonus syndrome (also known as "dancing eyes syndrome" or "myoclonic encephalopathy of infants"). There is usually an acute onset, with ataxia, vomiting, and irritability which can make examination difficult. It usually occurs as a paraneoplastic phenomenon of occult neuroblastoma or as a postinfectious encephalopathy. Adrenocorticotrophic hormone (ACTH) or steroid therapy can have a dramatic short-term effect on reducing the symptoms in some children, but the opsoclonus and other cerebellar signs may become steroid-dependent and re-emerge on attempts to wean the child, or during an intercurrent illness.

Regardless of the short-term response, children with opsoclonus often have long-term developmental problems, including motor and cognitive handicaps.[17] Subtle saccade dysmetria may also persist. Currently, immunoglobulin therapy appears to be promising.[18]

# References

1 Harris CM, Jacobs M, Shawkat F, Taylor D. The development of saccadic accuracy in the first 7 months. *Clin Vis Sci* 1993; **8**: 85–96.

2 Atkinson J. Development of optokinetic nystagmus in the human infant and monkey infant. An analogue to development in kittens. In: Freeman RD, ed. *Developmental Neurobiology of Vision*. New York: Plenum Press, 1979: 227–87.

3 Demer JL, von Noorden GK. Optokinetic asymmetry in esotropia. *J Ped Ophthalmol Strab* 1988; **25**: 286–92.

4 Timms C, Shawkat F, West P, Harris CM. The relationship between binocular function and monocular optokinetic symmetry. *Transactions of the VIIIth International Orthoptic Congress* 1995: 217–21.

5 Casteels I, Harris CM, Shawkat F, Taylor D. Nystagmus in infancy. *Br J Ophthalmol* 1992; **76**: 434–7.

6 Kushner BJ. Infantile uniocular blindness with bilateral nystagmus. *Arch Ophthalmol* 1995; **113**: 1298–1300.

7 Leigh JR, Zee DS. *The Neurology of Eye Movements*, 2nd edn. Philadelphia: FA Davis, 1991.

8 Harris CM. Other eye movement disorders. In: Taylor DSI, ed. *Paediatric Ophthalmology*, 2nd edn, Chapter 40.2. Oxford: Blackwell Scientific Publications, 1997.

9 Harris CM, Shawkat F, Russell-Eggitt I, *et al.* Intermittent horizontal saccade failure ("ocular motor apraxia") in children. *Br J Ophthalmol* 1996; **80**: 151–8.

10 Arnoldi KA, Tychsen L. Prevalence of intracranial lesions in children initially diagnosed with disconjugate nystagmus (spasmus nutans). *J Paed Ophthalmol Strab* 1995; **32**: 296–301.

11 Wattam-Bell J, Braddick O, Atkinson J, Day J. Measures of infant binocularity in a group at risk for strabismus. *Clin Vis Sci* 1987; **1**: 327–36.

12 Shawkat FS, Harris CM, Taylor DSI, *et al.* The optokinetic response differences between congenital profound and non-profound unilateral visual deprivation. *Ophthalmology* 1995; **102**: 1615–22.

13 Shawkat FS, Harris CM, Taylor DSI, Kriss A. The role of ERG/VEP and eye movement recordings in children with ocular motor apraxia. *Eye* 1996; **10**: 53–60.

14 Tressider J, Fielder AR, Nicholson J. Delayed visual maturation: ophthalmic and neurodevelopmental aspects. *Dev Med Child Neurol* 1990; **32**: 872–81.

15 Lambert SR, Kriss A, Taylor D. Delayed visual maturation. A longitudinal clinical and electrophysiological assessment. *Ophthalmology* 1989; **96**: 524–9.

16 Harris CM, Kriss A, Shawkat F, *et al.* Delayed visual maturation in infants: a disorder of figure–ground separation? *Brain Res Bull* 1996; **40**: 365–9.

17 Papero PH, Pranzateilli MR, Margolis LJ, *et al.* Neurobehavioural and psychosocial functioning of children with opsoclonus–myoclonus syndrome. *Dev Med Child Neurol* 1995; **37**: 915–32.

18 Pless M, Ronthal M. The treatment of opsoclonus–myoclonus with high dose intravenous immunoglobulin. *Neurology* 1996; **46**: 583–4.

# 16 Albinism

STEPHEN CHARLES

Albinism is the term used to describe a heterogeneous group of inherited disorders characterised by skin hypopigmentation and ocular abnormalities including nystagmus and reduced visual acuity.[1] Traditionally, albinism has been broadly divided into two groups on the basis of clinical features:

- Oculocutaneous albinism, characterised by hypopigmentation of hair, skin and eyes.

- Ocular albinism, where hypopigmentation appears confined to the eyes.

Albinoidism describes conditions where there is congenital hypomelanosis, but where visual acuity is normal and there is no nystagmus. Recently, molecular genetic studies have allowed more precise classification of albinism related to the underlying molecular pathology.

## Melanogenesis, ocular features and classification

### Melanogenesis

Melanocytes are exclusively responsible for melanin production, or melanogenesis, which occurs in the skin, hair bulbs, uvea, and ocular pigment epithelium. Melanocytes of the skin, hair bulbs and iris stroma are derived from the neural crest, whereas the pigment epithelial layers of the iris, ciliary body and retina are derived from the outer layer of the optic cup (neuroectoderm). Melanin is synthesised in cytoplasmic organelles called melanosomes. Maturation of melanosomes occurs in four stages: stage 1 and 2 premelanosomes acquire melanogenic enzymes but contain no melanin; melanogenesis begins in stage 3 premelanosomes and is completed in fully pigmented stage 4 melanosomes.

There are two major forms of melanin: black-brown eumelanin and yellow-red pheomelanin. Biosynthesis of both eumelanin and pheomelanin begins with the conversion of the substrate L-tyrosine to L-dihydroxyphenylalanine (DOPA) and then L-DOPAquinone. Both steps are catalysed by the enzyme tyrosinase. DOPAquinone is a very reactive compound that rapidly enters the eumelanin or pheomelanin pathway. Tyrosinase is the major regulator of the eumelanin pathway but other enzymes and factors are also involved, including tyrosinase-related protein 1 (TRP-1) and TRP-2. No enzyme control of pheomelanin synthesis has been described.

### Ocular features

Ocular features are similar irrespective of the type of albinism.[1] There is nystagmus, reduced visual acuity, iris translucency, reduced fundus pigmentation, foveal hypoplasia and decussation defects at the optic chiasm demonstrated by visual-evoked potential (VEP) studies (Table 16.1). Strabismus, refractive errors and anomalies of the anterior segment of the eye, such as posterior embryotoxon, are common.

Affected infants with all types of albinism are slow to see and may appear blind in the early post-

Table 16.1   Ocular features of albinism

Reduced visual acuity
Nystagmus
Iris translucency
Fundus hypopigmentation
Foveal hypoplasia
Decussation defect at the optic chiasm

natal period. Roving eye movements are seen initially, changing to a pendular, horizontal nystagmus during the first year. The nystagmus is often jerky on lateral gaze, and reduces in intensity with age. Visual acuity is usually reduced to the level 6/24 to 6/60. Near vision tends to be better and many young albinos can read small print unaided. Irides have a grey or light-blue colour although in some types of albinism there may be sufficient pigmentation so that irides appear brown. Iris translucency is a particularly important sign (Figure 16.1): using retroillumination the iris and globe diffusely transilluminate due to hypopigmentation of the pigment epithelia. In the fundus, the choroidal vasculature is visible through the hypopigmented retinal pigment epithelium (Figure 16.2). Choroidal vessels may be visible in the macular area (macular transparency), although there may be sufficient macular pigment in some cases to mask the choroid. Foveal hypoplasia is always present with absence of the normal hyperpigmentation of the foveal region, foveal pit and normal foveal

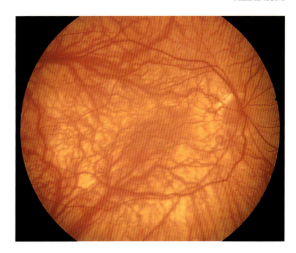

Figure 16.2   Fundus photograph in OA1 showing prominent choroidal vessels, macular translucency and foveal hypoplasia. (Reprinted from: Charles SJ, Green JS, Grant JW, Yates JRW, Moore AT. Clinical features of affected males with X-linked ocular albinism. *Br J Ophthalmol* 1993; **77**: 222–7, with permission)

avascular zone. Retinal vessels may cross the putative foveal area.

There are several mechanisms responsible for poor vision in albinism. Although nystagmus clearly limits vision, psychophysical testing indicates that visual resolution in albinos is limited by factors other than nystagmus alone. Foveal hypoplasia may be the major cause of poor vision but other structural abnormalities such as optic nerve head dysplasia are sometimes seen. In all forms of albinism reduced visual acuity may broadly be related to the degree of ocular hypopigmentation[1] although there may be exceptions: oculocutaneous albinism has been reported with macular transparency and normal visual acuity.

**Classification** (Figure 16.3)

Albinism has been classified by clinical assessment of the amount, type and distribution of pigment, mode of inheritance, and biochemical analysis of tyrosinase activity.[1] Tyrosinase activity has been assessed by the hair bulb incubation test where intact hair bulbs from affected individuals are incubated in tyrosine and then examined by

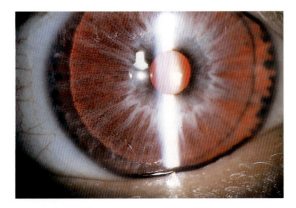

Figure 16.1   Marked iris translucency in OCA1A. Note visible lens and ciliary processes through translucent iris

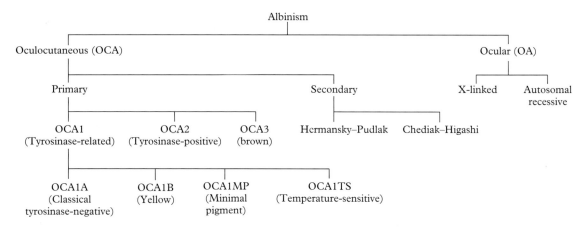

Figure 16.3    Classification of albinism

microscopy for the production of pigment. The tyrosinase assay is used in research but has limited use in current clinical practice. With the advent of molecular biology, the underlying molecular pathology of different types of albinism is being elucidated.[2,3] Although clinical assessment remains paramount, mutation analysis will allow more specific classification in the future.

Albinism is broadly divided into:

- Oculocutaneous (OCA)

- Ocular albinism (OA)

This basic division is useful although certain oculocutaneous albinos may have significant amounts of pigmentation and ocular albinos may have pigmentation in the normal range but reduced relative to unaffected siblings. Albinism is linked with visual pathway abnormalities which are discussed later in the chapter.

## Oculocutaneous albinism

Oculocutaneous albinism (OCA) may be divided into two groups: in one, the primary defect lies in melanogenesis and the melanocyte (*primary* OCA) and in the other albinism is secondary to abnormal biogenesis of intracellular organelles common to a variety of different cell types, including melanocytes (*secondary* OCA). Primary OCA includes those types where tyrosinase activity is

reduced or absent (tyrosinase-related OCA; OCA1), those with normal tyrosinase activity (tyrosinase-positive OCA; OCA2), and other types, such as brown OCA (OCA3). Secondary OCA includes systemic diseases such as Hermansky–Pudlak syndrome and Chediak–Higashi syndrome. Inheritance is almost exclusively autosomal recessive. Whether another form, *autosomal dominant* OCA, is a distinct form, is debatable.

### Primary OCA

#### OCA1: tyrosinase-related OCA

This wide phenotypic variation in tyrosinase-related OCA is divided into four types.[3]

The tyrosinase gene (*TYR*) has been mapped to chromosome 11 (11q14–21) and many *TYR* mutations have been found in patients with OCA1. In Caucasians, no single mutant *TYR* allele accounts for a significant fraction of the total: therefore, in the absence of parental consanguinity most patients are compound heterozygotes for different mutant alleles. This explains the range of different phenotypes, depending on the amount and type of residual tyrosinase activity.[3]

#### OCA1A (classical tyrosinase-negative OCA)

This has no tyrosinase activity and no melanin formation with only immature stage 1 and 2 melanosomes present. Patients have white hair and pale skin throughout life. Visual acuity is usually 6/60 or worse. There is complete trans-illumination of the iris, giving a "pink-eyed" appearance, with severe photophobia.

## OCA1B (yellow OCA)

These individuals, originally described in Amish families, have little or no pigment at birth but increasing pigmentation with age, the hair becoming yellow-red and the skin a yellow-cream colour. Hair bulbs of patients with yellow OCA have tyrosinase but with very low activity.

## OCA1MP (minimal pigment OCA)

This has been described where individuals have no skin or eye pigmentation at birth but minimal amounts of pigment develop in the iris in the first decade of life.[4] Acuity is usually 6/60. Tyrosinase activity is very low or absent. It is not entirely clear if this is a truly distinct type of OCA1 and, if it is, whether "platinum" OCA may represent the same phenotype.

## OCA1TS (temperature-sensitive OCA)

This has recently been described, due to a temperature-sensitive abnormality of tyrosinase with very low activity at 35°C, but no activity at higher temperatures. Melanin production is therefore dependent on the skin temperature in each area of the body. Patients have white skin, blue irides and white axillary and scalp hair but lightly pigmented arm hair and dark brown leg hair. This is the human equivalent of tempera-ture-related forms of albinism seen in the Siamese cat and the Himalayan mouse.

## OCA2: tyrosinase-positive OCA

This is the commonest form of albinism, with normal tyrosinase activity. Affected individuals are indistinguishable from tyrosinase-negative cases at birth, with white hair and pink skin. However, there is increasing pigmentation with age, so that the hair may become yellow or light brown, with freckles and pigmented naevi and there may be slight tanning. There is a high degree of phenotypic variability, especially between different racial groups. An African tyrosinase-positive albino may develop more darkly pigmented hair and skin than a normal blond Caucasian. Fundus pigmentation may develop consistent with skin colour and acuity tends to be a slightly better than OCA1, from 6/18 to 6/60.

OCA2 is associated with mutations of the P gene (15q11–13), which codes for a transmem-brane polypeptide thought to be involved in melanosomal tyrosine transport.[2,3]

## OCA3: brown OCA

Brown OCA has been described in Africans and Afro-Americans as a variety of OCA with less photosensitivity and more pigmentation than African OCA2 albinos. There is light-brown skin and hair and blue-grey transilluminating irides, with some degree of retinal pigmentation.[5] Acuity ranges from 6/18 to 6/60. Tyrosinase activity is normal. Melanosome maturation is affected: some melanosomes are pigmented and fully matured but many have minimal amounts of melanin suggesting that they were arrested in an early premelanosomal stage. Red (or rufous) OCA is a rare form of albinism described in natives from Africa and New Guinea with mild nystagmus, rela-tively good acuity (6/6 to 6/36) and a reddish tint to the hair, skin, irides and fundus. In both inher-itance is autosomal recessive.

A mutation in the tyrosinase-related protein-1 gene, (TRP-1) located at 9p23, has been found in an individual with brown OCA. It is proposed that TRP-1 acts as a regulatory protein in eume-lanin production, affecting tyrosine hydroxylase activity of tyrosinase. Mutations may produce brown rather than black eumelanins. Red OCA appears to be an allelic variant of OCA3 as muta-tions of the TRP-1 gene have been identified in affected individuals.

## Autosomal dominant OCA

Several families have been described with OCA and autosomal dominant inheritance. It is not yet clear if this is indeed a distinct entity or whether it is due to tyrosinase mutations in affected individuals in several sequential generations.

## Secondary OCA

### Hermansky–Pudlak syndrome

Hermansky–Pudlak syndrome is an autosomal recessive condition characterised by OCA, a bleeding disorder and a ceroid storage disease. It is an uncommon cause of OCA but is particularly prevalent in the Puerto Rican population. Affected individuals may present to a dermatologist or haematologist with a bruising tendency, or to an ophthalmologist with albinism and nystagmus.[6] The bleeding disorder is usually mild with bruising, epistaxis or gingival bleeding, but occasionally severe haemorrhage resulting in death can occur. Examination of platelets shows a reduction in storage granules (or dense bodies) associated with a deficiency of serotonin, adenine nucleotides and calcium in the platelet. This results in abnormal platelet aggregation and increased bleeding time. The most severe problems are related to the abnormal deposition of a ceroid-lipofuscin material in the lungs (causing pulmonary fibrosis), gastrointestinal tract (causing a granulomatous colitis), and kidneys, (causing renal failure).

There is great variability of pigmentation: affected individuals may be severely hypopigmented, similar to OCA1, or almost normal. Visual acuity also varies but is usually around 6/60. Uveal pigmentation may be variable but there is usually fundus hypopigmentation. Decussation defects are demonstrated by VEP. Tyrosinase activity may be low to normal.

The *HPS* gene is localised to chromosome 10q23.1–q23.3.[7] The gene product is a novel transmembrane protein that is likely to be a component of multiple cytoplasmic organelles and is apparently crucial for their normal development and function.

### Chediak–Higashi syndrome

Chediak–Higashi syndrome is a rare autosomal recessive condition where OCA is associated with susceptibility to infection and the presence of giant peroxidase-positive granules in peripheral blood leucocytes. Affected children often die in the first few years of life due to infection and few survive to adulthood. Inheritance is autosomal recessive. The phenotype is variable: hypopigmentation may be mild and only noted when compared with other normal family members. The skin may have patches of slate-grey pigmentation and the hair light brown to blond. Ocular features are typical of other types of albinism, with nystagmus, iris translucency, foveal hypoplasia and decussation defects but their systemic disease overshadows their ophthalmic problems.

The *CHS* gene has been localised to chromosome 1q42.1–q42.2. The gene product is unknown but it is thought to be involved in normal functioning of intracellular organelles, including lysosomes and melanosomes.

## Ocular albinism

Ocular albinism (OA) is divided into two major types on the basis of inheritance:

- X-linked
- Autosomal recessive

### X-linked ocular albinism

X-linked ocular albinism (XLOA, OA1) is also known as Nettleship–Falls XLOA since Nettleship described a form of nystagmus affecting males with X-linked inheritance[8] and subsequently Falls described the fundus appearance characteristic of the female carrier state.[9] In affected males with XLOA, skin and hair pigmentation is essentially normal but the characteristic ocular features of albinism are found. Acuity is 6/36 or better.[10] Decussation defects are present at the optic chiasm. In black patients, the diagnosis may be difficult: there may be hypopigmented patches on the skin but iris translucency is absent with normal fundus pigmentation and foveal hypoplasia may be the only consistent ophthalmoscopic abnormality.

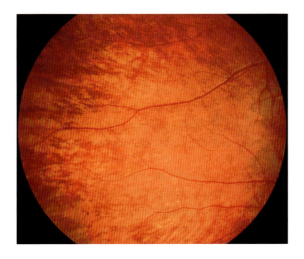

Figure 16.4 Fundus photograph of OA1 carrier female showing typical mud splattered fundus. (Reprinted from: Charles SJ, Green JS, Grant JW, Yates JRW, Moore AT. Clinical features of affected males with X-linked ocular albinism. *Br J Ophthalmol* 1993; 77: 222–7, with permission)

Skin histology in affected males shows abnormal giant melanin granules[11] termed "macromelanosomes", indicating that the effects of the condition are not confined to the eyes. Macromelanosomes are not specific to XLOA and may also be found in Chediak–Higashi syndrome, Hermansky–Pudlak syndrome, naevus spilus, neurofibromatosis and xeroderma pigmentosum, but not in normal skin. Carrier females have normal vision but may be identified by iris translucency and a characteristic mud-splattered fundus appearance (Figure 16.4).[9,12] Macromelanosomes may be present on skin biopsy.[12] Some obligate carriers are described with an entirely normal ophthalmic examination. In rare cases, carriers show reduced visual acuity and nystagmus, so-called "manifesting heterozygotes." Many cases of XLOA are initially wrongly diagnosed as idiopathic congenital nystagmus. XLOA should be suspected in all male infants with nystagmus: examination of the mother, even in the absence of a family history, may enable diagnosis without the need for further examination.

The *OA1* gene locus has been localised to region Xp22.3 by linkage studies and the gene has been cloned. It is suggested that the OA1 gene product is a membrane protein, possibly involved in the formation/maturation of melanosomes.

**Autosomal recessive ocular albinism**

In some families, males and females are equally affected with a form of OA, and a number of isolated cases of OA have been observed in females indicating autosomal recessive inheritance. In autosomal recessive ocular albinism (OAR), females show the same ocular features as affected males with XLOA: they do not have the characteristic XLOA-carrier fundus. Skin and hair pigmentation is in the normal range. Tyrosinase activity is normal. Skin examination shows normal melanosomes without macromelanosomes.

Mutations of the *TYR* and *P* gene have been found in some cases of OAR, indicating that at least some cases are really mild forms of OCA1B or OCA2. OAR is therefore a heterogeneous group of conditions, resulting from mutations of the *TYR*, *P* polypeptide and perhaps other genes involved in pigmentation.

**Visual pathway abnormalities in albinism** (see Chapter 3)

All albino mammals have an abnormal projection of the optic pathways. In normally pigmented humans, nerve fibres of the temporal retina remain uncrossed and project to the ipsilateral hemisphere whereas fibres from the nasal retina decussate in the optic chiasm. The majority of fibres from the temporal retina subserve the central 20° of the nasal field. In albinos, the majority of fibres from the temporal retina are misrouted to cross in the optic chiasm (Figure 16.5), and only 10–20% of fibres remain uncrossed, as opposed to 45% in normals. Therefore each occipital cortex receives a monocular projection of the central visual field rather than corresponding images of the contralateral visual field. This misrouting is demonstrated by

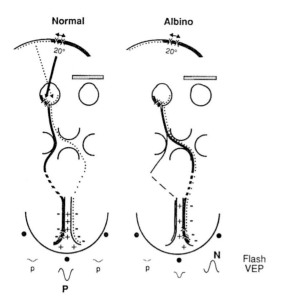

Figure 16.5    Diagram of visual pathway from one eye in a normal control and an albino. In the albino, temporal retinal fibres subserving the nasal field from the fixation point to an eccentricity of 20° project anomalously to the contralateral hemisphere. VEP shown using 'negative upwards' convention. (Reprinted from: Russell-Eggitt I, Kriss A, Taylor DSI. Albinism in childhood: a flash VEP and ERG study. *Br J Ophthalmol* 1990; 74: 136–40, with permission.)

visual evoked potential (VEP) studies where there is hemispheric asymmetry to monocular stimulation which reverses when the other eye is stimulated. VEP abnormalities in albinism may be best elicited by flash stimulation in children[13] but by the pattern onset VEP in adults.[14] VEP has therefore become an important investigation in the assessment of the child with nystagmus. The electroretinogram shows larger a-waves, and shorter a- and b-wave latencies. This may be accounted for by the stronger effects of flash stimulus on the albino eye, with light transmission through the translucent iris, and greater fundal reflectance and light scatter because of lack of retinal pigment absorption.

### Pigment and the developing visual system

Pigment has an important role in the normal development of the visual system. Normal central pathways may be produced in albino mice by the introduction of a functional tyrosinase transgene confirming the relationship between the albino gene and pathway abnormality.[15] It was thought that pigment was important in axonal guidance since part of the primitive eye stalk appeared to be transiently pigmented in mice and rats,[16] with axons preferring melanin-free zones. However, other studies have not supported this finding and the precise role of pigment in chiasmal development remains poorly understood.[17]

Normal foveal development involves peripheral migration of inner retinal layers to form the foveal pit, with central migration of cone photoreceptors, increasing foveal cell density. In the albino, no such migration occurs so that foveal cones remain spaced apart and the foveal pit is absent. The aetiology is not understood.

### Management

The albino infant may appear not to see, and parents should be warned that normal visual maturation may be delayed. Refractive errors are common, particularly astigmatism, and the early correction of refractive errors should be considered to maximise visual potential.

Tinted lenses may provide symptomatic relief of photophobia. In many albinos reading vision is good but some patients may be helped by a strong reading addition or telescopic low visual aids. Most children are able to be educated in an ordinary school environment.[18]

Strabismus is common, but early surgery to promote stereopsis is not indicated although cosmetic squint surgery may be considered later.

In the tropics, lack of pigment predisposes albinos to development of malignant skin tumours. This is a particular problem in African albinos where death from squamous cell carcinoma is common. Skin protection using barrier creams, hats, long-sleeved shirts and long trousers, together with regular dermatological assessment, is to be encouraged.

## Genetic assessment and counselling

A formal genetic assessment is important and a detailed family tree may reveal the mode of inheritance. Once the diagnosis is established, parents may be helped by genetic counselling, with particular reference to the risk of having further affected children.

The overall prevalence of albinism worldwide is estimated to be 1 in 20 000, but there is a wide variation between different types and in different racial groups. In Africa and the African American population, OCA2 is the most common form, but in Caucasian populations OCA1 and OCA2 appear to be equally frequent.[3] Ocular albinism is less common with a prevalence of 1 in 50 000.[19]

Prenatal diagnosis, based on fetoscopy and fetal scalp biopsy (OCA1), fetal sexing (XLOA) and more recently molecular genetic techniques (OCA1, XLOA) have been used. Some clinicians may feel that the relatively mild and stationary nature of albinotic conditions compared to other inherited conditions should not warrant prenatal diagnosis. The ultimate decision should remain with the parents, but it is crucial that adequate genetic counselling is available, and that counsellors and parents have access to comprehensive information about the condition.

## References

1 Kinnear PE, Jay B, Witcop CJ Jr. Albinism. *Surv Ophthalmol* 1985; **30**: 75–101.
2 Carden SM, Boissy RE, Schoettker PJ, Good WV. Albinism: modern molecular diagnosis. *Br J Ophthalmol* 1998; **82**: 189–95.
3 King RA, Hearing VJ, Creel DJ, Oetting WS. Albinism. *The Metabolic and Molecular Bases of Inherited Disease.* New York: McGraw-Hill, 1995; 4353–92.
4 Summers CG, King RA. Ophthalmic features of minimal pigment oculocutaneous albinism. *Ophthalmology* 1994; **101**: 906–14.
5 King RA, Lewis RA, Townsend D, *et al.* Brown oculocutaneous albinism: clinical, pathological and biochemical characterization. *Ophthalmology* 1985; **92**: 1496–1505.
6 Summers CG, Knobloch WH, Witcop CJ, King RA. Hermansky–Pudlak syndrome: ophthalmic findings. *Ophthalmology* 1988; **95**: 545–54.
7 Oh J, Bailin T, Fukai K, *et al.* Positional cloning of a gene for Hermansky–Pudlak syndrome, a disorder of cytoplasmic organelles. *Nature Genetics* 1996; **14**: 300–6.
8 Nettleship E. On some hereditary diseases of the eye. *Trans Ophthalmol Soc UK* 1909; **29**: 57–198.
9 Falls HF. Sex-linked ocular albinism displaying typical fundus changes in the female heterozygote. *Am J Ophthalmol* 1951; **34**: 41–50.
10 Charles SJ, Green JS, Grant JW, *et al.* Clinical features of affected males with X-linked ocular albinism. *Br J Ophthalmol* 1993; **77**: 222–7.
11 O'Donnell FE Jr, Hambrick GW, Green WR, *et al.* X-linked ocular albinism; an oculocutaneous macromelanosomal disorder. *Arch Ophthalmol* 1976; **94**: 1883–92.
12 Charles SJ, Moore AT, Grant JW, Yates JRW. Genetic counselling in X-linked ocular albinism: clinical features of the carrier state. *Eye* 1992; **6**: 75–9.
13 Russell-Eggitt I, Kriss A, Taylor DSI. Albinism in childhood: a flash VEP and ERG study. *Br J Ophthalmol* 1990; **74**: 136–40.
14 Apkarian P. A practical approach to albino diagnosis: VEP misrouting across the age span. *Ophthal Paed Genetics* 1992; **13**: 77–88.
15 Jeffrey G, Schutz G, Montoliu L. Correction of abnormal retinal pathways found with albinism by introduction of a functional tyrosinase gene in transgenic mice. *Devel Biol* 1994; **166**: 460–4.
16 Silver J, Sapiro J. Axonal guidance during development of the optic nerve. The role of pigmented epithelia and other extrinsic factors. *J Comp Neurol* 1981; **202**: 521–38.
17 Jeffrey G. The retinal pigment epithelium as a development regulator of the neural retina. *Eye* 1998; **12**(3b): 499–503.
18 Taylor WOG. Visual disabilities of oculocutaneous albinism and their alleviation. *Trans Ophthalmol Soc UK* 1978; **90**: 423–45.
19 O'Donnell FE Jr, Green WR. The eye in albinism. *Clinical Ophthalmology.* Philadelphia: JB Lippincott, 1989.

# 17  The phakomatoses

NICOLA RAGGE

The phakomatoses (from the Greek *phakos* meaning "birthmark") are a collection of hereditary disorders united by distinctive neurologic and dermatologic manifestations. They include neurofibromatosis types 1 and 2, tuberous sclerosis, von Hippel–Lindau disease, Sturge–Weber syndrome, ataxia-telangiectasia (Louis–Bar syndrome), and Wyburn–Mason syndrome.[1] Although there are some overlapping clinical features, such as renal cysts in both tuberous sclerosis and von Hippel–Lindau disease, and café au lait patches and neurofibromas in the neurofibromatoses, they are distinct diseases genetically.

Other related haemangiomatous syndromes include Klippel–Trenaunay–Weber syndrome and cutis marmorata telangiectatica. In both Klippel–Trenaunay–Weber syndrome (naevus flammeus of the face and extremities associated with hypertrophy of the underlying soft tissues and bone) and cutis marmorata telangiectatica with associated naevus flammeus, there may be congenital glaucoma.

This chapter, however, will focus on the neurofibromatoses, tuberous sclerosis, von Hippel–Lindau disease and Sturge–Weber syndrome.

## The neurofibromatoses

The neurofibromatoses, which mainly refer to types 1 and 2, have in common multiple tumour types, including neurofibromas, central nervous system tumours, and dermatological features.

Developmental abnormalities such as hamartomas also occur, implying an important role of the normal NF genes in development. In keeping with many dominantly inherited conditions, there is high intrafamilial variability. The mechanism for this is still unclear, although epigenetic mechanisms are likely to be very important.

## Neurofibromatosis type 1

Neurofibromatosis type 1 (NF1) or von Recklinghausen disease is an autosomal dominant condition affecting 1 in 2000 to 1 in 4000 of the population.[2,3] The principal external features of NF1 are café au lait patches, freckling, multiple cutaneous and subcutaneous neurofibromas and iris hamartomas. The main complications arise from neurofibromas (together with their malignant counterpart, neurofibrosarcomas), central nervous system tumours (including gliomas and ependymomas), phaechromocytomas, and a multitude of developmental anomalies such as bony abnormalities in the sphenoid and tibial pseudoarthrosis. As well as the classic neurologic malignancies of NF1, patients with NF1 may also be at increased risk of developing other malignancies seen in the non-NF population, for example acute non-lymphocytic leukemia, Wilms' tumour, and rhabdomyosarcoma.

### Clinical findings

The National Institutes of Health (NIH) has drawn up inclusional criteria for the diagnosis of NF1 (Table 17.1). In addition to these defining

Table 17.1  Diagnostic criteria for neurofibromatosis 1

The diagnostic criteria are met if a person has two or more of the following:

- Six or more café au lait macules over 5 mm in greatest diameter in prepubertal persons and over 15 mm in greatest diameter in postpubertal persons
- Two or more neurofibromas of any type or one plexiform neurofibroma
- Freckling in the axillary or inguinal regions
- Optic glioma
- Two or more iris hamartomas (Sakurai–Lisch nodules)
- A distinctive osseous lesion such as sphenoid dysplasia or thinning of long bone cortex with or without pseudoarthrosis
- A first-degree relative (parent, sibling, or offspring) with neurofibromatosis 1 by the above criteria

Table 17.2  Complications of neurofibromatosis 1

Nervous system
  Plexiform neurofibromas
  Spinal neurofibromas
  Gliomas
  Optic pathway gliomas
  Other orbit tumours
  Neurofibrosarcoma
  Aqueductal stenosis
  Cerebrovascular abnormalities
  Intellectual handicap
  Seizures
  Coordination problem
  EEG abnormality

Skeleton
  Scoliosis
  Pseudoarthrosis of distal long bone
  Lateral thoracic meningocele
  Lambdoidal suture defects
  Sphenoid wing dysplasia
  Pectus excavatum
  Genu valgum/varum

Skin
  Café au lait patches
  Hyperpigmentation overlying plexiform neurofibromas
  Other hyperpigmentation
  Hypopigmentation
  Axillary or inguinal freckling
  Other freckling
  Neurofibromas, cutaneous or subcutaneous
  Juvenile xanthogranuloma

Genitourinary Tract
  Neurofibromas
  Pelvic rhabdomyosarcoma

Eye
  Iris hamartoma (Sakurai–Lisch nodules)
  Prominent corneal nerves
  Glaucoma

Endocrine system
  Phaeochromocytoma
  Duodenal carcinoid
  Premature or delayed puberty

Cardiovascular system
  Renal artery stenosis
  Cerebrovascular disease
  Angiomas

Respiratory system
  Neurofibromas of oral cavity, larynx, mediastinum

Gastrointestinal system
  Visceral neurofibromas
  Colon ganglioneuromatosis
  Abdominal pain

Haematopoietic system
  Atypical forms of childhood leukaemia
  Increased risk of acute lymphoblastic leukaemia and Hodgkin's lymphoma

Adapted from Riccardi[3] and Huson.[2]

features, however, a plethora of other clinical complications are commonly and variably present (Table 17.2). Life expectancy is reduced due to an increased risk of malignancies and NF1-related complications.

**Skin signs**  The skin hyperpigmentation in NF1 occurs in several forms, notably café an lait patches, freckling and diffuse hyperpigmentation. Multiple café au lait patches are present in over 99% of individuals with NF1, and can range in size from a few millimetres to many centimetres in diameter. They are often the presenting feature of the disease. Larger areas of hyperpigmentation may outline an underlying plexiform neurofibroma, and over the spinal region may signify underlying spinal cord involvement. Freckling is present in 70–80% of individuals with NF1 by adulthood.

**Neurofibromas**  There are four types of neurofibromas:[3]

- Cutaneous

- Subcutaneous

- Nodular plexiform

- Diffuse plexiform

The cutaneous neurofibromas develop towards the end of the first decade, in early puberty, during pregnancy, or occasionally after trauma to the skin. The earlier in life they develop, the more likely they are to be prolific. They are initially sessile but later often become pedunculated.

The other types of neurofibromas include subcutaneous neurofibromas, nodular plexiform neurofibromas (which involve major nerve plexuses), and the diffuse plexiform neurofibromas (which encompass all the other types and insinuate into the tissue planes).

Malignant transformation can occur in all types of neurofibromas, and presents as pain, increasing tumour size and focal neurological deficit. The overall risk of neurofibrosarcoma to the NF1 patient is about 5%, but occurs more commonly in deeply located neurofibromas.

**Neurological complications** Mild mental retardation and/or learning difficulties appear to affect about 30–45% of individuals with NF1, independent of the severity of disease. Some of this is related to neurological complications including hydrocephalus, gliomas, irradiation, aqueductal stenosis, and other cerebral malformations. Mental retardation is more likely to occur in those individuals with a microdeletion of chromosome 17, including those with a Noonan phenotype or Watson syndrome (a disease characterized by café au lait patches, mental retardation and pulmonary stenosis, thought to be allelic to NF1). Many young individuals with NF1 display "bright spots" in the brain parenchyma on T2-weighted magnetic resonance imaging (MRI) scans. Typically located in the basal ganglia and internal capsule, they are also seen in the midbrain, pons, cerebellar peduncles, and subcortical white matter. They may correspond to areas of dysplastic glial proliferation and aberrant myelination and their clinical significance and possible association with tumour development and intellectual impairment is unclear.

### Ophthalmic findings

Iris hamartomas (Sakurai–Lisch nodules) are one of the cardinal features of NF1 and are present in the majority of adults with NF1 (see below) (Figure 17.1). Other anterior segment manifestations of NF1 include: prominent corneal, conjunctival and ciliary nerves; congenital ectropion uveae; angle anomalies; posterior embryotoxon; buphthalmos or later-onset glaucoma, especially in association with an ipsilateral plexiform neurofibroma of the eyelid or ectropion uveae; heterochromia iridis; iris mammillations; neurofibromas of conjunctival and ciliary nerves; and anterior subcapsular cataract.

Posterior segment manifestations include: hamartomas of the optic disc, retina and choroid; retinal haemangioma; congenital hypertrophy of the retinal pigment epithelium; myelinated nerve fibres; sectoral retinitis pigmentosa; and cone–rod dystrophy. Multiple choroidal hamartomas, which appear as multiple, small pigmented, circumscribed lesions together with hypopigmented areas may occur. The histology reveals a diffusely thickened choroid with many ganglion cells, nerve fibres and "ovoid bodies", consisting of hyperplastic Schwann cells. Choroidal naevi and melanoma have been described in increased numbers in NF1, although these may be coincidental findings since these conditions are relatively common. Combined pigment epithelial and retinal hamartomas have been described, but are more a feature of NF2.

**Gliomas of the optic pathways** Optic pathway gliomas (OPGs) can occur as isolated

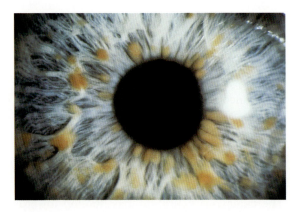

Figure 17.1  Multiple iris hamartomas in NF1

findings or in association with NF1, when they tend to present earlier. The frequency of gliomas of the anterior visual pathway in NF1 is around 15–19%, with about a third of these being symptomatic.[4,5] Frequencies as high as 70% have been quoted depending on the clinical setting and the inclusion of minor optic nerve thickening seen on MRI. OPGs in NF1 are often multicentric or bilateral and are then diagnostic of NF1. Screening for gliomas and watching for progression is difficult in the young age group: visual acuity, colour vision, optic nerve head appearance, MRI, electrodiagnostic testing and visual fields are used in combination. OPGs involving the chiasm are often complicated by precocious puberty.

OPGs can display features that are highly suggestive of NF1. Tubular expansion of the optic nerves, often with lengthening and kinking and extension to include the chiasm (Figure 17.2) and even optic tracts are highly characteristic of NF1 gliomas. Computed tomography (CT) and MRI demonstrate double-density tubular thickening of fusiform tumours of the optic nerve. On T2-weighted MRI, a zone of high intensity surrounds a central low-density core, representing the optic nerve. The high-intensity area appears to correspond to the pathological finding of perineural arachnoidal gliomatosis characteristic of NF1 gliomas.

There is a controversy as to whether OPGs represent truly invasive astrocytomas or whether they are hamartomas. Invasiveness and prognosis are related to position of the tumour and histological grade. In general, anterior gliomas, i.e. those located in the optic nerves alone, tend to have a more benign histology and are less invasive. This type tends to predominate in NF1, when patients are more likely to suffer more serious complications from other intracranial tumours.

**Iris hamartomas**   Iris hamartomas (Sakurai–Lisch nodules) are one of the diagnostic features of NF1 (Figure 17.1) and are present in up to 95–100% of adults with the disease.[6] They are not, however, exclusive to NF1 and have also been

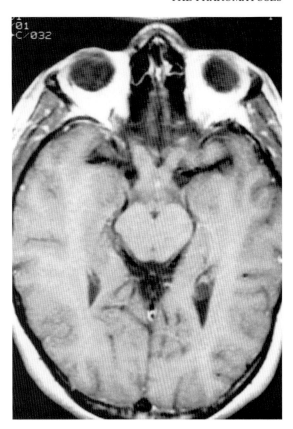

Figure 17.2   T1-weighted MRI scan of chiasmal glioma in patient with NF1. (Courtesy of Ms N Ragge)

reported in Watson syndrome, NF2, Cushing disease, and rarely in "normal" individuals. In blue and green irides, they appear as pale-to-medium brown, fluffy elevations, and in dark brown irides they are cream coloured, dome-shaped and well defined. They vary in size and number from a single, tiny lesion to numerous, large nodules up to 2 mm in diameter. They are distributed in a random fashion on the anterior surface of the iris and occasionally just in the angle.

Histologically, they consist of a condensation of spindle cells of melanocytic origin on the anterior iris surface. They are not usually detectable at birth, but increase in prevalence with age so that by the age of 5 years almost 50% of children demonstrate them. Thereafter, they can be seen in 75% of 15-year olds and 90% of 25-year olds, increasing to almost 100% thereafter. Rarely they can be the only sign of NF1.

**Orbitotemporal neurofibromatosis** Orbital involvement, generally referred to as orbitotemporal neurofibromatosis, may occur as part of generalized NF1, when it is often familial, or as a separate syndrome. A neurofibroma may involve the orbit, eyelids, and temporal area, and may even extend intracranially. Proptosis of the globe can occur and there may be associated buphthalmos and optic nerve compression. The skeletal changes include partial or total absence of the greater wing of the sphenoid, with resultant prolapse of the temporal lobe into the orbit. Pulsating exophthalmos or rarely enophthalmos may occur.

### Genetics of NF1

NF1 is an autosomal dominantly inherited disease with highly variable expression. About 30% of all cases represent new mutations. However, in terms of genetic counselling it is important to examine parents and other family members to determine if subtle signs of NF1 are present before deciding that the individual is likely to have a new mutation. It is not unusual for a parent to have subtle signs of NF1, for example, iris hamartomas alone and a child with a full picture of NF1. In this case, of course, the recurrence risk would be 50%. It is now possible to perform prenatal diagnosis in families with affected individuals using closely linked or intragenic markers for the *NF1* gene. Screening for mutations in the *NF1* gene on a large scale is not yet feasible.

The *NF1* gene is located on the chromosome 17q11.2. It is a large gene, containing at least 56 exons (coding portions) and is expressed ubiquitously, but especially in neurons, Schwann cells and oligodendrocytes in association with microtubules. It appears to act as a classical tumour suppressor gene like retinoblastoma. Mutations occur in both alleles of the *NF1* gene in tumours in NF1 patients. The *NF1* gene product neurofibromin may have three specific functions: the regulation of cellular oncogenes (*ras*) which are important in cell-cycle regulation and therefore growth and differentiation; microtubular function; and involvement in phosphorylation-mediated signal-transduction pathways. Early treatment approaches to prevent tumour development in NF1 are being developed based on the use of farnesyl transferase inhibitors which prevent the farnesyl transferase-mediated membrane association of *ras*. This would in theory inhibit the malignant potential of *ras*-activated cells.

### Management of NF1

The management of NF1 is mainly concerned with the early detection and treatment of complications of the disease and advice regarding presymptomatic screening of relatives. The patient and their family are best managed by a multidisciplinary team involving a geneticist, paediatrician, surgical specialist, ophthalmologist, and genetics counsellor as appropriate to the complications. For a detailed review of management of the paediatric patient with NF1, the reader is referred to the articles by Riccardi.[3,7]

## Neurofibromatosis type 2

Neurofibromatosis type 2 (NF2) is a dominantly inherited disorder characterised by the development of bilateral vestibular schwannomas ("acoustic neuromas") and multiple central nervous system tumours including meningiomas, gliomas, ependymomas and schwannomas.[3,8] NF2 has only been defined as an entity distinct from NF1 in the last fifteen years, following mounting clinical and genetic evidence. NF2 is a much rarer disease than NF1, with a prevalence of 1 in 33 000 to 1 in 40 000.[9]

### Clinical findings

The hallmark of NF2 is the presence of bilateral vestibular schwannomas (Figure 17.3) which occur in 85% of patients. The NIH criteria[10] are summarised in Table 17.3. Spinal tumours are a frequent manifestation of NF2. Although NF1 and NF2 are separate diseases genetically, some clinical features overlap, which has led to much of the confusion over the years. Overall, the skin manifestations of NF2 tend to be less prolific than NF1. For example, it is rare

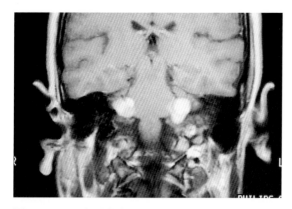

Figure 17.3 Gadolinium-enhanced T1-weighted MRI scan of bilateral vestibular schwannoma in NF2. (Courtesy of Ms N Ragge)

to find an NF2 patient with more than five café an lait patches although there may be larger and atypical café au lait patches. Cutaneous and subcutaneous neurofibromas are found in NF2, but not usually in abundance as in NF1. Cutaneous and subcutaneous schwannomas are found in NF2, but not NF1. The problem is that some NF2 patients can fulfil the current criteria for the diagnosis of both NF2 and NF1 if they have two of the following: cutaneous neurofi-bromas, six café au lait patches, more than two iris hamartomas or a CNS glioma. Definitive genetic studies will clarify this group of individuals with overlapping features.

Schwann cell tumours of the central nervous system are the commonest type of tumour in NF2. In addition to vestibular schwannomas

Table 17.3 Diagnostic criteria for neurofibromatosis 2[10]

The diagnostic criteria are met if a person has either of the following:
• Bilateral VIIIth nerve masses seen with appropriate imaging techniques (for example, computed tomographic or magnetic resonance imaging)
• A first-degree relative with neurofibromatosis 2 and either unilateral VIIIth nerve mass or two of the following:
  Neurofibroma
  Meningioma
  Glioma
  Schwannoma
  Posterior capsular cataract or lens opacity at a young age

these include other cranial nerves, mainly Vth, IXth and Xth, spinal root and intramedullary schwannomas. Other tumours include multiple meningiomas (Figures 17.4a–d and 17.5), and gliomas, which although of low histological grade can cause devastating disease if located in the brainstem or spinal cord. Deep plexiform neurofibromas occur as in NF1 and can lead to neurological dysfunction and malignant degeneration. Patients with NF2 also show calcified subependymal deposits, probably sited within glial hamartomas, and bilateral choroid plexus calcification. As in NF1, there is huge variability in expression of the disease phenotype between individuals with NF2, both in terms of tumour type and location and the clinical severity of disease. However, there may be a mild and severe phenotype that breeds true within families.

Vestibular schwannomas are often the greatest source of morbidity in NF2. Individuals with NF2 most commonly present with hearing loss, sometimes with tinnitus or unsteadiness, in their teens or twenties. By this time the vestibular schwannomas have reached a significant size and are technically harder to remove while preserving hearing and facial nerve function. Pre-symptomatic diagnosis would be of great benefit and allow early screening for tumours. Since dermatological features are often subtle, ophthalmic examination can be of great value in early diagnosis.

**Ophthalmic findings**

Over 80% of NF2 patients have ocular abnormalities.[11] Around 70–80% of individuals have early-onset lens opacities, characteristically posterior subcapsular and capsular cataract and cortical cataract.[11,12] The plaque-like capsular opacities and dense posterior, central cortical cataract cause most visual loss; however, the lens opacities can be difficult to detect unless the pupil is dilated. The presence of other developmental abnormalities including Mittendorf dot (a remnant of the hyaloid system), embryonal cataract and persistent hyperplastic primary vitreous in some individuals, suggests that there

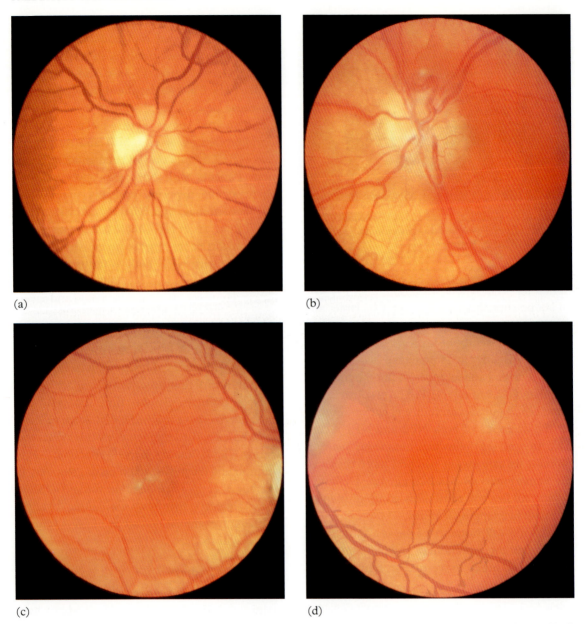

(a)

(b)

(c)

(d)

Figure 17.4    Right and left fundi of patient with NF2 who developed optic nerve sheath meningiomas. Both discs are pale and swollen (a) and (b) and there are small retinal hamartomas at the posterior pole (c) and (d)

may be a spectrum of changes of a developmental nature at the posterior lens pole in NF2. Other anterior segment findings include conjunctival masses, hypertrophied corneal nerves, and iris hamartomas.

Moderately severe visual loss in NF2 is more commonly due to intracranial and optic nerve sheath meningioma than to cataracts. Other causes of visual loss include retinal abnormalities, such as retinal hamartomas and epiretinal membranes, chronic papilloedema, amblyopia secondary to childhood ocular motor paresis or strabismus, and corneal scarring.[11] Retinal hamartomas can occur in up to 23% of individuals with NF2 (Figure 17.4). These include small hamartomas located near the disc, macula

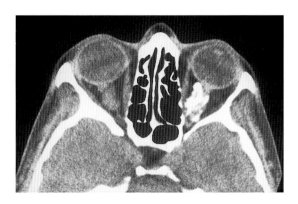

Figure 17.5  CT scan of same patient as in Figure 17.4 showing calcified, thickened left optic nerve and thickened right optic nerve

or in the periphery, combined pigment epithelial and retinal hamartomas (CPERH), and optic disc gliomas. Epiretinal membrane formation, which is also seen in NF2, may be part of the spectrum with CPERH. Occasionally vitreo-retinal degeneration and retinal detachment can occur. Other reported findings include retinal haemangioblastomas, medullated nerve fibres, choroidal naevi, uveal melanoma, and choroidal hamartomas.

Ocular motor pareses occur in over 10% of children with NF2 and strabismus is common.

### Genetics of NF2

In 1993, the gene for NF2 was cloned and the gene product "merlin" or "schwannomin" was characterised as a 595 amino acid protein.[13,14] The term "merlin" was used by one group to denote the NF2 gene product as a moesin-, ezrin-, radixin-like protein (see below) that may play a role in mediating interactions between the cell membrane and the cytoskeleton.[14] The name "schwannomin" was used by another group to denote its role in the production of schwannomas (similar to "neurofibromin" in NF1).[13]

Tightly linked DNA markers can now be used for presymptomatic diagnosis of NF2 in large pedigrees. However, sporadic cases comprise one-third to one-half of all NF2 patients. As a result, segregation analysis is not possible for many at risk individuals, and at present direct mutation screening cannot detect all mutations. Thus clinical examinations continue to be important in diagnosis. Audiological testing may detect an early sensorineural hearing loss, but MRI with Gadolinium-enhanced DTPA is required for definitive diagnosis or exclusion of small vestibular schwannomas. Current recommendations for at-risk relatives (before the availability of a genetic diagnostic test) are that subjects should be seen on a two-yearly basis from 10 to 16 years of age and then on a yearly basis until 50 years, when screening may be ceased if the subjects remain asymptomatic.

## Von Hippel–Lindau disease

Von Hippel–Lindau disease (VHL) is a classical inherited tumour suppressor gene syndrome predisposing affected individuals to haemangioblastomas of the retina and central nervous system, renal cell carcinoma, phaechromocytoma, and renal, pancreatic and epididymal cysts.[15] The incidence is 3 in 100 000. There is almost complete penetrance by the age of 60 years. Renal cell carcinoma is the most common cause of death, and median survival is reduced to 49 years.

### Clinical findings

The diagnostic criteria and clinical features of VHL are summarised in Tables 17.4 and 17.5. The cumulative risk of an individual with VHL developing a retinal haemangioblastoma, cerebellar haemangioblastoma, and renal cell carcinoma at age 30 years are 44%, 38% and 5%, respectively. This increases to 84%, 70%, and 69%, respectively, by age 60 years.

Table 17.4  Criteria for diagnosis of von Hippel–Lindau disease

---

- Isolated cases
  Two or more haemangioblastomas (retinal or CNS) or a single haemangioblastoma in association with a visceral manifestation, e.g. pancreatic, renal, epididymal cysts or renal carcinoma
- Familial cases
  Single haemangioblastoma or visceral complication

---

Table 17.5    Clinical features of von Hippel–Lindau disease

| Clinical feature | Maher *et al.* study[19] | Neumann *et al.* study[20] | Mean age at diagnosis (years)[19] |
|---|---|---|---|
| Retinal haemangioblastoma | 50% | 52% | 25 |
| Cerebellar haemangioblastoma | 50% | 43%* | 29 |
| Spinal cord haemangioblastoma | 13% | | 34 |
| Renal cell carcinoma | 28% | 25%** | 44 |
| Phaeochromocytoma | 7% | 35% | 20 |

*includes all CNS haemangioblastoma
**includes renal cysts and cancer
Adapted from Maher[15]

## Ophthalmic findings

Retinal haemangioblastomas are the most common presenting findings in patients with VHL.[16] Between 25% and 80% of patients with retinal haemangioblastomas will have VHL. The younger the age at presentation with a retinal haemangioblastoma, the greater the likelihood of VHL. All patients with a retinal haemangioblastoma and their first-degree relatives should be screened for VHL. Multiple retinal haemangioblastomas are diagnostic of VHL as are a single retinal haemangioblastoma and a first-degree family member with any of the manifestations of VHL.

Clinically, the retinal and optic nerve head haemangioblastomas of VHL can be divided into two types: endophytic and exophytic.

- Endophytic lesions are elevated red vascular tumours arising from the superficial retina or optic disc and growing into the vitreous (Figure 17.6a,b). Larger peripheral tumours often have a feeding arteriole and draining venule. Smaller tumours consist of a net of dilated capillaries and can be best viewed on fluorescein angiography or angioscopy (Figure 17.7a,b). Visual loss results from exudative or traction retinal detachment, vitreous haemorrhage, macular oedema, epiretinal membrane formation or macular holes. Vascular hamartomas, which are characterised by small moss fibre-like, minimally elevated vascular lesions in the superficial retina usually adjacent to a retinal vein, have also been described.

- Exophytic haemangioblastomas are less common and arise from the outer retinal

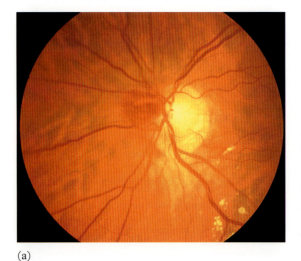

(a)

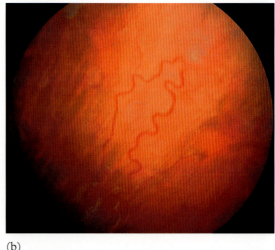

(b)

Figure 17.6    Optic nerve (a) and peripheral retinal haemangioblastoma (b) in VHL disease

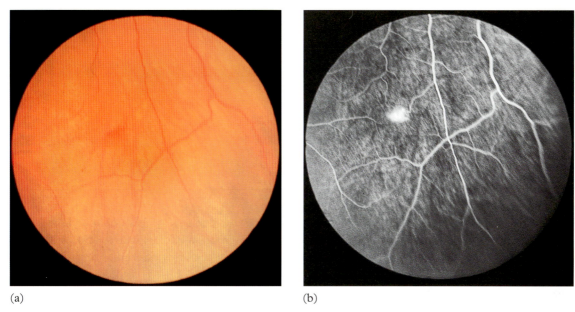

(a)  (b)

Figure 17.7   (a) Fundus photograph and (b) fluorescein angiogram of small peripheral angioma detected during screening in VHL disease

layers, often in the peripapillary area. They should be differentiated from peripapillary neovascularization, juxtapapillary choroiditis, and papilloedema. More posterior optic nerve haemangioblastomas may present as a progressive optic neuropathy or a chiasmal syndrome.

The retinal, optic nerve and central nervous system vascular tumours are indistinguishable in histologic appearance and are best classified as haemangioblastomas. They consist of vascular endothelial-lined channels separated by vacuolated "foam" cells. The tumours are comprised of three main cell types: endothelial cells, pericytes and lipid laden interstitial stromal cells – the "foam" cells. In contrast to the normal situation, the tumour endothelial cells are fenestrated, explaining the high prevalence of exudation from these vascular tumours.

The management of retinal haemangioblastomas depends on their location and size. They are often not symptomatic until serious damage occurs due to complications such as haemorrhage, retinal detachment or macular oedema. Spontaneous regression of retinal haemangioblastomas has been described, but is exceptional.

Generally, haemangioblastomas progressively enlarge, hence the advantage of early detection and prophylactic treatment. Small peripheral tumours are best treated with argon laser photocoagulation sometimes enhanced by fluorescein to improve uptake. Cryotherapy can be applied to larger peripheral tumours.

## Genetics of VHL

The gene for VHL disease is located on chromosome 3p25–p26. The VHL protein appears to be able to move between the nucleus and cytosol, forming specific multiprotein complexes in the cytoplasm. It may control a cellular transcription factor, Elongin (SIII), which interacts with RNA polymerase II.

## Screening and presymptomatic diagnosis

The early diagnosis of complications in VHL, such as retinal haemangioblastomas and renal cell carcinoma leads to reduced morbidity and mortality. The Cambridge screening protocol is given in Table 17.6. Gd-DTPA MRI in two separate sessions is the most useful way of

Table 17.6  Recommended Cambridge screening protocol for von Hippel–Lindau disease[19]

---

Affected patient
  Annual physical examination and urine testing
  Annual indirect ophthalmoscopy and slit-lamp biomicroscopy
  MRI or CT of brain every three years to age 50 and every five years thereafter
  Annual renal ultrasound
  24-hour urine collection for vanillyl mandelic acids

Relatives at risk
  Annual physical examination and urine testing
  Annual indirect ophthalmoscopy and slit-lamp biomicroscopy from age 5 years
  MRI or CT of brain every three years from age 15 to 40 years and then every five years until age 60
  Annual renal ultrasound scan with abdominal CT scan every three years from age 20 to 65 years
  24-hour urine collection for vanillyl mandelic acids

---

screening for brain and spinal cord haemangioblastomas. Linkage studies allow presymptomatic diagnosis and appropriate screening in selected families. Mutation analysis is now possible in about 75% of families.

## Tuberous sclerosis (Bourneville disease)

Tuberous sclerosis, now referred to as the tuberous sclerosis complex (TSC), is a disorder characterised by the development of hamartomatous tumours in multiple organ systems from all primary germ layers. It has an incidence of 1 in 10 000. The classic Vogt triad of seizures, mental retardation and facial angiofibromas is only present in a minority of patients, but is diagnostic when present. The most recent diagnostic criteria divide clinical and radiographic findings into primary, secondary and tertiary diagnostic features[17] (Table 17.7). Patients will be given a definite diagnosis of tuberous sclerosis if they either have one primary feature, two secondary features, or one secondary plus two tertiary features. Probable tuberous sclerosis is diagnosed in the presence of either one secondary plus one tertiary feature, or three tertiary features. Patients are tuberous sclerosis suspects if they have either one secondary feature or two tertiary features.

### Clinical findings

The classical skin lesions are the hypopigmented macules, best detected with Wood's light, and present in 86% of individuals with TSC, facial angiofibromas, and subungual fibromas. Facial angiofibromas are small, often confluent, red, raised nodules and may be treated by repeated dermabrasion. Typical locations are the nasolabial folds, the malar areas, and on the chin. Individual tumours are composed of hyperplastic connective and vascular tissue. Fibrous forehead plaques and shagreen patches are considered secondary diagnostic criteria. Shagreen patches are confluent areas of skin tumour with a waxy, yellowish brown or flesh-coloured appearance and are most often present on the forehead, back or legs. Ashleaf spots and confetti skin lesions are considered tertiary diagnostic criteria. Other secondary and tertiary features are listed in Table 17.7.

All patients with TSC have central nervous system involvement, but the extent and severity of symptoms is highly variable. The most typical MRI abnormality on neuroimaging is a high signal lesion involving the cerebral cortex that corresponds to the cortical hamartoma (tuber). T2-weighted images are helpful in detecting cortical tubers, while subependymal nodules, which are often seen lining the IIIrd ventricle are better demonstrated with T1-weighted images. Giant cell astrocytomas of the brain occur in 2% of patients. The tubers of TSC occur predominantly at the grey–white matter interface. They are characterised by loss of normal cortical cytoarchitecture and the presence of abnormal neurones and glial cells.

Table 17.7   Diagnostic criteria for tuberous sclerosis complex

| Diagnostic features | Confirmation |
|---|---|
| *Primary features* | |
| Facial angiofibromas (adenoma sebaceum) | Clinical |
| Multiple ungual fibromas | Clinical |
| Cortical tuber | Histological |
| Subependymal nodule or giant-cell astrocytoma | Histological |
| Multiple calcified subependymal nodules protruding into the ventricle | Radiographic |
| Multiple retinal astrocytomas | Clinical |
| | |
| *Secondary features* | |
| Affected first-degree relative | |
| Cardiac rhabdomyoma | Histological or radiographic |
| Other retinal hamartoma or achromic patch | Clinical |
| Cerebral tubers | Radiographic |
| Non-calcified subependymal nodules | Radiographic |
| Shagreen patch | Clinical |
| Forehead plaque | Clinical |
| Pulmonary lymphangiomatosis | Histological |
| Renal angiomyolipoma | Histological or radiographic |
| Renal cysts | Histological |
| | |
| *Tertiary features* | |
| Hypomelanotic macules | Clinical |
| "Confetti" skin lesions | Clinical |
| Renal cysts | Radiographic |
| Randomly distributed enamel pits in deciduous and/or permanent teeth | Clinical |
| Hamartomatous rectal polyps | Histological |
| Bone cysts | Radiographic |
| Pulmonary lymphangiomatosis | Radiographic |
| Cerebral white-matter "migration tracts" or heterotopias | Radiographic |
| Gingival fibroma | Clinical |
| Hamartoma of other organs | Histological |
| Infantile spasms | Clinical |

About 40% of patients with TSC are mentally subnormal. Sixty percent of patients have seizures. The severity of seizures correlates with the degree of mental retardation. Patients who have seizures in the first year of life are usually more severely affected. In infancy patients may have myoclonus, infantile spasms, and hypsarrhythmias on electroencephalography (EEG). Some patients are autistic or may display hyperactive or self injurious behaviour. Obstructive hydrocephalus may occur secondary to the brain lesions.

## Ophthalmologic findings

The optic nerve and retinal tumours of TSC were first described by Van der Hoeve.[1] Two morphologic types of retinal astrocytic hamartomas have been recognised (Figure 17.8a,b):

- A more common, relatively flat and translucent, soft-appearing lesion usually located in the peripheral fundus.

- An elevated, nodular, and calcific mulberry-like lesion typically located in the posterior pole adjacent to the optic nerve.

An intermediate type of lesion with features of both types may also be encountered.

Most retinal tumours are static in size and appearance. Some, however, grow and become calcific with time. Occasional complications include vitreous haemorrhage, retinal detachment or glaucoma. Release of granules into the vitreous has been described, but there is never malignant degeneration. Other ocular findings include peripheral depigmented or hyper-pigmented RPE lesions of the retinal pigment epithelium, atypical colobomata, optic atrophy,

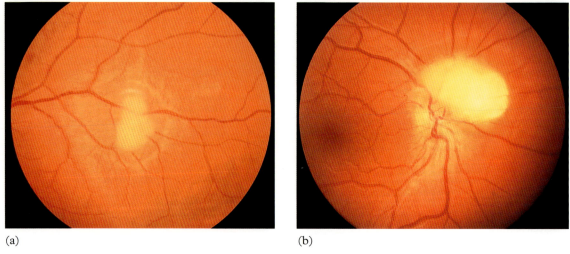

(a)          (b)

Figure 17.8 Peripheral (a) and peripapillary (b) astrocytic hamartoma in TSC

eyelid angiofibromas, white patches of the iris or eyelashes, and strabismus.

## Genetics of tuberous sclerosis

Tuberous sclerosis complex (TSC) is inherited in an autosomal dominant fashion with a rate of about 60% new mutations. The trait is highly penetrant with a moderate variability in symptoms within families. Two different genes (*TSC1* and *TSC2*) each account for about 50% of cases of TSC with an indistinguishable phenotype. *TSC1* maps to 9q34 and *TSC2* to 16p13.3, contiguous to the gene for adult polycystic kidney disease. The TSC2 protein product, tuberin, has a region of homology to the *Rap1* activator *Rap* 1-*GAP* and is presumed to function as a tumour suppressor gene. The 9q gene has yet to be cloned.

Genetic counselling may be difficult in some families with TSC where some relatives have soft clinical signs of the disease but do not fulfill the minimal diagnostic criteria. In the absence of DNA testing, an extensive screening protocol with cutaneous, neuroradiological, cardiac, renal, and ophthalmological evaluations should be used to screen first-degree relatives before counselling is given. Even if extensive screening of parents is negative, a recurrence risk of 2% in subsequent pregnancies should be given. Prenatal diagnosis is now possible using mutation analysis of the *TSC2* gene. Foetal ultrasonography and MRI studies have also been used to detect cardiac and brain tumours, but their sensitivity and specificity are suboptimal.

## Sturge–Weber (encephalotrigeminal angiomatosis)

Sturge–Weber syndrome is characterised by the classic triad of naevus flammeus (port-wine stain) of the face, leptomeningeal angiomatosis with cerebral gyriform calcifications, and choroidal haemangioma with or without glaucoma. It is important to note over 85% of patients with facial port-wine stain do not have brain or eye problems. The presence of the haemangioma, however, prompts the investigation for ocular or brain pathology. Not all patients have all three components of the syndrome, but two are required for the diagnosis. There are no patients with neurologic and ocular disease without a cutaneous haemangioma.

## Clinical findings

The facial angioma occurs along the distribution of the ophthalmic, maxillary, and rarely, mandibular divisions of the trigeminal nerve. It may extend into the region of the upper cervical nerves. The lesion usually stops along the facial midline but may cross it. The flat angioma, which consists of dermal ectatic capillary to venular-sized blood vessels, may become nodular or verrucous with age. The port-wine stain does not regress or respond to steroids, but is currently treated successfully with the carbon dioxide laser.

The central nervous system vascular malformations are most often confined to the pial vessels of the occipitoparietal area. The slow flow of blood through these vessels leads to hypoxia, encephalomalacia, cortical atrophy, and subsequent calcification. The majority of patients have intracranial calcifications with a characteristic "tram-line" pattern. About 80% of patients with Sturge–Weber syndrome develop focal or generalised seizures because of CNS involvement. The presence of seizure activity in the first year of life is a poor prognostic factor and is often associated with developmental delay and sometimes hemiplegia or hemianopsia. Medical therapy for the seizures is often disappointing and a number of medications may be used concurrently without success. Excision of the involved cortical areas, or even a hemispherectomy have been used with encouraging results in these situations.

**Ophthalmologic findings**

Congenital glaucoma in Sturge–Weber syndrome is almost always associated with involvement of both lids and the areas of distribution V1 and V2 branches of the trigeminal nerve by the port-wine stain. In one study, up to 71% of patients with Sturge–Weber syndrome developed glaucoma, which occurred before age 2 years in two-thirds of cases.[18] Episcleral haemangiomas were present in 69% of patients and choroidal haemangiomas in 55%. In general, the more extensive the haemangioma, the more severe the glaucoma and the earlier its presentation. The proposed mechanisms for the development of glaucoma include: (1) outflow

obstruction because of abnormal angle development and vascularization of the iris; (2) elevated episcleral pressure with reduced outflow; (3) secondary angle closure in older patients with choroidal haemangioma, retinal detachment and neovascular glaucoma; (4) hypersecretion of aqueous humour; (5) hyperpermeability of blood vessel walls of choroidal haemangioma; and (6) adult open-angle glaucoma mechanisms.

Although the corneal diameter is enlarged, there are usually no horizontal breaks in Desçemet's membrane. Gonioscopy and histopathologic studies reveal an angle pattern suggestive of goniodysgenesis in infantile cases: the uveal meshwork is thick; the scleral spur is poorly developed; the iris insertion may be high; and there may be a Barkan's membrane. There may also be vascularization of the angle and trabecular meshwork. The histopathologic changes of the anterior chamber angle in older patients are similar to those of open-angle glaucoma.

The glaucoma generally is resistant to topical medical treatment. However, medications may be useful in maintaining good control of the intraocular pressure after surgery. Goniotomy or trabeculotomy in infants, and trabeculotomy with or without trabeculectomy in older children and adults, have been used in patients with Sturge–Weber syndrome with varying degrees of success. Surgery may be complicated by intraoperative serous choroidal detachment and occasionally by suprachoroidal haemorrhage. It is hence reasonable to start patients with Sturge–Weber syndrome on topical beta-blockers and carbonic anhydrase inhibitors as soon as their glaucoma is diagnosed. If the intraocular pressure is controlled, surgery may be avoided or delayed. If the pressure remains elevated, a goniotomy or a trabeculotomy is most likely the initial procedure of choice. Filtering procedures with or without antimetabolites could be performed next.

Choroidal cavernous haemangiomas are usually diffuse in Sturge–Weber syndrome. They are most often located temporal to the optic disc and are most elevated in the macular area. Haemangiomas do not cause any visual disturbances early in life but may lead to the late development of overlying retinal cystoid changes or exudative retinal detachment. Other ocular findings in Sturge–Weber syndrome include heterochromia iridis, conjunctival angioma, dilatation of episcleral vessels and retinal aneurysms associated with an arteriovenous angioma of the thalamus and midbrain. Visual field defects may be present in patients with occipital lobe meningeal involvement and cortical atrophy.

## Genetics and pathogenesis of Sturge–Weber syndrome

Sturge–Weber syndrome is not inherited. The primary lesion in Sturge–Weber may be either a defective structural differentiation of the vascular wall and persistence of the sinusoid embryonic vascular bed in the region of angiomatosis or a defective migration and differentiation of the pro- and mesencephalic neural crest leading to abnormal proliferation of blood vessels and goniodysgenesis.

## References

1 Van der Hoeve J. Eye diseases in tuberous sclerosis of the brain and in Recklinghausen's disease. *Trans Ophthal Soc UK* 1923; **43**: 524–41.
2 Huson S. Clinical and Genetic Studies of von Recklinghausen Neurofibromatosis. Edinburgh: University of Edinburgh: 1989, MD thesis.
3 Riccardi VM. *Neurofibromatosis: Phenotype, Natural History, and Pathogenesis*, 2nd edn. Baltimore, MD: Johns Hopkins University Press, 1992: 498.
4 Lewis RA, Gerson LP, Axelson KA, *et al.* Von Recklinghausen neurofibromatosis. II. Incidence of optic gliomata. *Ophthalmology* 1984; **91**: 929–35.
5 Listernick R, Charrow J, Greenwald M, Mets M. Natural history of optic pathway tumors in children with neurofibromatosis type 1. *J Pediatr* 1994; **125**: 63–6.
6 Ragge NK, Falk RE, Cohen WE, Murphree AL. Images of Lisch nodules across the spectrum. *Eye* 1993; 7: 95–101.
7 Riccardi V. Type 1 neurofibromatosis and the pediatric patient. *Curr Prob Ped* 1992; **22**: 66–106.
8 Mulvihill JJ, Parry DM, Sherman JI, *et al.* Neurofibromatosis 1 (Recklinghausen disease) and neurofibromatosis 2 (bilateral acoustic neurofibromatosis) – an update (NIH conference). *Ann Int Med* 1990; **113**: 39–52.
9 Evans DRG, Huson SM, Donnai D, *et al.* Clinical study of type 2 neurofibromatosis. *Quart J Med* 1992; **84**: 603–18.
10 Consensus Development Panel. National Institutes of Health Consensus Development Conference Statement on Acoustic Neuroma, December 11–13, 1991. *Arch Neurol* 1994; **51**: 201–7.
11 Ragge NK, Baser ME, Klein J, *et al.* Ocular abnormalities in neurofibromatosis 2. *Am J Ophthalmol* 1995; **120**: 634–41.
12 Bouzas EA, Freidlin V, Parry DM, *et al.* Lens opacities in neurofibromatosis 2: further significant correlations. *Br J Ophthalmol* 1993; 77: 354–7.
13 Rouleau GA, Merel P, Lutchman M, *et al.* Alteration in a new gene encoding a putative membrane-organizing protein causes neurofibromatosis type 2. *Nature* 1993; **363**: 515–21.
14 Trofatter JA, MacCollin MM, Rutter JL, *et al.* A novel moesin-, ezrin-, radixin-like gene is a candidate for the neurofibromatosis 2 tumor suppressor. *Cell* 1993; **72**: 791–800.
15 Maher ER. Von Hippel–Lindau disease. *Eur J Cancer* 1994; **30A**: 1987–90.
16 Moore AT, Maher ER, Rosen P, *et al.* Ophthalmological screening for von Hippel–Lindau disease. *Eye* 1991; **5**: 723–8.
17 Roach C, Smith M, Huttenlocher P, *et al.* Diagnostic criteria of tuberous sclerosis complex. *J Child Neurol* 1992; 7: 221–4.
18 Sullivan T, Clarke M, Morin J. The ocular manifestations of Sturge–Weber syndrome. *J Pediatr Ophthalmol Strab* 1992; **29**: 349–56.
19 Maher ER, Yates JR, Harris R, *et al.* Clinical features and natural history of Von Hippel–Lindau disease. *Quart J Med* 1990; 77: 1151–63.
20 Neumann HPH, Lips CJM, Hsia YE, Zbar B. Von Hippel–Lindau syndrome. *Brain Pathol* 1995; **5**: 181–93.

# 18 Visual pathway disorders

JOHN ELSTON

Of the large number of pathological processes that may affect the visual pathways in infancy and childhood, two major categories of disorder can be recognised. In the first only, vision is affected. These children may be referred to the ophthalmologist from primary healthcare workers, for example general practitioners, health visitors, orthoptists or optometrists. They present with physical signs noted by the parents or carers, or occasionally detected by screening. Examples are the apparently blind infant, with or without nystagmus or the school child observed to be having visual difficulties. Such children may also present with squint or proptosis. In the second category, as well as visual difficulties other problems are present or have developed. Examples are developmental delay or regression, unsteadiness, weakness, lethargy or fits. Dependent upon the major symptomatic impact of the underlying disorder, these children may be referred directly to the ophthalmologist, or be tertiary referrals for diagnostic evaluation from pediatricians or other colleagues.

In both groups, visual symptoms are unusual. Up to the age of 10 years or so, children rarely complain of reduced, or even total loss of vision in one eye, and bilateral visual loss may not be symptomatic until very advanced. Congenital and early acquired homonymous visual field defects are always asymptomatic.

## Evaluation

Considerable time and patience is needed to evaluate a child with deteriorating vision. The pregnancy, birth and family history and general, physical and intellectual development are all relevant and should be enquired after. Specific symptoms that should be asked for in older children include headache, double vision, and pain on eye movement.

It is important to have some measure of visual function at the first clinic visit against which to gauge progress. This will be either linear Snellen acuity, letter matching or grating acuity dependent on the age of the child. Colour vision can be measured with Ishihara plate numbers, or in preverbal children by tracing the "snake" in the plates at the back of the book. Afferent pupillary function is difficult to assess in children because accommodation is difficult to reliably control. With experience and sympathy it is usually possible to elicit useful Goldmann visual fields from the age of about five or six years even in sick children. Ocular alignment and eye movements are relatively easy to test and may be very helpful diagnostically.

The optic discs should be examined through dilated pupils, by direct and indirect ophthalmoscopy. In young children the importance of the diagnostic information that may be available from dilated fundoscopy (for example, retinal haemorrhage in non-accidental injury) outweighs any neurological contraindication to pupillary dilatation. The refraction is useful in evaluating optic disc size and shape, and may be a useful clue, for example high hypermetropia in Leber's amaurosis. The optic disc is relatively colourless in neonates and young children, and unless there is a clear difference in colour between the two optic discs, it is difficult to be dogmatic about atrophy. Attention should be focused on differences between the nerve fibre layer of the retina of the two sides. The inner limiting membrane in infancy and childhood is highly reflective, and if the nerve fibre layer is defective, prominent reflections can be seen surrounding the retinal blood vessels.

Topographical localisation of pathology is inevitably more difficult in children than in adults. Most children with visual pathway problems will need to be referred for investigation. It is important to have ready access to neuroimaging, and to be able to discuss the clinical problem with a neuroradiological colleague before ordering the test. Finding time to discuss the films directly with the radiologist, and if appropriate other colleagues, e.g. a neurosurgeon or oncologist, is educational and fosters a collaborative approach. Visual electrophysiology is also an essential investigation of children with suspected visual pathway disease and it is important that the visual science department is able to offer a full diagnostic evaluation including pattern electroretinograms (PERG), flash electroretinography (FERG), and flash and pattern visual-evoked potentials (see Chapter 3).

The child's management may involve arranging a consultation, sometimes at very short notice, with a pediatrician, a neurosurgeon or a geneticist. A network of sympathetic colleagues interested in the management of these children should be established.

The child's parents will be anxious and often frightened. It may fall to the ophthalmologist to make the diagnosis of a life-threatening condition, such as intracranial tumour. This is a highly unusual situation in ophthalmology and requires tact, sympathy, and time. A trainee must involve a senior colleague at the earliest opportunity. The family of a child newly diagnosed with a visual pathway disorder may well need considerable support from the social work department.

# Congenital disorders of the optic nerve

## Optic nerve hypoplasia

If bilateral and severe, optic nerve hypoplasia presents in infancy with little or no visual response, roving conjugate eye movements sometimes with bursts of abnormal fast eye movements ("nystagmus") superimposed.[1] If the hypoplasia is less severe, and particularly if it is asymmetrical or unilateral, the child may present with a squint, or with one of the associated abnormalities (see below).

Damage to the developing optic nerve occurs in the first or early in the second trimester. Optic nerve hypoplasia occurs in the foetal alcohol syndrome. No other definite causes have been established, but there is an association with low maternal age and possibly maternal diabetes mellitus.

If the hypoplasia is severe, the abnormality of disc size is easy to identify. The same applies if it is unilateral or very asymmetric. However minor degrees of hypoplasia are difficult to detect. It is useful to try to identify the scleral rim. There is often a peripapillary choroidal/retinal defect exposing the sclera around the rim which may mimic optic atrophy. The choroidal/retinal edge may be pigmented (double-ring sign) (Figure 18.1a,b).

There may be an associated brain maldevelopment. This may be severe and widespread or localised, for example septo-optic dysplasia or even isolated growth hormone deficiency. One or both optic nerves may be hypoplastic or dysplastic in children with developmental tumours affecting the anterior visual pathways, such as craniopharyngioma.

Children with both unilateral and bilateral optic nerve hypoplasia are at increased risk of endocrine disturbances, particularly growth hormone deficiency and referral to a pediatric neurologist is indicated in all cases. Neuroradiologic imaging is helpful in identifying any associated central nervous system abnormalities. Cortical visual-evoked potentials may give useful information about the long-term visual prog-

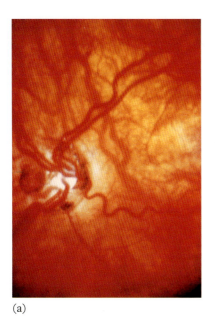 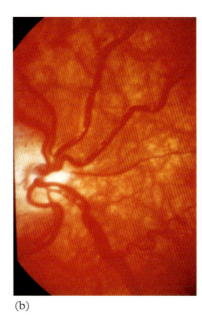

Figure 18.1 Both optic discs are hypoplastic; the left (a) has peripapillary pigmentation (double-ring sign). (Courtesy of Mr J Elston)

(a)  (b)

nosis. The parents will need appropriate counselling support and advice particularly about the education of a child with severely impaired vision.

## Optic nerve coloboma

Coloboma is due to a failure or abnormality of closure of the foetal fissure of the optic cup. The coloboma may be confined to the optic nerve head, or involve the iris and retina in isolation or combination. The eye may be small (microphthalmos). The abnormality may be unilateral (unusual) or bilateral, but asymmetric. Presentation is therefore with an abnormality of appearance of the eye or eyes, squint or failure of visual development. The condition may occasionally be autosomal dominant, with variable penetrance. It is usually sporadic with no identifiable cause.[2]

There is a spectrum of optic disc appearance, with associated retinal abnormality. The visual potential of the eye will be determined by whether or not the macula is involved and the severity of the optic nerve abnormality. The retina may be detached or become detached at a later stage and a specialist vitreoretinal opinion will be required in these cases. Spontaneous re-attachment may occur.

A number of systemic developmental associations are recognised. These include:

- CHARGE association. The acronym stands for *c*oloboma, *h*eart defect, *a*tresia choanae, *r*etarded growth and development, *g*enital anomalies, *e*ar anomalies and deafness. A child's parents will need to be questioned with these possibilities in mind and may need to be referred on because of other problems.

- Tracheo-oesophageal fistula (TOF). An infant with coloboma and feeding difficulties should be referred to exclude this abnormality. More usually a child with a known TOF is referred because of concerns about vision which may be due to coloboma.

- Chromosomal disorders. Children with a number of rare chromosomal disorders presenting to pediatricians with other problems may be found to have optic disc colobomas.

Visual function will need to be maximised in the conventional way with spectacle correction of any refractive error and treatment of amblyopia. In school-age children the peripatetic teacher for the visually handicapped may need to be involved, and in some cases registration as partially sighted or blind may be appropriate. Because of the genetic implications of the diagnosis both parents must be examined to exclude minor degrees of iris, optic nerve or retinal coloboma.

### Optic disc dysplasia

The condition most commonly presents with squint due to an associated anisometropia often with astigmatism.[3] One or both optic discs is found to be tilted or segmentally hypoplastic (Figure 18.2a,b). The association of unilateral high myopia with myelinated retinal fibres and a relative afferent pupillary defect is part of this spectrum of disorder. The morning glory optic disc anomaly is a unilateral disturbance of optic nerve head development. The disc is abnormally large with blood vessels radiating from it and a central proliferation of glial tissue with a persistent hyaloid artery (Figure 18.3). The retina may be detached, or become detached later.

The aetiology of this spectrum of optic nerve dypsplasia is unknown. However children with congenital or developmental tumours involving the anterior visual pathways (e.g. craniopharyngioma) may be found to have segmental disc hypoplasia. In most cases conventional management of any associated amblyopia and refractive error is all that is required. Neuroimaging is indicated if any aspect of visual function deteriorates.

### Congenital atrophy

Congenitally atrophic optic discs are normal size and the damage to the developing axons has occurred late in the second or in the third trimester. The damage may be to either the anterior or posterior visual pathways, in the latter case transsynaptic degeneration accounting for the atrophy. Children with congenital optic atrophy usually have multiple neurological and developmental problems but may be referred by a pediatrician for an opinion on visual development. Neuroimaging will usually have been carried out already, but cortical visual-evoked potentials (including hemifield stimulation) may be helpful in predicting visual function.

## Acquired disorders of the optic nerve

### Papilloedema

Papilloedema is not in itself usually symptomatic. Occasionally with a very rapid and sustained rise in intracranial pressure, for

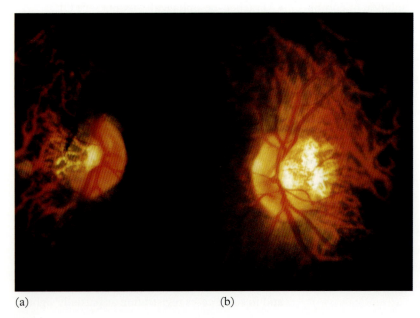

(a)　　　　　　　　　(b)

Figure 18.2 The optic discs show segmental hypoplasia; the visual acuity was good, but the visual field was constricted nasally. (Courtesy of Mr J Elston)

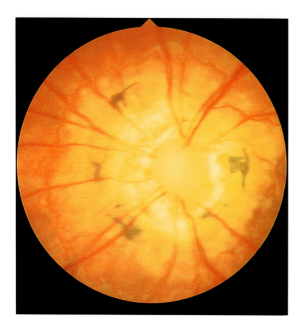

Figure 18.3    Morning glory disc

previous episodes of papilloedema and some-times to chiasmal compression from an expanded IIIrd ventricle, may mean disc swelling is subtle or absent. Symptoms, such as deterioration in visual function, diplopia, headache, neck ache, backache or unsteadiness are an important guide to shunt blockage.

Persistent raised intracranial pressure may occur in childhood secondary to cerebral venous sinus thrombosis. This can be caused by blood dyscrasias, severe dehydration or middle-ear infection. Idiopathic intracranial hypertension may also occur in childhood.

The physical signs will be dependent upon the rate of rise of intracranial pressure, its height and chronicity. Chronic papilloedema may be associated with retinal haemorrhages and exudates (Figure 18.4a,b,). Asymmetric or unilateral papilloedema can be due to an anatomical variant protecting the retrolaminar blood supply to one optic nerve. Unilateral or bilateral VIth nerve palsy may be found as a non-localising sign. Ocular motor signs may be important in topographical localisation, for example skew deviation in posterior fossa tumours.

A child presenting with papilloedema needs urgent neuroimaging as this will determine whether the appropriate referral is directly to a paediatric neurosurgeon or neurologist.

example following cerebral venous sinus thrombosis, vision may deteriorate acutely bilaterally. More often, the raised intracranial pressure will be symptomatic, though often non specifically (headaches, etc.) in which case the child may be referred to an ophthalmologist. Serious intracranial disease such as posterior fossa tumours may present in this way to the ophthalmologist. In hydrocephalus, optic atrophy, consecutive to

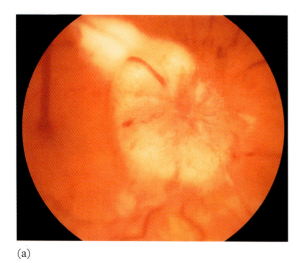

(a)

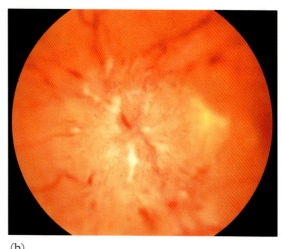

(b)

Figure 18.4    Chronic papilloedema with marked disc swelling, haemorrhages and exudates

## Optic disc swelling in the absence of raised intracranial pressure

Some children referred with suspected intracranial pressure do not have true papilloedema secondary to raised intracranial pressure but other conditions which lead to blurring of the disc margins. Optic disc drusen are often buried in children and the optic discs appear swollen without the characteristic drusen on the surface of the disc (Figure 18.5a–c). The optic disc vasculature may show aberrant branching and drusen can usually be clearly demonstrated on ultrasound or high-resolution computed tomography (CT) scanning of the optic nerve head.[4] Rarely, optic nerve drusen, particularly if evident on the disc in childhood, indicate a low-grade

optic neuropathy which can be compressive, for example, due to fibrous dysplasia involving the optic canal.

High hyperopia in childhood may be associated with very small crowded optic nerve heads which mimic disc swelling. This may cause problems in diagnosis, especially when the child has presented with headache and malaise. The presence of spontaneous venous pulsatation of the central retinal vein and the lack of haemorrhages adjacent to the disc margin are helpful in excluding papilloedema but where there is doubt about the benign nature of the optic disc appearances, neuroradiological imaging may be necessary.

Arterial hypertension may present in childhood with optic disc swelling. As with adults,

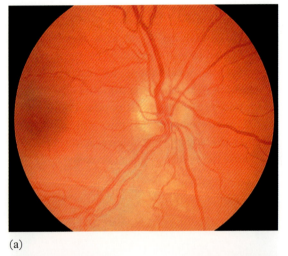

(a)

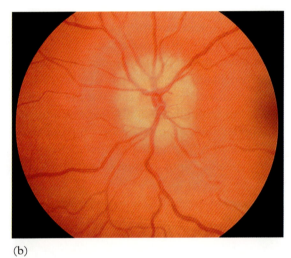

(b)

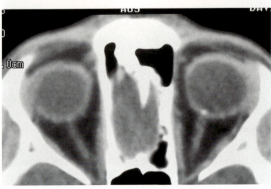

(c)

Figure 18.5 Bilateral disc swelling (a) and (b) in a 10-year-old girl due to buried optic disc drusen seen on CT scan shown in (c)

there is a risk of infarcting the disc if the blood pressure is lowered too quickly. Optic disc swelling occurs in optic neuritis in childhood but is accompanied by visual loss and evidence of optic neuropathy.

## Optic atrophy

Optic atrophy is a physical sign, not a diagnosis. It may be unilateral or bilateral, partial or complete and, if bilateral, symmetric or asymmetric. There are obviously many possible causes including perinatal hypoxic/ischaemic insults, trauma, compression of the anterior visual pathways, chronically raised intracranial pressure and metabolic disorders. Optic atrophy may also be inherited, usually as an autosomal dominant trait[5] with variable clinical expression (Figure 18.6a–d).

In children with hydrocephalus, progressive optic atrophy may be the only sign of shunt blockage as sometimes symptoms of visual disturbance or headache may be absent. The ventricles are rigid and scanning may not show much, if any, increase in size when the shunt is blocked. Ophthalmologists should have a low threshold for referring these children for

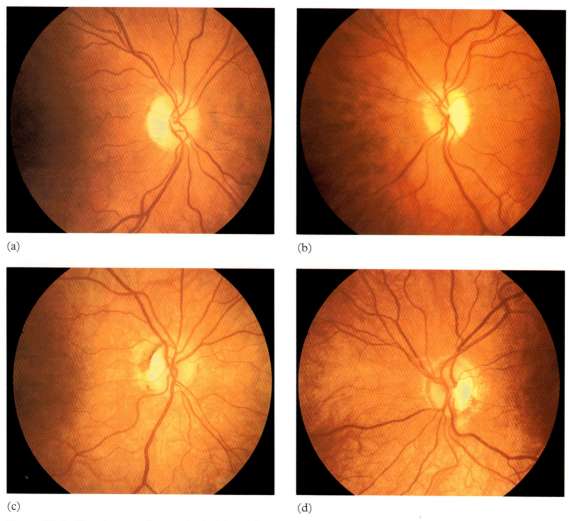

(a)

(b)

(c)

(d)

Figure 18.6   Dominant optic atrophy in (a) and (b) a 12-year-old girl and (c) and (d) her mother (b). Note the characteristic temporal pallor

intracranial pressure monitoring, if there is a suggestion of increasing optic atrophy, reduced visual function or onset of strabismus.

Most children with optic atrophy have an established cause for the visual pathway damage, for example hydrocephalus, visual pathway tumour or history of an ischaemic hypoxic insult in the perinatal period. Children with optic atrophy without any clear associated risk factors, particularly those with recent onset of visual deterioration, require urgent investigation including neuroradiologic imaging.

## Optic neuritis

In the first decade, this characteristically presents with acute severe bilateral reduction of vision over 24 to 48 hours sometimes to no perception of light. Retrobulbar pain or headache may be a feature. The visual-evoked potential (VEP) shows reduced amplitude with very prolonged latencies. Recovery of visual function is usually also relatively rapid but continues over several days or weeks.[6]

*Unilateral optic neuritis* can occur in the first decade in association with neurotropic virus infection (for example, chickenpox) and with juxtapapillary toxoplasmosis. Rarely, sphenoidal sinusitis can cause a retrobulbar neuritis.

In *bilateral optic neuritis*, disc swelling is invariably present with dilated pupils and afferent defects. There may be some cells in the vitreous, but no retinal vascular changes. With the resolution of the disc swelling, optic atrophy develops, but recovery of excellent visual function is the rule. The aetiology is unknown. There is no association with multiple sclerosis. However, unilateral or bilateral sequential optic neuritis in older (teenage) children may be associated with multiple sclerosis. In the vast majority of children there will be no associated systemic findings.[6,7]

All children presenting with optic neuritis will need neuroimaging (MRI) and cerebrospinal fluid (CSF) examination. Blood tests to exclude a specific cause are indicated and include mito-

chondrial DNA examination to look for Leber's hereditary optic neuropathy (LHON), which can present in the first decade. Children with acute bilateral simultaneous optic neuritis should be treated with systemic steroids, which appear to speed the resolution. This is particularly valuable if vision is reduced to very low levels.

## Optic nerve glioma (see Chapter 17)

Optic nerve glioma may present with proptosis or squint in the first decade, but is often asymptomatic especially in neurofibromatosis type 1 (NF1). The eye is usually also displaced downwards and often laterally. Eye movements, particularly elevation, are reduced. The optic disc may be chronically swollen, with a relative afferent pupillary defect. In the absence of proptosis, the disc is more commonly atrophic.[8] Visual acuity may be relatively well maintained, even in the presence of chronic disc swelling or atrophy. Towards the end of the first decade, Lisch nodules can be seen on the iris in NF1.

Sporadic optic glioma is a more aggressive tumour in childhood than that occurring with NF1. Serial documentation of visual function is important in deciding if intervention is indicated. Apart from acuity, colour vision and visual fields should be measured. Optic disc photographs are useful. MRI is needed to show the extent of the glioma which in NF1 may well be bilateral, and involve the chiasm either in continuity with one or both nerves or independently.

Children with optic nerve glioma should to be managed in collaboration with a paediatriac oncologist and with input from clinical geneticists. Sporadic optic glioma confined to the intraorbital nerve, and showing rapid growth or causing blindness, should be excised with preservation of the globe. In neurofibromatosis, the glioma is more indolent and may regress spontaneously. Chemotherapy may be indicated where there is evidence of tumour enlargement and deteriorating visual function in a functioning eye.

## Trauma

Optic neuropathy may occur in closed head injury by transmission of force from the frontal/temporal region to the optic canal. The damage may be due to focal peri- or intraneural hemorrhage, and there is usually no fracture. Recovery is unpredictable and no specific treatment is of proven value.

The visual pathways may be severely damaged in non-accidental injury. Shaking injury in infants causes retinal hemorrhage (Figure 18.7), and postmortem, haemorrhage into the optic nerve sheath is very common.[9] There may be damage to the posterior visual pathways and visual cortex from shearing injury or ischaemia. Optic atrophy is a common sequel.

Accurate documentation of the ophthalmological findings is essential in cases of suspected non-accidental injury and all cases must be seen by a consultant. Epileptic fits or attempts at resuscitation do not cause a haemorrhagic retinopathy. Accidental head trauma should not be considered to have done so unless it was very severe (e.g. road traffic accident) and independently verifiable.

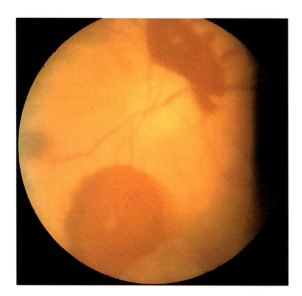

Figure 18.7 Retinal and preretinal haemorrhages in an infant with non-accidental (shaking) injury

## Leber's hereditary optic neuropathy

Although this characteristically presents in the second or third decades, it may occur in the first and may not be symptomatic until the second eye is involved. In the acute stages, there is evidence of optic disc swelling which is replaced by profound atrophy as the swelling resolves. A boy presenting with optic atrophy of uncertain aetiology should always be tested for the mitochondrial DNA mutations known to cause the condition. Appropriate genetic counselling will be needed.[10]

## Miscellaneous conditions involving the retina/optic nerve

The anterior visual pathways may be damaged by a number of disorders presenting primarily to pediatricians. Ophthalmological features may provide a clue to the underlying diagnosis. In other cases, the underlying disorder will be known or suspected and the child referred for visual assessment. Examples are as follows:

- Neurometabolic disorders, e.g. Batten disease, mucopolysaccharidoses and adrenoleukodystrophy. Note that biotinidase deficiency (which is treatable) may present with ataxia and poor vision due to optic atrophy.

- Mitrochondrial cytopathy.

- Leukaemic infiltration/deposit involving the optic nerve.

- Radiation optic neuropathy. This may occur following radiotherapy targeted particularly in the parasellar region in the management of, for example, craniopharyngioma or germ cell tumour. The occurrence is not strictly dose dependent and it is more likely to occur if the visual pathways are already severely compromised. Vision deteriorates rapidly, usually approximately nine months after the treatment. Hyperbaric oxygen therapy may retrieve some visual function.

In otherwise unexplained cases of optic atrophy, the possibility of genetically determined (dominant) optic atrophy should be considered and the parents and child examined for the characteristic nerve fibre defect in the retina, which involves the papillomacular bundle. Visual acuity in this disorder is usually stable in childhood but may deteriorate in late adult life. The possibility of secondary optic atrophy due to a primary retinal abnormality should also be excluded.

## Disorders of the chiasm

Chiasmal disorders may present in infancy as a blind or very poorly seeing baby with nystagmus or present in older children with progressive visual failure.[11] A variety of disorders may affect the chiasm (Table 18.1). See-saw nystagmus is pathognomonic of chiasmal disease but is uncommon. More commonly, the nystagmus is atypical and acquired after a period of normal ocular motor function. All infants with nystagmus acquired after four months of age should have MRI scanning to exclude chiasmal disease. The underlying pathology may be chiasmal dysplasia or more commonly a congenital cyst or tumour involving the chiasm. Acquired or progressive chiasmal disease in older children tends to present late, with severely affected vision. Dependent on the underlying problem, other symptoms such as headache or growth failure may predominate. Parasellar disease may present as a sensory exotropia if vision is more severely affected in one eye.

Children with NF1 may develop a chiasmal glioma (see Chapter 17). The glioma may be extensive, involving both optic nerves and tracts (Figure 18.8).

External chiasmal compression by craniopharyngioma and germ cell tumours may present to the ophthalmologist with visual failure (Figure 18.8). Granulomas, including Langerhans cell histiocytosis and infections, particularly tuberculosis, may also involve this region. The chiasm may be damaged in closed head trauma or by an expanding IIIrd ventricle in communicating hydrocephalus.

Visual acuity is often severely reduced at presentation. Colour vision is also often affected. A bitemporal or other chiasmal/parasellar field defect will be present but may be difficult to demonstrate in a young child. The optic discs

Table 18.1   Chiasmal disorders in childhood

Developmental defects
  Absence of chiasm (achiasmia)
  Chiasmal misrouting in albinism

Tumours
Intrinsic:    Chiasmal glioma
Extrinsic:    Craniopharyngioma
            Dysgerminoma
            Metastatic disease

Inflammatory disorders
  Langerhans' cell histiocytosis
  Sarcoidosis

Trauma

Other uncommon disorders
  Hydrocephalus with distended IIIrd ventricle
  Tuberculosis

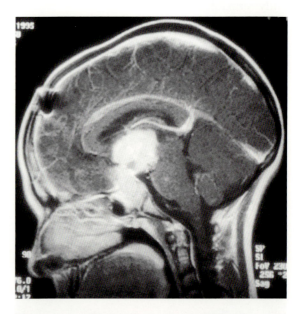

Figure 18.8   Germ cell tumour involving chiasm and adjacent visual pathways in an 8-year-old girl who presented with rapidly progressive visual failure. The biopsy site can be seen. (Courtesy of Mr J Elston)

may be dysplastic (see above) or show swelling and/or pallor. Damage to nearby structures, particularly the hypothalamus and pituitary may be found. Growth failure or decline is especially common.

An MRI will be needed to determine appropriate referral. The visual function should be documented and an attempt made to measure the visual fields. Optic disc photographs are useful in monitoring progress.

## Retrogeniculate disorders

Severe visual deficit from posterior visual pathway pathology may present in infancy with poor or absent fixation, an exotropia and no purposive eye movements. Nystagmus is usually absent but intermittent abnormal fast eye movements may be seen. In cases due to prenatal (or perinatal) damage (e.g. hypoxia or haemorrhage) other neurological signs, particularly signs of cerebral palsy, may dominate the clinical picture. A single lesion causing congenital unilateral retrochiasmal damage will not cause symptoms and is usually discovered by chance. Acquired unilateral pathology may present with other symptoms such as raised intracranial pressure.

Visual function will depend on the nature and extent of the underlying pathology.[12,13] Optic atrophy occurs with posterior visual pathway damage if it occurs prenatally or in the early postnatal period. MRI scanning may be helpful in determining the stage of development at which the injury to the developing brain took place. Isolated unilateral or bilateral occipital lobe dysplasia may occur. Developmental vascular anomalies, such as arteriovenous malformation may not be symptomatic until the first or second decade or even later. Trauma, both accidental and non-accidental, may also be responsible. Near drowning and carbon monoxide poisoning may both be associated with selective damage to the occipital cortex. Closed head trauma may be followed by transient complete blindness, with substantial recovery of vision within hours and continuing over weeks. Other causes of damage include tumours and complicated migraine.

Many children with symptomatic disorders involving the retrochiasmal visual pathways have other developmental and neurological problems, and these cases will be referred from neurologists or paediatricians for an assessment. Cortical visual-evoked potentials with hemifield stimulation may be useful in assessing visual function in older children but often the long-term visual prognosis is difficult to predict in early infancy. The prognosis is best in those infants with relatively well preserved VEP responses and those in whom the visual pathways are structurally normal on CT or MRI scanning.[12] Most infants with cortical visual impairment show gradual improvement in visual function often over many months and even years.[13] Visual perceptual problems are often a prominent feature and may only be discovered after a careful history is taken.[14] It is uncommon for complete blindness to occur so it is important not to be too pessimistic with parents at the initial consultation. The parents should be encouraged to continue to stimulate the child to use any residual visual function by using very large brightly coloured toys or coloured lights as appropriate. A referral to the peripatetic teacher for the visually impaired at an early stage is useful and, although in most cases there is no treatment available, parents value the opportunity to have their child reassessed in the eye clinic periodically to measure progress.

## Delayed visual maturation

Delayed visual maturation is in part a diagnosis of exclusion and can only reliably be made in retrospect once an infant with poor vision shows evidence of normal development of visual function. Affected infants present in the first six to eight weeks of life, when an infant is noticed by the parents to have no eye contact or visual interest. The condition may occur in isolation or may be seen in infants with systemic illness, or non-specific developmental delay. It commonly occurs in otherwise normal infants with ocular and/or visual pathway disorders, for example, ocular or oculocutaneous albinism.

Clinical examination reveals poor visual function either in isolation or with the associations noted above. The site of the dysfunction in the developing visual system is unknown. The electroretinogram (ERG) and VEP are usually normal unless the infant has other ocular or systemic abnormalities.[15]

The major differential diagnosis is from cortical visual impairment. If the electrodiagnostic investigations are normal and general development is also normal, improvement in visual function may be expected. The parents may be given a cautiously optimistic prognosis and further investigation is not necessary unless the expected visual recovery does not occur. Spontaneous improvement in vision usually starts at about twelve to fifteen weeks of age. If electrophysiology is abnormal and/or other developmental problems are suspected the child will need neuroimaging and referral to a paediatric neurologist.[16]

## Functional visual loss

Characteristically, vision in both eyes is affected towards the end of the first or beginning of the second decade; it occurs more commonly in girls than boys. The child may complain of reading difficulties. Poor acuity may have been detected at a routine school eye test, or a visit to the opticians, sometimes arranged because of a complaint of headache or poor school performance. Usually there is an obvious mismatch between the level of measurable visual function and the child's activities. Visual fields may be inconsistent, and constricted or show spiralling. There are no abnormal physical signs. The child is often indifferent to the concern that the poor vision is causing parents and doctors.[17]

It may be possible to coax the child towards or up to normal levels of visual acuity by the use of low-power cylindrical plus lenses or rotating cylindrical lenses to cancel one another out.

However, the inability to do so does not rule out the diagnosis. Full cycloplegic refraction is important, with correction of any refractive error. Retinal disorders, for example X-linked retinoschisis or early Stargardt disease can present a very similar picture, without obvious physical signs, and full electrophysiological investigation is important. This should include a flash and pattern ERG and pattern VEP (see Chapter 3). A large mismatch between the visual function recorded with the pattern VEP and the visual acuity is helpful in confirming the diagnosis. In the absence of a cause for the poor vision, it is worth interviewing the parents without the child present, to see if a simple explanation for the problem such as bullying or family difficulties can be determined. In some cases, paediatric psychiatric help may be required. Most cases resolve spontaneously within a few months.

## Management of children with visual pathway disorders

Although most children with visual pathway damage causing visual impairment will not be amenable to specific treatment, it is important to offer children and their parents regular follow-up appointments so that progress can be assessed and the parents are afforded an opportunity to raise any questions or concerns. The extent of the visual deficiency may not be appreciated until the child starts school. Correction of refractive errors, the provision of low visual aids, where appropriate, and the management of amblyopia can be carried out at these regular visits. The surgical correction of any unsightly strabismus may also be helpful.

The ophthalmologist should ensure that information about the child is shared with other colleagues, including paediatric neurologists, community paediatricians and peripatetic teachers for the visually impaired. A number of organisations have valuable services for visually impaired children and their parents.

The local authority will have specialist teachers in the education department and rehabilitation workers in the social services department to give information, assessment, advice and instruction. The Royal National Institute for the Blind (RNIB) has regional advisers for education and can be consulted about financial benefits, leisure activities and computer technology. There are a number of voluntary organisations for the visually impaired who can give information and support (see Appendix).

# References

1 Roberts-Harry J, Green SH, Willshaw HE. Optic nerve hypoplasia: associations and management. *Arch Dis Child* 1990; **65**: 103–6.
2 Warburg M. Classification of microphthalmos and coloboma. *J Med Genet* 1993; **30**: 664–9.
3 Brodsky MC. Optic disc dysplasia. *Surv Ophthalmol* 1994; **39**: 89–112.
4 Friedman AH, Beckermann B, Gold DH, *et al.* Drusen of the optic disc. *Surv Ophthalmol* 1977; **21**: 373–90.
5 Votruba M, Carter AC, Holder GE, *et al.* Clinical features in affected individuals from 21 pedigrees with dominant optic atrophy. *Arch Ophthalmology* 1998; **116**: 351–8.
6 Taylor D, Cuendet F. Optic neuritis in childhood. In: Hess RF, Plant GT, eds *Optic Neuritis.* Cambridge: Cambridge University Press, 1986: 73–85.
7 Steinlin MI. Eye problems in children with multiple sclerosis. *Paediatr Neurol* 1995; **12**: 207–12.
8 Dutton J. Gliomas of the anterior visual pathways. *Surv Ophthalmol* 1994; **38**: 427–52.
9 Budenz PL, Farber NG, Mirchandany HG, *et al.* Optic nerve haemorrhages in abused infants with intracranial injuries. *Ophthalmology* 1994; **101**: 559–65.
10 Newman N, Lott M, Wallis D. The clinical characteristics of pedigrees of Leber's hereditary optic neuropathy with the 11 778 mutation. *Am J Ophthalmol* 1991; **111**: 750–63.
11 Taylor D. Chiasmal defects. In: Taylor D, ed. *Paediatric Ophthalmology.* Oxford: Blackwell Scientific Publications; 1996: 719–30.
12 Dutton G, Ballantyne J, Boyd G, *et al.* Cortical visual dysfunction in children: a clinical study. *Eye* 1996; **10**: 302–9.
13 Huo R, Burden SK, Hoyt CS, Good WV. Chronic cortical visual impairment in children: aetiology, prognosis, and associated neurological deficits. *Br J Ophthalmol* 1999; **83**: 670–5.
14 Dutton GN. Cognitive visual dysfunction. *Br J Ophthalmol* 1994; **78**: 723–6.
15 Lambert SR, Kriss A, Taylor D. Delayed visual maturation. A longitudinal clinical and electrophysiological assessment. *Ophthalmology* 1989; **96**(4): 524–8.
16 Hoyt CS, Good WV. Visual factors in developmental delay and neurological disorders in infants. In: Simons K, ed. *Early Visual Development: Normal and Abnormal.* New York: Oxford University Press, 1993: 505–12.
17 Kathol RG, Cox TA, Corbett JJ, Thompson HS. Functional visual loss. Follow-up of 42 cases. *Arch Ophthalmolol* 1983; **101**(5): 729–35.

# Appendix   Parent support groups and organisations for the visually impaired

**British Retinitis Pigmentosa Society**
PO Box 350
Buckingham
MK18 5EL
Tel: 01280 860363

**Contact a Family**
170 Tottenham Court Road
London
W1P 0HA
Tel: 020 7383 3555

**Council for Disabled Children**
8 Wakley Street
London
EC1V 7QE
Tel: 020 7843 6000

**LOOK (National Federation of Families with Visually Impaired Children)**
Queen Alexandra College
49 Court Oak Road
Harborne
Birmingham B17 9TG
Tel: 0121 428 5038

**LOOK Scotland**
Contact: George Chree
15 West Park Avenue
Inverbervie
Angus

Scotland
DD1 OTY
Tel: 01561 362347
E mail: GCHREE2709@aol.com

**National Library for the Blind**
Cromwell Road
Bredbury
Stockport SK6 2SG
Tel: 0161 494 0217

**Retinoblastoma Society**
St Bartholomew's Hospital
West Smithfield
London
EC1A 7BE
Tel: 020 7600 3309
Website: www.rbinfo@rbsociety.org.uk

**Royal National Institute for the Blind**
224 Great Portland Street
London
W1N 6AA
Tel: 020 7388 1266
Website: www.rnib.org.uk
E mail: Jhowell@rnib.org.uk (Website editor)

**Scope (formerly the Spastics Society)**
12 Park Crescent
London
W1N 4EQ
Tel: 020 7636 5020

**Sense – the National Deafblind and Rubella Association**
11–13 Clifton Terrace
Finsbury Park
London
N4 3SR
Tel: 020 7272 7774

**Sense Scotland**
5th Floor Finnieston Street
Clydeway Centre
Glasgow G3 8JU
Scotland
Tel: 0141 221 7577

**Toxoplasmosis Trust**
61–71 Collier Street
London
N1 9BE
Tel: 020 7713 0663

**Vision Aid**
22a Chorley New Road
Bolton
Lancashire
BL1 4AP
Tel: 01204 531882

# Index

Page numbers in *italics* refer to tables and boxes, those in **bold** refer to figures

ectropion 155
electrical activity 40–1
electro-oculogram 26–7
electronystagmography 194, 195
electrophysiological tests
　advantage of 17, 26
　clinical indications 29
　optic nerve function 33–6
　retinal function 29–33
　types 26–9
　visual cortex function 33–6
ELISA 68
encephalotrigeminal angiomatosis *see* Sturge-Weber
　syndrome
endogenous endophthalmitis 90
endophytic lesions 216
endothelial dystrophies 75–6
enterococci 68
entropion 155
environmental influences 54
eosinophilic granuloma 172
epiblepharon 154
epibulbar dermoids 56
epicanthic folds 155
epidemic keratoconjunctivitis 65–6
epidemiology, defined 1
epidermolysis bullosa 71
epiphora, congenital 162–3
epithelial dystrophies 71, 72
erythema multiforme
　clinical features 70–1
　pathogenesis 71
　precipitating factors 70
　treatment 71
esodeviations 177–80, 197
established trachoma 64
exodeviations 48, 181–2
exophoria 181
exophytic haemangioblastomas 216–17
Expanded Programme of Immunisation 10
exudative retinal detachment 141
eye examinations 14–25
eye movement
　disorders 191–9
　examinations 21
eye reversal 45–6
eyelid disorders 154–61

facial angiofibromas 218
facial defects 55, 169
familial adenomatous polyposis coli 122
familial exudative vitreoretinopathy 125–6, **127**
family members, examinations 24
Farnsworth D15 test 19

Fasanella Servat procedure 157–8
fibrillin gene 117
fibrous dysplasia 171
filtration surgery 84, 97, 105
fixation, quality of 16
flash electroretinogram 27–8
fleck retina syndromes 139–40
Fleischer ring 77
Flexner-Wintersteiner rosettes 144
fluorometholone 84
folic acid 118
folinic acid 88
forced choice preferential looking 16–17
foscarnet 89
foveal hypoplasia 101, 201
foveal pit formation 39, **40**, 206
Fox Pentagon procedure 159
Frisby test 21, **22**
frontalis sling 157, 159
5–fluorouracil 97, 105, 106, 107–8
Fuch's heterochromic cyclitis 86
fundoscopy 23
fundus, glaucoma 101

galactosaemia 114
gamma-aminobutyric acid (GABA) 42, 51
ganciclovir 89
gaze-paretic nystagmus 196
gelatinous drop-like dystrophy 74–5
genes, eye development 53–4
genetic control, visual development 39–40
genetic counselling 5, 148, 207
genetic eye disease 4–5
genitourinary abnormalities 57
ghost vessels 85
giemsa staining 65, 66, 68
glaucoma
　amblyopia 110
　assessment 98–102
　cataracts 116, 117
　clinical presentation 92–3
　incidence 92
　iris maldevelopment 57
　JIA 83, 84
　medical therapy 102–3
　occlusion 110
　presentation *94*
　pupil-block 120
　refractive correction 110
　service team *98*
　surgical therapy 103–10
　treatment 102
　types 93–8
glutamate 42, 51